The Doctor of Nursing Practice and the Nurse Executive Role

Al Rundio, PhD, DNP, RN, APRN, CARN-AP, NEA-BC, DPNAP
Associate Dean for Post Licensure Nursing
Programs: RN to BSN Program; Graduate Nursing
& Doctoral Programs & CNE
Clinical Professor of Nursing
College of Nursing and Health Professions
Drexel University
Philadelphia, Pennsylvania

Virginia Wilson, MSN, RN, NEA-BC, NE-BC
Clinical Assistant Professor
Director, Innovation and Intra/Entrepreneurship
MSN Program
College of Nursing and Health Professions
Drexel University
Philadelphia, Pennsylvania

 Wolters Kluwer

Philadelphia · Baltimore · New York · London
Buenos Aires · Hong Kong · Sydney · Tokyo

Acquisitions Editor: Shannon W. Magee
Product Development Editor: Maria M. McAvey
Developmental Editor: Pamela Goehrig Thomson
Editorial Assistant: Zachary Shapiro
Production Project Manager: Alicia Jackson
Design Coordinator: Holly Reid McLaughlin
Manufacturing Coordinator: Kathleen Brown
Senior Marketing Manager: Mark Wiragh
Prepress Vendor: Absolute Service, Inc.

9 8 7 6 5 4 3 2 1

Printed in China

Library of Congress Cataloging-in-Publication Data

The doctor of nursing practice and the nurse executive role / [edited by] Al Rundio, Virginia Wilson.
    p. ; cm.
  Includes bibliographical references and index.
    ISBN 978-1-4511-9517-0 (paperback)
  I. Rundio, Al, editor. II. Wilson, Virginia, 1953- , editor.
  [DNLM: 1. Nurse Administrators. 2. Nursing, Supervisory. 3. Leadership. 4. Nurse's Role. WY 105]
  RT89
  362.17'3068—dc23
                            2014033415

RRS1409

Contributors

Joseph Anton, RN, MSN
Vice President of Emergency Medicine
Thomas Jefferson University Hospitals
Philadelphia, Pennsylvania

Jean Barry, PhD, RN, NEA-BC
Associate Professor of Nursing
Kirkhof College of Nursing
Grand Valley State University
Allendale, Michigan

Joan Rosen Bloch, PhD, CRNP
Associate Professor
College of Nursing and Health Professions
School of Public Health
Drexel University
Philadelphia, Pennsylvania

Elizabeth A. Gazza, PhD, RN, LCCE, FACCE
Associate Professor of Nursing
School of Nursing
University of North Carolina Wilmington
Wilmington, North Carolina

Diane F. Hunker, PhD, MBA, BSN, RN
Director of Nursing Programs
Doctor of Nursing Practice Program Coordinator
Associate Professor
Department of Nursing
Chatham University
Pittsburgh, Pennsylvania

William J. Lorman, PhD, MSN, PMHNP-BC, CARN-AP
Vice President, Chief Clinical Officer
Livengrin Foundation, Inc.
Bensalem, Pennsylvania
Assistant Clinical Professor
College of Nursing and Health Professions
Drexel University
Philadelphia, Pennsylvania

Faye A. Meloy, PhD, MSN, MBA
Associate Dean
Pre-Licensure Nursing Programs
Drexel University
Philadelphia, Pennsylvania

Sally K. Miller, PhD, FNP-BC, AGACNP-BC, AGPCNP-BC, FAANP
Clinical Professor
College of Nursing and Health Professions
Drexel University
Philadelphia, Pennsylvania

Carol Patton, Dr. PH, RN, FNP-BC, CRNP, CNE
Associate Clinical Professor
College of Nursing and Health Professions
Drexel University
Philadelphia, Pennsylvania

Seun O. Ross, DNP, MSN, RN, CRNP-F, NP-C, NEA-BC
Senior Director
Patient Care Services
MedStar Harbor Hospital
Baltimore, Maryland

Foreword

These are exciting times for one to be in nursing. Who ever dreamed that one day we would have a practice doctorate?

Nursing has certainly advanced from an educational perspective over time. We remember well the days that when a nurse had a baccalaureate degree, he or she was a step ahead of everyone else. Now, the Bachelor of Science in Nursing (BSN) degree is generally required in order for a nurse to get employed.

The Institute of Medicine report on *The Future of Nursing* (2010) has advanced the cause. This report calls for the doubling of nurses with a doctoral degree by the year 2020. The reality is that those nurses with a doctoral degree still average about 1% to 2% of the general nursing population. Academia wants nursing educators to have a doctorate. Many service settings are also demanding this credential.

There was a problem in that those nurses, who practice as an advanced practice nurse or a nurse executive, did not want to pursue a research doctorate because they are rooted in the world of practice. When the American Association Colleges of Nursing conceived the idea of a practice doctorate, the needs of such nurses were met. The practice doctorate has taken flight like no other program has. Who ever thought that within a few short years there would be well over 300 Doctor of Nursing Practice (DNP) programs up and running in the United States?

Even though the practice doctorate has taken off, this does not underscore the need for more nurses who also seek a research doctorate, namely, the Doctor of Philosophy (PhD).

If one makes a comparison of the PhD versus the DNP, the PhD nurse generates primary research and new knowledge to change the world around us; the DNP nurse translates the evidence from primary research into the world of practice in order to improve care to the patients that are served. Many term this translational research. There is an entire body of knowledge developing that is exploring the area of implementation science, that is, implementing the evidence to see the effect on patients. What an exciting time for both the PhD-prepared and the DNP-prepared nurse.

The primary role of a nurse executive is to improve the care to patients from a systems perspective as well as balance the inherent costs, which continue to grow. Nurse executives are in a pivotal position to effect change in care delivery models that are both cost-effective and efficient as well as assure the provision of quality care to the patient.

The net effect of the Patient Care and Affordable Care Act (2010) will be a reformed health-care delivery system. Because the United States is primarily an intervention system, this Act will change the focus of care delivery to a primary care system that focuses on prevention and integrated health systems rather than an intervention system. Who else is better prepared on the topics of prevention and education other than nurses? This reformed delivery system will also require significant policy changes. Ethical issues are going to have to be dealt with, for example, the concept of futility. The DNP-prepared nurse executive will be able to provide administrative oversight for such a reformed delivery system.

This book is the first of its kind to really address the DNP nurse executive. This book brings together a cadre of nurse executives, who are well-known in their field. Key topics currently facing the nurse executive as well as topics that are more futuristic are addressed in this book. This is a wonderful book for nurse executives, nurse educators, and others who want to learn more about the contemporary nurse executive role.

Our hope is that you find this book a useful tool in your arsenal of literature on executive leadership and management.

Al Rundio
Ginny Wilson

Acknowledgments

We would like to acknowledge the following individuals for their support of our work on this book:

Dr. Gloria F. Donnelly, PhD, RN, FAAN, Dean of the College of Nursing and Health Professions, Drexel University, Philadelphia, PA, for her unwavering support and commitment of our scholarly endeavors.

To all of the contributors of this book. We would not have such a book without the dedication, commitment, and expertise of our contributors. They have devoted much time out of their busy schedules to help us accomplish our goals of producing such a text.

To Anna Pohuly and Fred Anderson, Administrative Assistants to the Associate Deans at Drexel University, for their unwavering administrative support during the writing of this book.

To the many health-care and educational institutions that have allowed us to practice administration. There is no better experience than the "lived experience."

To the American Nurses Credentialing Center (ANCC) Knowledge Center for allowing us to educate and prepare many nurse executives for certification as an executive.

And to anyone whom we may have missed in writing these acknowledgments. Our belief is that life is about relationships and connectedness. There have been many such individuals who have contributed to our development as nurse executives. We sincerely thank them.

Al Rundio
Ginny Wilson

Contents

Contents

Nurse Executive Leadership

Al Rundio

INTRODUCTION

Doctor of Nursing Practice (DNP) programs have proliferated the past few years in the United States. The proliferation of such programs demonstrates that nursing is a practice discipline and that clinicians as well as nurse executives can benefit from such a degree as well as contribute to improved patient care outcomes within various health-care systems.

According to Fitzpatrick and Wallace (2009), the DNP is necessary secondary to the complexity of the health-care system, increased diversity of patients and staff, the focus on improved outcomes, enhanced technology and application of such technology, and advanced aging of the U.S. population.

According to Chism (2010), the DNP clinical practice–focused doctorate needs to be grounded in clinical practice and demonstrate how research has an impact on practice. Rather than conducting primary research, the practice doctorate translates research into practice with the ultimate goal of achieving improved patient outcomes. Nurse executives with a DNP are in a pivotal role to affect such change and improvement in care through the reshaping of the health-care delivery system in our nation.

The American Association of Colleges of Nursing (2006) defined eight essentials for DNP programs. Essential II is the following: Organizational and systems leadership for quality improvement and systems thinking leadership is essential to the improvement of health-care delivery systems with a resultant increase in the quality of care that is provided to patients. The following section highlights some key aspects of leadership.

LEADERSHIP

There is no doubt about it—those facilities that have excellent leaders excel. The recent downturn in our economy provides excellent examples of the facilities that embrace change and survive and those that have succumbed to the economy secondary to maintaining the status quo.

There are several leadership theories that one can explore. The reality is that most great leaders embrace various leadership theories. Some leaders are born great. All leaders have essential traits that make them successful as a leader. Yet, others are transformational in nature where they transform the entire culture of an organization as well as the organization itself.

Leadership Is an Art: Leadership Theory and Style

As a former vice president (VP) of nursing in a community hospital, new legislation was passed that recognized advanced practice nurses (APNs). This legislation provided prescriptive practice to APNs. I felt that it was vitally important that APNs be appropriately credentialed on the hospital's medical staff. This would assure that the medical staff could work collaboratively with these newly credentialed practitioners. I had to convince several people in the organization that this idea of medical staff credentialing for APNs warranted discussion, and we should investigate the possibilities of making this happen. The VP of medical affairs kept stalling the issue, always placing it on a "back burner."

Finally, I felt that I had had enough of the stall tactics, so 1 day, I advised him that if something was not done, I would have to sue him and the hospital for restraint of trade. I also discussed this with the chief executive officer (CEO) of the organization. The issue was discussed that month at the hospital board meeting with the board of governors voting to appoint an ad hoc committee to study the issue. The VP of medical affairs and I, as well as the other board members, were appointed to this committee. It took nearly 2 years of education and discussion, but finally, this committee unanimously recommended to the full board of governors that APNs should be credentialed on the hospital's medical staff. The board of governors unanimously approved this. Several years later, many APNs have and continue to be credentialed on this hospital's medical staff.

Sometimes, leadership involves stepping out of the box where it is safe. Sometimes, it is where one becomes somewhat aggressive in nature to accomplish what is needed for the organization and nursing. Leadership is also a commitment to one's value system.

Leadership is integral to the functioning of any organization. It is important to understand that leadership and management are not necessarily the same entity, yet they are implicitly intertwined. The corollary is that if you manage well, you also must be leading well.

There have been many theories studied on the topic of leadership. Today, we recognize how vital good leadership is to the survival of any organization. This is quite evident in health care. With dollars allocated to health care being continually compressed and the nursing shortage escalating, excellent leadership is certainly needed in our health-care delivery systems. As a DNP, the highest educational credential for practicing clinicians and nurse executives, it is essential to embrace the concept of leadership. Only through excellent leadership can nursing move forward in contributing to improved outcomes of care for our patients.

The following describes 10 management/leadership "pearls" to make one successful as a leader. These 10 management/leadership pearls can help you on your journey to successful leadership and management.

At age 26 years, I was offered a supervisory position in an emergency department (ED). I was eager to become a nursing manager: It was a career move that I had worked for, and I was excited that it finally had happened.

Here are some key concepts I have learned in the years since that first job. These 10 pearls can help you on your journey to successful leadership and management.

1. **Build trust.** This simple concept is vitally important. When staff members trust their manager, they will move mountains and do almost anything to help accomplish the organization's goals and objectives.

As a new manager, I wanted to change things overnight. I had come from an ED assistant charge nurse position on the 3 to 11 p.m. shift, and I wanted to make the new hospital a carbon copy of the old one. My rationale was that if it worked at the old hospital, it would work at the new one. I learned differently early on. The patients were different. The cultures of both institutions were different. I should have just observed, and I should have become better acquainted with the staff before implementing many changes. The staff did not even know me. How could they trust me?

2. **Never ask someone to do something that you have not done yourself.** I learned this when I was 17 years old and employed after school as a shoe salesman for a major shoe chain. I was the new kid on the block.

One day when I went to work, Sam, the assistant manager, asked me to weed the tarred parking lot. Everyone loved it when Sam was working because he was a great guy who treated everyone fairly, but he was always joking around. So I asked him if he was serious about his request. I was dressed in a suit, and weeding certainly was not a part of my job description. Sam told me that it was my turn. He went on to say that he had done it himself many times before and he would never ask someone to do something he had not done himself. So, reluctantly, I headed to the parking lot and did the weeding. But from then on, I watched to see if Sam really lived what he told me. I saw Sam shampoo carpets and do many other chores. He did do whatever he asked someone else to do.

Sam's actions garnered trust and demonstrated to the rest of the employees that he knew what it was like to be in the trenches. One reason I feel that I was so successful as a VP of nursing was that I had started as an orderly in the operating room (OR). I knew what it was like to do a shave preparation, transport a patient, and mop the OR floor.

3. **Delegate.** A manager and leader cannot do it all, so it is important to learn delegation skills early on. Delegation frees leaders and managers to do what they should be doing best, that is, leading the organization in the right direction and managing the staff so that organizational goals and objectives are accomplished.

4. **Replenish your cup.** I learned this skill when I took a VP of nursing position. I lived and breathed my job and placed family second to it. I had reached my ultimate goal, so I wanted to be successful. A Catholic priest, our hospital chaplain at that time, became a good friend. One day, he came to my office and asked me to go to the community center for a workout and a swim. During our swim, he told me that people cannot give to others if they do not take care of themselves first. "You have to learn how to take time for yourself and replenish and refill your cup before you give to others," he said.

Other great nursing leaders I know feel the same way. They all say that they work hard, but they play equally as hard. Replenishment for me comes in the form of workouts at the gym, long bike rides, and rock concerts. Replenishment comes to different individuals in different forms, but it is an extremely important concept to embrace and live.

5. **Learn Politics 101.** Nurses tend to be apolitical. Most do not even like the word *politics*; it is necessary to be politically correct to advance your agenda as well as that of nursing. For example, as a VP of nursing, I had to use agency nursing for a short time to stabilize staffing and ultimately contribute to retention of staff by providing safe staffing ratios. Agency nursing costs more than regular staffing. This was the first time that the hospital was using agency nurses, and finance division was really concerned about the additional cost.

So I went out of my way to bond with key individuals in the finance division. When the chief financial officer asked that I play golf with him at the annual hospital golf tournament, I graciously accepted the invitation. Now, I hate golf. It is not a fast enough sport for me. Nevertheless, I had a friend who taught me how to play golf in 10 days so that I would be ready for the tournament and would not look like a total idiot. I played an entire round of golf. Finance became an ally, and I was able to make many positive changes in nursing as a result of this one political move. I will never compromise my value system for politics, but nurses need to become more politically astute to advance nursing.

6. **Master change.** There is no doubt about it, change never stops in health care. A colleague said that managing today is like managing in white water; change is constant. If organizations are going to survive, then change must be a constant, and leaders and managers need to embrace this concept.

7. **Take risks.** Nothing ventured, nothing gained. Analyze the situation. If it looks good and your gut tells you to proceed, then take the risk. Do not panic if you fail. You can succeed at everything. If you do not take a risk, you will not grow. Learn from risk taking, and do it whenever you can.

8. Be a leader. Leaders do the right thing. At times, this may not make them popular. Leaders need to do what needs to be done, and this may mean sticking to their guns. As one colleague told me, if it is lonely at the top, then that is a sign of good leadership.

9. Be willing to give up things to advance your career. As leaders and managers, we may manage our department or service extremely well and implement many positive changes. If an opportunity comes up, it may involve giving up what we are currently leading and managing for a promotion. Do not hold on; just let go and relish in the fact that you have an opportunity to develop in new and exciting ways. This contributes to our growth and development as leaders and managers.

10. Practice the piano. Consistently practice the nine management pearls for success. Just as one would ready a piano concerto for a recital, practicing these pearls until they are perfected can lead to true success.

From nurse.com. Copyright 2005 Gannett Healthcare Group. All Rights Reserved.

Through several case studies provided in this chapter, the reader explores different aspects of transformational leadership. The goal is that these case studies will bring some "life" to leadership.

LEADERSHIP EXAMPLES

Leading Change: Implementation of a Nursing Informatics System

CASE SCENARIO

1

I was a new VP of nursing at an acute care community hospital. The year after my appointment, the hospital was on a survey by The Joint Commission on Accreditation of Healthcare Organizations.

I had prepared and accomplished a lot for this survey. For example, I had implemented new criterion-based performance descriptions and evaluations for all staff levels; had written a new philosophy statement for the nursing division; and had revised the quality improvement program, including the committee composition.

The country was experiencing a nursing shortage, much like the one that we are currently experiencing.

I will never forget the nurse surveyor from The Joint Commission. She was educationally focused and nursing process-oriented. She was on a mission. For her, the nursing process was a hammer that slammed home the importance of registered nurses (RNs) completing initial patient assessments. She contended, "This is what RNs can use to justify their role. What we do differently from LPNs or other health-care providers is the initial nursing assessment, which must be done by an RN, and the plan of care for the patient." From this particular nurse surveyor, we received a type I contingency that reflected a deficiency in how we used the nursing process.

The contingency came as no surprise. Back then, everything seemed to be a problem for our education department. For example, the nursing process was not being done because the staff lacked education supporting it. We had discussed the issue at the nursing quality improvement committee. We had implemented a vast education program. We then monitored compliance. We were dismayed when compliance barely improved from the initial survey. That is when it hit me. We were not dealing with a staff education or compliance issue. The problem was much simpler. Nurses in acute care did not value the nursing process because we basically functioned in a medical model. The nurses could not see what the nursing process did to improve patient care. Practicing in the midst of a staffing shortage, why do something if it did not improve care? And was not it my role as VP of nursing to get rid of any work that had no effect on patient care? It became apparent to me that we had a systems problem and what really was needed was a systems change, a new way of thinking that would let the system dictate the process.

I used that negative survey as a catalyst to obtain funding for a nursing informatics system where the documentation was based on standards of nursing practice. The system based the plan of care on the nursing process without the nurses realizing it was a care plan and that it involved the nursing process. Effective informatics systems in nursing become so interwoven into everyday care that they become invisible to the user. They become decision support models for the care delivery system.

Our organization implemented ExcelCare, a system that incorporated 200 medical-surgical standards of nursing care. We formed a committee of staff nurses and clinical nurse specialists who tailored these standards to the nursing practice at our institution. The standards were based on research in the literature. For example, I remember changing the standard for circling cast drainage because a nurse researcher had concluded that neurovascular checks on an extremity were more effective than circling the cast drainage. This system achieved 100% compliance with the nursing process because the documentation system was based on units of care, the nursing practice standards. Selected units of care were individualized for each patient and formed an individualized plan of care. In the computer system, nurses documented against the units of care selected for the patient. Care dramatically improved at the organization.

The staff was committed to the system. For instance, when the computer system crashed 1 day, nurses just could not go back to handwritten documentation. We had started with a computer illiterate staff, and now everyone loved the system. The system became so effective that the hospital still uses it today, almost 15 years later. It is one of my legacies at that hospital.

▶ **Discussion Questions**

1. How does your organization implement change?
2. In assessing your organization, how many problems are directly related to the actions of people compared with a problem in the system?

3. Can you identify a major issue that requires the change process in your organization?
4. Can you list two practices that you feel are mundane and should be changed in your organization?

▶ **Answers**

1. Most change can be explained by current theories. For example, Kurt Lewin, a noted change theorist, describes three steps in the change process: (1) unfreezing, where the organization senses a need for change; (2) movement, where a change agent has been selected and the process of implementing the change begins; and (3) refreezing, where the new change becomes imbedded into the organization's routine. Occurring daily, change is inherent in today's management. As one nurse manager recently stated, "Managing change is like rowing in white water. It is constant."
2. Most problems in organizations result from variation in a particular system rather than problems with specific individuals. Most problems in organizations require a change in the system, so that human beings can do the correct things.
3. You should be able to identify a few processes that could be improved by change within your own organization.
4. Take a look at practices that evolve into rituals over the years. Oftentimes, such practices require change based on current standards of practice.

▶ **Issues**

1. The nursing process
2. Systems theory and change theory
3. Standards of care
4. Quality improvement
5. Leadership
6. Staff involvement
7. Nursing informatics

Ethical Leadership: Leaders Do the Right Things

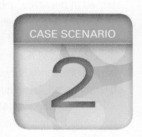
CASE SCENARIO
2

On the job, Jane had a special friend who no one else had. She was the assistant director of adolescent services at a residential chemical dependency treatment center, a private, for-profit residential facility with 42 adolescent and 18 adult resident beds—60 inpatient residential beds. Jane was responsible for day-to-day management and operations of the adolescent unit.

Jane owed her job to the CEO and owner of the center, with whom she had a personal friendship. This relationship sometimes spilled over into the management arena at the center.

The 42 female and male residents housed in the adolescent unit ranged from ages 13 to 18 years. The average length of stay was 6 to 9 months. Treatment at this facility focused on the 12-step philosophy of Alcoholics Anonymous. Residents attended both individual and group education and counseling sessions. Although treatment also focused on basic life skills, residents attended 2 hours of school each day and enjoyed an active leisure activity program.

John was the director of the leisure activities program at the center. An avid sportsman, he planned many outside and off-site activities for the adolescent residents. Thirty-year-old John reported to Jane, who was 49 years old.

Jane developed a crush on John. He just brightened her day. As for John, he had a lot to gain from his association with Jane, even though he did not like her sometimes quirky pursuit (e.g., 1 day she lifted her blouse up to expose her breasts during a meeting with him). Nevertheless, Jane made sure he had a company credit card. She would authorize hours of overtime for him and just about anything else he wanted for his program. One day, Jane's behavior deteriorated. Although noted for mood swings, Jane appeared exceptionally depressed. She seemed so distraught at the daily treatment team meeting that the clinical director approached her to see what was wrong. Oddly, she stated, "It's one of my better days. Everything's fine." The clinical director left early that day to attend an outside meeting, but on his return trip home, the human resource (HR) director paged him. She advised him that a serious incident had transpired that day—six staff members had witnessed Jane trying to engage John in heavy petting in the adolescent community room in front of about 15 adolescent residents. When John asked her to stop, she responded, "I bet Mark won't mind," pointing to a 15-year-old adolescent resident who had a sexual abuse history. Then Jane went and sat on Mark's lap.

When Mark started shouting, "Ms. Jane! Ms. Jane!" she whispered in his ear, "The louder you shout, the harder I'll sit on you." After a few moments, Jane got off of Mark's lap and went about her business as if nothing had happened. The clinical director advised the HR director that he would come right in to further address the incident in question.

Later that same day, John went to the HR director, with whom he shared that day's occurrence. He said he felt that Jane was sexually harassing him. After the clinical director arrived at the office, John was asked to put his story in writing.

The HR director then summoned Jane to her office, where she and the clinical director confronted her with the events of that day. She denied everything, even though the HR director advised her that six staff members had witnessed the occurrence. In light of the large discrepancy between her story and the accounts of the staff members, the clinical director asked, "As a director, how would you determine the truth here?"

Jane advised him to talk to John. "He will tell you the truth about what happened. He will prove my innocence," she said.

"What would you do if John confirmed the allegations and was even willing to place them in writing?" the clinical director responded. "If that is the case," Jane replied, "then I should be fired." And she was. The clinical director terminated her employment, stating that John had not only verbally confirmed the events of the day but had put his allegations in writing. After Jane left, the clinical director notified the Institute of Abuse and Neglect of the Division of Youth and Family Services about what had occurred that day at the center.

Discussion Questions

1. Was this situation handled properly or should it have been dealt with differently?
2. Should the employee have been terminated on the spot, or were there alternative courses of action?
3. What constitutes sexual harassment in the workplace?
4. What legal issues could evolve from this case?
5. When is the right time to report such cases to the appropriate authorities?

Answers

1. This situation was handled properly, as a prompt investigation by the appropriate responsible departments had occurred.
2. The employee could have been suspended pending more investigation. However, several witnesses saw what happened in this case so there was sound reason to terminate this employee as soon as possible.
3. Sexual harassment in the workplace can stem from any verbal and certainly any physical inappropriate conduct of a sexual nature. When verbal comments of a sexual nature disturb employees, then sexual harassment most likely exists.
4. Sexual harassment is the most apparent legal implication. The terminated employee could always claim wrongful discharge; however, this would be unlikely.
5. Whenever a suspect act has been committed, in this case, involving a vulnerable population of children, the appropriate authorities/agencies should be notified.

Issues

1. Sexual harassment in the workplace
2. Termination as a form of discipline
3. Case investigation
4. Legal issues related to sexual harassment in the workplace
5. Legal issues related to the protection of minor residents
6. When to report certain cases/events
7. Leadership in action—leaders do the right thing

Leading in Times of Crisis: Disaster Management

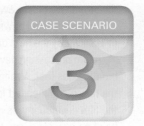

CASE SCENARIO

3

It was May in the early 1990s. I was a VP of nursing in a community hospital in southern New Jersey. Sigma Theta Tau was inducting one of my nursing directors in a Sunday afternoon ceremony.

The nursing directors had to rotate day-shift house coverage on weekends. The nursing director, who was joining Sigma Theta Tau, was scheduled to work the weekend day of her induction. She asked other directors to switch weekends with her, but no one could. When she came to me, I volunteered to cover for her. I felt that her participation in the induction ceremony was important.

That weekend was the weekend from hell. Anything and everything happened. On Saturday, a pediatric trauma patient arrived in our ED. His mother had been at a yard sale in a rural area that our hospital serviced. It was raining that day and the 6-year-old ran between parked cars into the street and was struck by an oncoming motor vehicle. The child arrived in our ED comatose. He was going to the OR with a three-member surgical team. Because one of my practice areas was the OR, I went there to assist the team of three surgeons who operated on this child at the same time. Pediatric trauma and such a procedure were rare events at our facility. The case lasted a rather long time, but finally, the child was stabilized, transferred to our critical care unit, and then air lifted to the regional trauma center. The child had initially been brought to our facility because the helicopter was not running at the time of the accident due to inclement weather.

The evening nursing supervisor relieved me that day at 1 p.m., but she never saw me until 7 p.m. that evening.

The next day, Sunday, was a quiet day, quite the opposite of the previous day. I planned to go to lunch that day at 11:45 a.m. and then meet the evening supervisor at 1 p.m. for report. I hoped to be home by about 1:30 p.m. It was a perfect day, that is, until I went on the elevator to the second floor where the cafeteria is located.

As I came off of the elevator, the radiology secretary was running down the hallway. She yelled to me, "Al, get downstairs immediately. There is a terrible smell in radiology." I hit the "B" key for the basement, where radiology was located. As the elevator door opened, I could smell something like chlorine gas. I proceeded down the hallway where the smell was coming from, but the smell overcame me and I had to exit the area because I felt like I was going to pass out.

The smell was picked up by the air handling system in the new 101-bed patient tower, and bromide gas was quickly being dispersed throughout a major part of the hospital. Although the ink was not yet dry on our internal disaster plan (now crisis management plan), I declared an internal disaster. I was fortunate that I was the one who chaired the committee that had drafted this document so I was familiar with its content and could activate the plan. All of the patients in the tower were moved laterally to the cafeteria within 20 minutes. Every diabetic patient received medications and meals. Every chart was transferred to the holding area. No employees or patients were injured. Pediatric and obstetric patients were wheeled down the street two blocks away from the nursing home that the hospital owned and operated.

I was on a local news station that evening, and the hospital story was on the back cover of *USA Today* the next day.

A film processing developer unit sitting idle in a special procedures room had caused the bromide gas leak. While this room was being renovated, the company that manufactured the unit recommended leaving the film developer solution intact. The rationale was that if the film developer was removed while the machine was idle, the tubing would dry rot and be of no use. However, the gas in the film developer eroded the tubing and released a bromide gas. The Occupational Safety and Health Administration (OSHA) read the story in *USA*

Today and saw the local news the evening of the event. This incident triggered an OSHA inspection. Learning never ceases when one is in management.

▶ **Discussion Questions**

1. Can you identify a crisis situation where you had to be the leader? If so, what style of leadership did you use during the situation?
2. Are you familiar with your facility's crisis management plans?
3. Why would OSHA investigate such an incident?

▶ **Answers**

1. Most leaders tend to use an autocratic approach. Situational theory best fits such incidents, where one leads according to the situation at hand.
2. Every facility should have some sort of disaster plan. Plans should address both external disasters and internal disasters. Many facilities combine both in their plans, and others have two separate plans. Disaster plans need to be practiced. For example, one recommendation is that every facility conducts at least two mock disasters annually. A current disaster plan is so important because no one can anticipate what might actually occur during a real disaster.
3. OSHA's primary role is to protect workers. In fact, the organization initially came into being to protect workers from chemicals and other similar agents. Because the disaster in this scenario involved a chemical gas, OSHA would be interested to see if there were any injuries, especially to employees. The right-to-know laws and the Medical Safety Data Sheets (MSDS) are examples of OSHA standards.

▶ **Issues**

1. Patient safety
2. The Joint Commission on Accreditation of Healthcare Organizations (JCAHO) standards
3. OSHA standards
4. Internal disaster management
5. Leadership during a time of crisis

Leading a Foundational Change: Transforming the Philosophy Statement of a Nursing Division

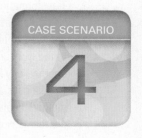

CASE SCENARIO

4

When I was a VP of nursing, I wanted the staff to understand and "live" the nursing philosophy in their employing organization. I was relatively new in the role and had begun the process of transforming the organization.

To some degree, transformational leaders need to "let go." They need to allow employees to grow and develop and take risks. Although difficult for some leaders, the effort can be well worth the end result. I, personally, have never liked how annual evaluations are completed. They seem so task-oriented, rote, and mundane. So, the first year I was in my role as VP, I decided to make the process more interesting. I added a step to the evaluation process. I asked each nurse manager to develop a philosophy statement for the division of nursing. The evaluation process would not be complete until I received their philosophy statement. This became important to them because the annual evaluation process was tied directly to merit raise for nurse managers. My goal was to review all of their statements and then synthesize one philosophy statement for our nursing division. In this way, all nurse managers would have input. An unexpected additional event occurred. The nursing managers decided that they would have their staff submit a philosophy statement appropriate for each nursing unit; for example, the detox unit philosophy statement would be somewhat different than the pediatric unit philosophy statement. One nurse manager went as far as to make the unit philosophy statement competitive. He elected to fund the cost of an annual national conference for the nurse who wrote the winning philosophy statement. He even took the winning philosophy statement and posted it so that the unit's philosophy statement was shared with all of the staff members.

I complimented the nurse manager on a job well done. He also did an excellent job on the philosophy statement that he had completed for his evaluation, even though at the start of the process, he had said he had no clue about what he was doing. Because he did not understand what a philosophy statement was, he had gone to a library to research the concept. He admitted that he had grown through the process.

Discussion Questions

1. Can you think of some ideas on how you can promote transformational leadership in your organization?
2. Does your organization employ the concepts of transformational leadership? If so, how are these concepts applied? If not, what model of leadership exists in your organization?
3. How are performance evaluations completed in your facility?
4. Can you identify a more innovative process for annual employee evaluations?

Answers

1. Transformational leadership can be promoted in an organization in many ways. Using Senge's approach that all organizations must be learning organizations is one way. Implementing the idea of quality circles, where the employees closest to the work unit use problem-solving techniques to improve work performance, is another way to implement transformational leadership. Encouraging employees to take risks and to transcend normal work performance expectations is another method. Implementation of a shared governance model of nursing care would be another way of encouraging transformational leadership.
2. This question has to be answered by you. You should try to identify if concepts of transformational leadership exist within your organization. If not, what style of leadership is apparent?

3. This question has to be answered by you. Most performance evaluations follow a criterion-based method of performance evaluation, that is, the employee is evaluated against predetermined criteria.
4. There are several ways of being innovative with performance appraisals. One way is to create self-evaluation assignments for the employees being evaluated, where the employees list goals and objectives each year and then evaluate themselves during their annual performance appraisal.

▷ Issues

1. Transformational leadership
2. Employee evaluation process
3. Risk taking
4. Philosophy statements for nursing
5. Self-actualization of employees

Leading a Renovation: Transforming the Physical Plant of Maternal–Child Health

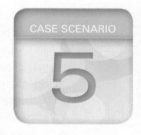
CASE SCENARIO
5

Empowerment of staff is inherent in the transformational leadership process. However, empowerment and the quality of work life it produces not only relate to the mental environment created by the nursing leader but also the physical workplace. Good architects recognize that those closest to the actual work usually create the best environment for practice.

Some hospital administrators wanted to renovate their pediatric and maternity nursing units into state-of-the-art facilities. They wanted the environment to not only benefit the patients but also the nurses who worked there. Nurse empowerment was a key philosophy of the nurse executive at this particular organization. So, it is no surprise when he empowered the maternal–child health nurse manager to take on the renovation and construction projects of the pediatric and maternity units.

The first aspect of the project involved the appointment of a project team, which was led by the respective nursing manager. The first charge to the team was to visit different units both within the state of New Jersey and neighboring states to obtain different ideas on how to proceed with a design. They visited hospitals in New Jersey and Pennsylvania.

In keeping with the hospital's location at the southern New Jersey shore, the nursing manager and her staff came up with the concept of mirroring the Ocean City boardwalk as the main theme for the pediatric unit. The unit design incorporated a lighthouse, built-in aquariums in the nursing stations, and erected rooms that replicated major shops on the Ocean City boardwalk. In fact, designs for the rooms were selected when respective vendors donated money to the pediatric unit. For example, the treatment room even had a friendly carousel horse in it because it was donated by the owner of one of the amusement piers on the boardwalk. This was all the idea of the nursing manager and her staff. The result was an outstanding, functional design. Success was obvious when adults requested that they be placed on this unit when admitted to the hospital (we all do have a child within us). The maternity unit took on a similar design. This unit, with staff involvement, incorporated the labor-delivery-recovery-postpartum (LDRP) concept of care and modeled their theme off of a Victorian bed and breakfast inn from Cape May, New Jersey. Again, the results were astounding. The patient volume doubled the first year that this unit was in operation.

The renovation of these two key nursing units in a community hospital setting just reinforced what nurse empowerment and transformational leaders can accomplish.

▶ **Discussion Questions**

1. What risks did the nursing leader take in this particular organization?
2. Do you think that the physical environment is important to the practice of nursing?
3. Does renovation of the physical environment contribute to improved morale and staff retention?

▶ **Answers**

1. The nursing leader took the risk of empowering a nursing manager who reported to him to take the lead role in a major construction project. Obviously, when delegating such an issue, the nursing leader believed that this nurse was competent and capable of handling such a task. Certainly, such a project could not be delegated to just anyone.
2. A physical environment that is conducive to both nurses and patients is important in the provision of quality patient care. Such environments not only incorporate aesthetics but also functionality so that nursing performs at its best. Form follows function, so to speak.
3. Renovation of the physical environment does contribute to improved morale and staff retention as long as nursing staff are involved in the process.

▶ **Issues**

1. Empowerment of staff
2. Transformational leadership
3. Construction codes
4. New roles for nursing

Leading Oneself: Transforming Oneself for the Future

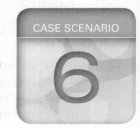

CASE SCENARIO

6

The future of health care and nursing is not guaranteed. One can never overprepare for evolving roles. Learning is lifelong, and education can come from formal college credit education or continuing education. Peter Senge states that organizations must be learning organizations to survive. He describes successful organizations as those organizations that are in a continuous learning mode.

A key component of any nurse leader's role is a vision of what the future holds. Some people claim this ability to be "visionary." Others obtain this vision by being active on state or regional committees and being tuned in to what is occurring in the world around them. This was the case with the nurse executive discussed here.

When looking at statistics of the elderly and where long-term care was heading in this nurse executive's state, it was apparent that more services for the elderly were in the future of his hospital's service area. Such services included assisted living, a new concept in his state. Another such service was subacute care within the hospital setting, where units were designed to help ill patients, who required intense therapy, with a quick transition from acute care units to a subacute nursing unit with less intense care provisions. From reviewing other states that had implemented such units, it was apparent that a licensed nursing home administrator had to oversee the operations of such units. Long-term care agencies had been threatened by the location of subacute units in acute care hospital settings. These agencies had lobbied successfully to at least mandate that a licensed nursing home administrator was involved.

The nurse executive believed that all nursing services within a hospital should report to the chief nursing officer within an organization. Recognizing what the future held, he decided to pursue appropriate licensure that would credential him as a licensed nursing home administrator. The process involved 100 continuing education units in long-term care; a 2,000-hour practicum in nursing home administration; and successful completion of a comprehensive national licensing examination in nursing home administration. The nurse executive did successfully accomplish these things before his hospital's subacute unit became operational. His goal of having hospital nursing units report to nursing was successful.

In transforming an organization, one oftentimes has to continually transform oneself in the process to contribute to the overall good of the entire organization. By doing this, administrators not only acquire talents and skills that will advance them in their current job role but also gain abilities that are transferable to other agencies and future employment.

Discussion Questions

1. In what way have you developed in order to transform yourself into a different role?
2. Had this nurse administrator not pursued continuing education as a licensed nursing home administrator, who would have managed the new subacute unit?
3. Where do you see the future of health care and nursing going?

Answers

1. Think about ways in which you have added to your own education and preparation for future roles. Where do you see yourself in 5 or 10 years? Are you prepared to take on different roles? Those who have several skill sets will be most employable in the future.
2. A licensed nursing home administrator would have to have been hired to manage this unit. This administrator may or may not have reported to the chief nursing

administrator. By securing a license as a nursing home administrator, the chief nurse administrator assured that this unit would report to nursing.

3. Take a look into the crystal ball. Review some current literature on the future of health care. Try to identify where you think the future of health care and nursing is headed.

▶ **Issues**

1. Transformational leadership
2. Licensure in nursing home administration
3. Elder care
4. Future issues in health care

REFERENCES

American Association of Colleges of Nursing. (2006). *The essentials of doctoral nursing education for advanced practice nursing.* Retrieved from http://www.aacn.nche.edu

Chism, L. A. (2010). *The doctor of nursing practice: A guidebook for role development professional issues.* Boston, MA: Jones and Bartlett.

Fitzpatrick, J. J., & Wallace, M. (Eds.). (2009). *The doctor of nursing practice and clinical nurse leader: Essentials of program development and implementation for clinical practice.* New York, NY: Springer.

Will Nursing Faculty Hinder or Facilitate Innovation in Nurse Executive DNP Students?

Joan Rosen Bloch

INTRODUCTION

The core question driving this chapter is how can nursing faculty inspire, educate, and empower nurse executive Doctor of Nursing Practice (DNP) students to grow professionally in directions needed for the American health-care system. Doctoral faculty must critically evaluate how the DNP educational journey provides added value to this unique student population of health-care leaders. Innovation is desperately needed to transform the American health-care system to improve the relatively poor health of the American people despite being the most expensive health-care system in the world (Institute of Medicine [IOM], 2013). How can doctoral nursing faculty and nurse executive students seize the opportunity of the DNP academic degree to bridge together nursing academe and practice at the highest levels?

DNP faculty have a unique opportunity to creatively design their DNP programs with curriculum and learning experiences that maximally enhance disciplinary empowerment and leadership among nurse executive DNP students. The educational journey, guided by the American Association of Colleges of Nursing (AACN) Essentials for Doctoral Education for Advanced Nursing Practice (American Association of Colleges of Nursing [AACN], 2006), can brilliantly foster mastery of

knowledge and practice scholarship for exemplar intra- and interdisciplinary collab-
orations needed for future innovation in health care. The DNP academic degree is
practice-focused. Nurse executive students seeking this terminal nursing degree have
a unique area of nursing practice: nursing and health-care leadership in complex
health-care systems. This necessitates a keen awareness on the part of DNP faculty
scholars who may have more experience with patient-level nursing practice and nursing research versus health systems and nurse executives in the real world of health-
care organizations. Thus, the purpose of this chapter is to provide some guidance
for DNP faculty and nurse executive DNP students such that the DNP journey is
optimized for all stakeholders. As suggested by the title, this chapter is intended to be
somewhat provocative. DNP faculty must think critically about DNP education for
nurse executive DNP students.

DNP education comes to nursing at a very exciting time. Just consider how
technology has exponentially changed health-care practices and systems. Providers
and administrators of health care have more data and knowledge than ever before.
Consider what this means for nurse executive DNP students, often stewards of
multiple regulatory requirements for data collection. The reality of synthesizing the
plethora of data into meaningful ways is extremely challenging. Will faculty expose
students to approaches to tackle such? Think about the endless opportunities of
synthesizing the plethora of data through a nursing lens using relevant theoretical frameworks to organize the plethora of knowledge into meaningful ways to
improve nursing practice and health-care systems. This chapter raises general pedagogical ideas to foster growth and innovation for DNP faculty and executive DNP
students. Tips are suggested along the way to consider for maximizing learning
opportunities. Solving complex health system problems that aim to improve health
outcomes necessitates broad new insights and understandings. Translating research
into practice paradigm shifts for DNP education. Statistical thinking is introduced
as a distinctive educational approach in doctoral nursing education. Nurse executive DNP students must know how to critically evaluate all the data that drives
health-care practice. Concluding this chapter is the author's personal story of how
she found her way to her doctoral education and her biases that directed the writing
of this chapter (see Box 1 on page 34).

PEDAGOGICAL UNDERPINNINGS FOR DNP FACULTY AND NURSE EXECUTIVE DNP STUDENTS

Good News: Controversies and Debate for the DNP Academic Degree

The AACN core competencies for DNP education (AACN, 2006) are clear, but that
is where the clarity ends. (See Table 2.1 on page 23 for the listing of AACN's eight
essentials for DNP education.) An ever-growing body of literature is appearing

to attempt to define what the DNP academic degree is or is not (Ketefian, 2013; Kupperschmidt, 2013; Melnyk, 2013; Nelson, Cook, & Raterink, 2013; Sebastian & White Delaney, 2013; Szanton, Taylor, & Terhaar, 2013). Some of the published literature attempt to clearly differentiate it from the Doctor of Philosophy (PhD) academic degree in nursing and prescribes specific categories of "projects" that DNP students should be engaged in which nomenclature to differentiate DNP from the PhD (Buchholz et al., 2013; Melnyk, 2013; Merrill, Yoon, Larson, Honig, & Reame, 2013; Szanton et al., 2013). However, the distinctions are not very clear, except for the distinct focus of the DNP degree is on nursing practice, not nursing research. Considering that the most seasoned faculty members, often those teaching DNP courses are far removed from practice, the nurse executive DNP students should be most empowered to know that they are the practice experts most familiar with the pressing practice challenges and problems. The health-care system is dynamic and ever-changing, and thus, the areas of need for nursing practice scholarship are most likely best known to those close to practice. Those seeking the DNP academic degree should be pushing the envelope for what they and their institutions need and how they direct their practice doctorate educational journey to develop their nursing scholarship.

Advanced practice nursing (APN) students motivated and passionate enough to seek a practice doctorate are able to push the direction of their doctoral work into unknown territories so nursing practice can contribute to its full maximum potential (IOM, 2011). Faculty must think broadly to help make that happen. Thus, it is not necessary to restrict where and what the nurse executive DNP students can or cannot do during doctoral work. These expert practitioners, the nurse executive DNP students, are quite accomplished leaders in their management and administrative roles. They will bring important *real-world* knowledge and insights unbeknown to faculty who, as mentioned earlier, are often far removed from practice. Nurse executive DNP students are in the thick and thin of multiple health-care system challenges. Through their doctoral journey in nursing, they are seeking new knowledge and ways of thinking to bring back to their nurse executive practice, with important doctorate credentials for their leadership positions. Will DNP faculty have the wisdom and ability to understand what a golden opportunity it is to have such DNP students? Although returning to the student role as an adult can be quite humbling, DNP faculty should be sensitive and realize the practice setting of the nurse executive DNP student is quite different than the nurse practitioner DNP student. Thus, the learning needs will vary because of the differences in their nursing practices. Because of current controversies and debates on what the curriculum and clinical practicum hours should look like, it means there is no one way for all DNP students. All have different APN practices back to their disciplinary home of nursing. Faculty must create opportunities to engage and listen carefully to the nurse executive DNP students to help guide them in having meaningful learning experiences during their DNP journey.

The DNP Degree: An Opportunity to Bridge Nurse-Academics with Nurse-Executives to Break Down Silos and Create Nursing Capital

Key in breaking down silos is opportunities of communication that facilitate developing and sustaining relationships. With nurse executives returning to nursing academia, the silo between the practice world of nursing and the academic world of nursing can be broken down. Perhaps for the first time in the history of nursing practice, science, and education, the profession of nursing is positioned to build *nursing capital* like never before. The author uses *nursing capital* in a similar fashion to the economic term *human capital* (Gopee, 2002; Heckman, 2000) but specific to nursing. Human capital, in general, refers to the collective knowledge, skills, and other assets defining the economic value individuals bring to the labor force. Education is a known investment in human capital that enhances economic productivity of the labor force (Heckman, 2000). Building professional nursing capital through advanced educational opportunities is a wise strategic move for the profession (Gopee, 2002). The fact that many nurse executives are seeking DNP degrees in the context of the thousands of nurses attending American Nurses Credentialing Center's annual Magnet conferences (American Nurses Credentialing Center [ANCC], 2014b) is particularly powerful for the professionalism of nursing practice. Nurse executives are often the key drivers actively enhancing nursing capital through leading their institution through the Magnet credentialing program. Likewise, many nurse executives are also returning to academic institutions for their terminal academic degree in nursing: the DNP (Kupperschmidt, 2013; Sonson, 2013; Swanson & Stanton, 2013). Directed by the core essentials for DNP education (AACN, 2006), these nurse executives will obtain enhanced knowledge and skills they will need to lead work environments where clinical scholarship thrives, a core essential of DNP education and Magnet recognition (ANCC, 2014a).

Through the ANCC's (a subsidiary of the American Nurses Association) website, the magnitude of what the Magnet credentialing is for the nursing profession is documented by the attendance at the annual conferences. In 2014, nearly 7,000 nurses came together in Orlando, Florida, to share evidence-based practices and address clinical scholarship and practice development (ANCC, 2014b). This is an important message for DNP faculty involved in teaching nurse executive DNP students. It is interesting to note that many nurse executive DNP students already have academic degrees from other disciplines (e.g., master of business administration [MBA], juris doctor [JD]). But, looking for more, despite their impressive leadership positions, they are returning to their disciplinary home of nursing for their terminal academic degrees, specifically in nursing practice.

Distance education creates an infrastructure for creating online learning communities among nurse executive DNP students. With sustained engagement as cohorts, journey together is a powerful way to build nursing capital just among nurse executive DNP students. Online technology provides an effective method for discourse, dialogue, and debate during the nurse executive DNP journey that bonds DNP students and DNP faculty in tremendously meaningful and productive ways. In safe learning environments, faculty have opportunities to push hard everyone's thinking in the current health-care system context, exploring multiple meanings and questions based on the plethora of knowledge that exists. Students and faculty learn from each other. With the DNP–PhD collaboration, there is great promise to advance nursing scholarship by continual flow of knowledge generation and translation to and from academia and practice (see Fig. 2.1).

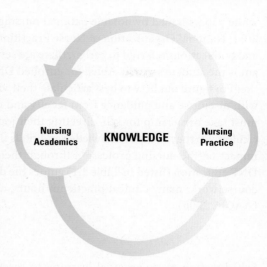

FIGURE 2.1. Knowledge generation and translation to and from academia and practice to improve patient care and health outcomes.

Learning by Design Pedagogy: What Should the Nurse Executive DNP Student Look Like at the Completion of Their Academic Degree?

Learning by design pedagogical approach guides educators to first identify what student outcomes should be before designing what to teach (Wiggins & McTighe, 2005). Thus, for DNP faculty and nurse executive DNP students, the question of what should high-level nurse executives look like at the end of the doctoral journey is an important one. A critical question is how to design doctoral learning experiences that further empower nurse executives to be the best leaders they can be. The American people desperately need critical input from the wisdom and perspectives of those leading others at the front lines of the health care. Nurse executive DNP students are leading the largest group of health-care workforce who are at the front lines.

Faculty need to question nurse executive DNP students why they are returning to academia and what they want to look like at the end of their journey. Faculty must also engage in this conversation among themselves during curriculum meetings. Many nursing faculty bring their own nursing lens from their own previous, and maybe even current, clinical practice experiences. Thus, there should be a broad range of practice perspectives. This is an ongoing and iterative process. Yet, as explained in the *learning by design* pedagogy (Wiggins & McTighe, 2005), without a vision of what the student should look like at the completion of the academic program, it is hard to create the appropriate educational program. Clearly with key, the white papers issued by notable national nursing organizations (AACN, 2006; IOM, 2011; National Organization of Nurse Practitioner Faculties [NONPF], 2010, 2013) and publications referred to earlier, there are several visions. However, most important is the student's vision. Thus, for enrolled DNP students, it will be important for them to figure out how to best articulate their vision. Surely, it is okay if changes are with discourse and guidance from faculty and other classmates. The DNP students must take ownership for self-directing their journey, within the context of the curriculum, so they seek the knowledge and skills that will enable them to broaden their impact on the nursing profession through their practice. The ACCN essentials for DNP education (listed in Table 2.1) guides the development of curriculum rich with course work, many clinical practicum hours, and a clinical scholarly DNP project (AACN, 2006).

Clinical Practicum Hours

Self-direction of experiential learning to meet the required clinical hours allows innovative ideas and opportunities. Each DNP student will have a different vision and the faculty challenge is to help push students to learning experiences that builds upon the strengths the DNP student brings to their doctoral studies. Table 2.2 lists questions for the nurse executive DNP students as they ponder potential opportunities for intra- and interdisciplinary learning experiences.

Thinking outside the Box

For this unprecedented educational and professional opportunity, there is *no* box— DNP faculty and nurse executive students must approach this journey with no predefined restrictors. Within the confines of the academic setting, all stakeholders need to think out of the box. DNP faculty should push DNP students' critical thinking, perhaps even if uncomfortable. At the doctoral level, discussions, in the classroom and outside the classroom, need to go beyond what nurses do, but to how nurses think. Faculty advisors should engage the DNP students in this conversation not just at the beginning of their doctoral journey but continuously. Engage all students in what and why they think about in their nurse executive positions and how their doctoral studies help or hinder their ideas. Ideally, at some part along the journey, the DNP students will engage the faculty member in core gaps in their knowledge about the problems they worry about in practice. Can these core gaps in knowledge be filled through existing theoretical structures of knowledge in the ways of knowing for clinical nursing scholarship?

What nursing and non-nursing theoretical frameworks guide their thinking? Which ones will they use to pursue their clinical scholarship? Faculty need to guide students to find theoretical frameworks that are conceptually and philosophically congruent to nurse executive DNP student's ways of knowing and thinking about nursing and the phenomenon they are concerned about. Knowing which theory to

TABLE 2.1. AACN's Eight Essentials of Doctoral Education for Advanced Nursing Practice

Essential I. Scientific Underpinnings for Practice

The DNP program prepares the graduate to:
1. Integrate nursing science with knowledge from ethics, the biophysical, psychosocial, analytical, and organizational sciences as the basis for the highest level of nursing practice.
2. Use science-based theories and concepts to:
   - determine the nature and significance of health and health care delivery phenomena;
   - describe the actions and advanced strategies to enhance, alleviate, and ameliorate health and health care delivery phenomena as appropriate; and
   - evaluate outcomes.
3. Develop and evaluate new practice approaches based on nursing theories and theories from other disciplines.

Essential II. Organizational and Systems Leadership for Quality Improvement and Systems Thinking

The DNP program prepares the graduate to:
1. Develop and evaluate care delivery approaches that meet current and future needs of patient populations based on scientific findings in nursing and other clinical sciences, as well as organizational, political, and economic sciences.
2. Ensure accountability for quality of health care and patient safety for populations with whom they work.
   a. Use advanced communication skills/processes to lead quality improvement and patient safety initiatives in health care systems.
   b. Employ principles of business, finance, economics, and health policy to develop and implement effective plans for practice-level and/or system-wide practice initiatives that will improve the quality of care delivery.
   c. Develop and/or monitor budgets for practice initiatives.
   d. Analyze the cost-effectiveness of practice initiatives accounting for risk and improvement of health care outcomes.
   e. Demonstrate sensitivity to diverse organizational cultures and populations, including patients and providers.
3. Develop and/or evaluate effective strategies for managing the ethical dilemmas inherent in patient care, the health care organization, and research.

Essential III. Clinical Scholarship and Analytical Methods for Evidence-Based Practice

The DNP program prepares the graduate to:
1. Use analytic methods to critically appraise existing literature and other evidence to determine and implement the best evidence for practice.
2. Design and implement processes to evaluate outcomes of practice, practice patterns, and systems of care within a practice setting, health care organization, or community against national benchmarks to determine variances in practice outcomes and population trends.
3. Design, direct, and evaluate quality improvement methodologies to promote safe, timely, effective, efficient, equitable, and patient-centered care.
4. Apply relevant findings to develop practice guidelines and improve practice and the practice environment.
5. Use information technology and research methods appropriately to:
   - collect appropriate and accurate data to generate evidence for nursing practice
   - inform and guide the design of databases that generate meaningful evidence for nursing practice
   - analyze data from practice
   - design evidence-based interventions
   - predict and analyze outcomes
   - examine patterns of behavior and outcomes
   - identify gaps in evidence for practice
6. Function as a practice specialist/consultant in collaborative knowledge-generating research.
7. Disseminate findings from evidence-based practice and research to improve healthcare outcomes.

TABLE 2.1. AACN's Eight Essentials of Doctoral Education for Advanced Nursing Practice (continued)

Essential IV. Information Systems/Technology and Patient Care Technology for the Improvement and Transformation of Health Care

The DNP program prepares the graduate to:

1. Design, select, use, and evaluate programs that evaluate and monitor outcomes of care, care systems, and quality improvement including consumer use of health care information systems.
2. Analyze and communicate critical elements necessary to the selection, use, and evaluation of health care information systems and patient care technology.
3. Demonstrate the conceptual ability and technical skills to develop and execute an evaluation plan involving data extraction from practice information systems and databases.
4. Provide leadership in the evaluation and resolution of ethical and legal issues within healthcare systems relating to the use of information, information technology, communication networks, and patient care technology.
5. Evaluate consumer health information sources for accuracy, timeliness, and appropriateness.

Essential V. Health Care Policy for Advocacy in Health Care

The DNP program prepares the graduate to:

1. Critically analyze health policy proposals, health policies, and related issues from the perspective of consumers, nursing, other health professions, and other stakeholders in policy and public forums.
2. Demonstrate leadership in the development and implementation of institutional, local, state, federal, and/or international health policy.
3. Influence policy makers through active participation on committees, boards, or task forces at the institutional, local, state, regional, national, and/or international levels to improve health care delivery and outcomes.
4. Educate others, including policy makers at all levels, regarding nursing, health policy, and patient care outcomes.
5. Advocate for the nursing profession within the policy and healthcare communities.
6. Develop, evaluate, and provide leadership for health care policy that shapes health care financing, regulation, and delivery.
7. Advocate for social justice, equity, and ethical policies within all healthcare arenas.

Essential VI. Interprofessional Collaboration for Improving Patient and Population Health Outcomes

The DNP program prepares the graduate to:

1. Employ effective communication and collaborative skills in the development and implementation of practice models, peer review, practice guidelines, health policy, standards of care, and/or other scholarly products.
2. Lead interprofessional teams in the analysis of complex practice and organizational issues.
3. Employ consultative and leadership skills with intra- and interprofessional teams to create change in health care and complex health care delivery systems.

Essential VII. Clinical Prevention and Population Health for Improving the Nation's Health

The DNP program prepares the graduate to:

1. Analyze epidemiological, biostatistical, environmental, and other appropriate scientific data related to individual, aggregate, and population health.
2. Synthesize concepts, including psychosocial dimensions and cultural diversity, related to clinical prevention and population health in developing, implementing, and evaluating interventions to address health promotion/disease prevention efforts, improve health status/access patterns, and/or address gaps in care of individuals, aggregates, or populations.
3. Evaluate care delivery models and/or strategies using concepts related to community, environmental and occupational health, and cultural and socioeconomic dimensions of health.

Essential VIII. Advanced Nursing Practice

The DNP program prepares the graduate to:

1. Conduct a comprehensive and systematic assessment of health and illness parameters in complex situations, incorporating diverse and culturally sensitive approaches.
2. Design, implement, and evaluate therapeutic interventions based on nursing science and other sciences.
3. Develop and sustain therapeutic relationships and partnerships with patients (individual, family or group) and other professionals to facilitate optimal care and patient outcomes.
4. Demonstrate advanced levels of clinical judgment, systems thinking, and accountability in designing, delivering, and evaluating evidence-based care to improve patient outcomes.
5. Guide, mentor, and support other nurses to achieve excellence in nursing practice.
6. Educate and guide individuals and groups through complex health and situational transitions.
7. Use conceptual and analytical skills in evaluating the links among practice, organizational, population, fiscal, and policy issues.

From American Association of Colleges of Nursing. (2006). *The essentials of doctoral education for advanced nursing practice.* Retrieved from http://www.aacn.nche.edu/publications/position/DNPEssentials.pdf

TABLE 2.2. Questions to Ponder When Nurse Executive DNP Students Begin to Design Clinical Practicum Learning Experiences

1. **Who and where is your dream team of leaders in health care?**
   a. One way to identify experts and leaders is to look for an IOM report (http://www.iom.edu/Reports/) on the topic of interest. The IOM gathers the nation's health-care leaders to write these reports. This is a good approach to find the experts that you should do literature searches.
   b. Another way is to go to websites of national organizations that are relevant to nurse executives because they are concerned with nursing practice aimed at improving quality of health-care systems and health-care outcomes. Some of these organizations include (1) Health Services and Resources Administration (HRSA), (2) Agency for Healthcare Research and Quality (AHRQ), (3) ANCC, (4) American Nurses Association (ANA), and (5) Institute for Healthcare Improvement (IHI).

2. **Can you create learning opportunities to spend time with identified health-care leaders?**
   a. How will you create a meaningful learning experience with focused objectives that will not burden the clinical preceptor or their organization?
   b. Can the AACN essentials for DNP educations guide how you write these objectives?

3. **How will exposure to these leaders broaden your knowledge and understandings of health care that can be translated into your nurse executive practice?**
   a. Use answers to the above question to develop your objectives.

4. **Health-care information technology (HIT) practicum: How can you expose yourself to cutting-edge technologies?**
   a. Can you design a practicum for experiential learning with a health systems HIT department? Could this provide you with more in-depth understandings of health information systems and how they can be used to capture nursing care inputs needed to optimize patient outcomes?
      1. Would it be helpful to see how HIT department and database operations actually get data for regulatory and administrative reports from information systems?
      2. What interoperability mechanisms exist or do not exist to maximize safety and quality for nursing and other health professionals at the point of care?
   b. Can you turn insights learned into manuscripts? This is a ripe area for nursing leadership—especially for DNP-PhD nurse and other interdisciplinary collaborators.

5. **Health-care data managers and analysts:** Would you want to get exposure to health-care analysts to strengthen your leadership abilities in understanding what data says or does not say? Can you create an "out of the box" experience? Remember, data drives resources (e.g., budgets for nursing).

TABLE 2.3. Tips: Choosing a Theory to Guide Nurse Executive DNP Scholarly Projects

1. Identify the key nursing practice issue/problem you wish to explore during your doctoral education.

2. Conduct preliminary library searches to see what is published.
   a. Search the relevant disciplines that you would expect to find publications. Do not forget databases for business and economics.
   b. Search for published reviews on the topic. Try using the words *review* or *systematic review* or *meta-analysis* to your search terms. Choose the most recent and read these first.

3. While reading the literature, take notes of the theoretical frameworks used to study this topic and the key constructs and variables under study.
   a. Decide if there are patterns of theories used for this topic and also if there are a pattern of constructs and variables measured when this topic is addressed and studied.

4. Nursing theory versus non-nursing theory?
   a. Pick the theory that *best fits and drives* the DNP scholarship project.
   b. There are four meta-concepts in nursing conceptual models: human beings, nursing, environment, and health (Fawcett, 2005). These are overarching, and many theories, whether they originate in nursing or not, are congruent and fit in to a larger conceptual model of nursing.
   c. For nurse executives concerned about with quality improvement and health outcomes, Donabedian's classic theories (Donabedian, 1981, 1984, 1986) should be studied. Most nursing theories do not address outcomes; thus, Donabedian's work is foundational in guiding health-care practice and research in health quality, outcomes, and policy.

use is not such a simple task, especially when there are so many health-related theories from a multitude of disciplines (Goodson, 2010). Table 2.3 outlines some tips to use when searching for a theory to use for DNP scholarly projects.

So What and What Next Questions

These are simple but important questions for faculty and DNP students to ask each other that hopefully will lead to engaged and challenging debates and conversations. Learning how to respectfully challenge and disagree by using cogent arguments is important. Health-care leaders, including nursing leaders in practice and academia, often use different language and have different agendas (Glazer & Fitzpatrick, 2013). Unifying language and agendas within the discipline first gives professional strength. Nursing academia through the DNP degree has created an innovative conduit, with great promise, to facilitate breaking down silos between leaders in nursing practice, education, and research. This conduit created between nurse executives and nurse researchers is critical during the DNP journey given that the profession of nursing has its own research institute at the National Institutes of Health (NIH), the National Institute of Nursing Research (NINR). Perhaps, critically valuable and a unique contribution of the DNP journey for the nurse executive DNP students is that their DNP journey will necessitate taking a pause in their successful and busy professional executive life to build on their successes with better understandings of nursing theory and science. Faculty must create safe and empowering learning environments to push the collective thinking to places where the nurse executive professionals have never been before. If faculty can truly create nonthreatening learning environments for the overworked, most likely stressed nurse executive DNP students, this DNP academic degree offers great promise for unpacking many black boxes in nursing processes and practices (Conn, 2012), thus paving the way for future innovation that will improve nursing practices and health-care outcomes.

TRANSLATING RESEARCH INTO PRACTICE TO IMPROVE HEALTH-CARE SYSTEMS AND HEALTH-CARE OUTCOMES: PARADIGM SHIFTS FOR DNP EDUCATION

Nursing scholarship of knowledge translation to practice for improving health-care systems and health outcomes demands a thorough understanding of essential aspects of the research process at the doctoral level (Buchholz et al., 2013). To translate research into practice requires expertise in appraising evidence presented either in published research reports or in the raw data generated by databases. Preparing practice scholars with DNP credentials will require an astute ability to interact with interdisciplinary colleagues about the evidence. Research designs, methods, and interpretation of data results using statistics are the same, no matter what discipline one is in.

Although the expected deliverables of the scholarly products expected from DNP students is a current topic of discussion (Kirkpatrick & Weaver, 2013; Melnyk, 2013; Nelson et al., 2013; Sylvia & Terhaar, 2014), it is clear that deliverables could be DNP projects that entail quality improvement, program evaluation, or secondary analyses retrieved from electronic health records. In the era of health-care reform in the United States, nurse executives educated at the most advanced level within the nursing profession will be the profession's key stakeholders in multidisciplinary collaborative teams (Swanson & Stanton, 2013). Acquiring new knowledge and analytical skills during the doctoral journey that is framed through the intersections of nursing science, nursing practice, interdisciplinary health-care science, and health-care practice is paramount.

A word of caution is warranted at this point. The Doctor in Public Health (DrPH) practice designed for health-care leaders shares salient similarities with the DNP. This is evident in Table 2.4. The information describing the DrPH programs were derived from websites (cited in the footnotes to Table 2.4). In Table 2.4, a glaring difference is that DrPH programs include *statistical thinking* in their curriculum (highlighted in the row that has grey shading). *Statistical thinking* is generally an unfamiliar term to nursing doctoral faculty. Exploring what it means raises important questions for doctoral education in DNP programs. Perhaps a paradigm shift for doctoral nursing education's approach to teaching and learning statistics should be considered. Thus, the construct of statistical thinking is addressed in the next section of this chapter.

TABLE 2.4. Similarities between Academic Practice Doctorate Programs for Executive Health-Care Leaders: Doctor of Public Health* and Doctor of Nursing Practice

	Doctor of Public Health*	Doctor of Nursing Practice
Marketing to what groups of students who seek health-care management and leadership positions	• Multidisciplinary • "Doctors ready to move into organizational leadership"* • Professionals seeking change*	Nurse executives
Seek students with proven or potential interest in leading health organizations.	Yes	Yes
Education addresses nursing leadership within the broader context of health-care systems.	• No • Curriculum seems to be centered in a medical model where nursing and what nurses do is invisible.	• Yes • Curriculum is nurse-centered in the larger multidisciplinary health-care context.
Improvement in quality health care incorporated into curriculum	Yes	Yes
Statistical thinking incorporated into curriculum	Yes	No
Integrated field experiences (e.g., required practice hours)	Yes	Yes
Emphasis on scholarship of application versus scholarship of discovery as in traditional Doctor of Philosophy (PhD) doctoral education	Yes	Yes
Writing of a "culminating project"	Yes	Yes

*Retrieved from the websites of Harvard's School of Public Health (http://www.hsph.harvard.edu/prospective-students/drph/) and Columbia University's Mailman School of Public Health (http://www.mailman.columbia.edu/academics/degree-offerings/phd-and-drph-programs).

Statistical Thinking: What Do the Data Really Mean?

Garbage in . . . garbage out
Figures can lie . . . and liars can figure
The devil is in the details

In a data-driven, highly regulated health-care industry, nurse executives are continually bombarded with data. Using data and other best evidence available to improve nursing practice, health-care systems, and the health outcomes is the ultimate goal. Interpreting what data really mean requires keen understanding of the data and how to interpret results that appear in reports that are then used to make important decisions. Measuring health-care use and outcomes can easily vary based on the measurement algorithms used, even when the same data are used. As an example, the author used three different measurement algorithms, including two frequently used indices, to compare adequacy of prenatal care use using the same dataset of one population. Based on the adequacy algorithm used, the results portrayed very different stories about prenatal care adequacy among the same population of mothers (Bloch, Dawley, & Suplee, 2009). Considering that federally funded programs depend on the results of such measures, this exercise in data analyses revealed clearly to these perinatal nurse scholars that secondary data analysis can definitively be worked to the agency's advantage. In this example, just the way the descriptive data were organized affected significance of the health outcome under study (neonatal brain injury among low-birth-weight infants). Thus, it would be prudent to ensure sufficient statistical training for nurse executive DNP students, so key questions of the data can be asked to determine what the data means or does not mean. For example, look at the chart in Figure 2.2. Although the chart in Figure 2.2 is very clear, the process of collecting all the data and analyses to get to that chart is not. The variables measured in the chart are important measures that are commonly reported for health-care systems and health outcomes. However, no assumptions should be made about the quality of the data, especially if serious decisions about allocation of resources based on this type of chart. For the nurse executive DNP student preparing to be a nursing practice scholar, one of the best skills that can be learned during doctoral studies is the analytical ability to confidently work with biostatisticians.

Very few PhD or DNP nursing students would ever get sufficient statistical training in their doctoral programs to collect, manage, and analyze the primary data that went into Figure 2.2. But all should get sufficient analytical knowledge to be able to ask core questions to scrutinize the data. But, for nurse executive DNP students, conceptual analytic knowledge to understand large datasets analyses is critical. Details of the data really do matter.

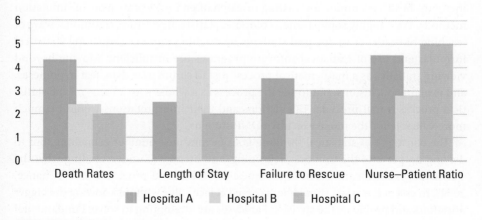

FIGURE 2.2. What do the data really mean?

For data that drives health-care policy in infinite number of ways, not paying close attention to understanding the small details about the data from the onset can lead to very big problems later on. This is ever so important in applying the scientific process to answer the "big questions" needed to improve health-care quality, safety, and outcomes in health care. Because the health-care industry is driven by data, there essentially is too much data and too much knowledge. Understandings of how to use the plethora of data in the context of all this knowledge are the key challenges. Answering the big questions with scientific rigor requires critical thinking about the relationships, meanings, and tremendous variation in the sea of data available for analysis. For nursing leaders, making sure *nurses* and *nursing processes* are not invisible in the data is paramount.

DNP educators and DNP students together have a window of opportunity to advance the profession by maximizing learning opportunities in statistical thinking. DNP faculty should look to how statistical thinking courses are taught in DrPH programs (see Table 2.4). Ideally, DNP faculty with advanced statistical modeling knowledge used in health service research can team teach with a biostatistician faculty member. The nurse-biostatistician team teaching approach can role model how this team approach would work in practice.

Statistical Thinking

Statistical thinking is not a familiar term in nursing education but perhaps should be. The statistics that health-care service researchers and epidemiologists perform are way more advanced than those taught in nursing doctoral programs. The nurse executive must have conceptual understandings of very advanced biostatistics that underpin the scientific processes used in the research reports published in the most respected interdisciplinary journals (e.g., *Health Services Research, The Milbank Quarterly, Journal of the American Medical Association* [*JAMA*]) that drive health-care practice. Health outcomes research often involves complex statistical modeling methods; health economic forecasting research often involves an array of simulation methods. With highly sophisticated computer statistical software, traditional ways of teaching biostatistics to doctoral students by teaching number-crunching statistical formulas and use of statistical software programs are insufficient. Moving beyond viewing statistics as a mathematical process just to summarize data, test hypotheses, and explain conclusions, but to see the process as a whole with a focus on the statistical processes that precedes calculations and their interpretations would be much more valuable for the nurse executive DNP student.

The construct of statistical thinking goes beyond just number crunching, but to delving deeper into the thinking, reasoning, and literacy of understanding what the statistical results mean in lieu of the questions asked and processes used (Chance, 2002). In essence, no data should be accepted at face value without knowing the bigger questions and problems the statistical analyses are attempting to solve. Fundamental to statistical thinking is the omnipresence of variation and understanding what processes produce, reduce, or explain the variability in reference to the big problems that are being asked of the data (Chance, 2002).

Process of Statistical Thinking: A Feedback Loop of Learning between Theory, Practice, and Data. All health-care executives, including nurse executives, are confronted with an overabundance of reports. Using an example of patient satisfaction reports, it is critically important for the nurse executive to think more deeply about the data and thoroughly understand what data was used to formulate these reports. Figure 2.3 illustrates the process of understanding the data from a statistical thinking approach. No explanation is needed to explain to nurse executives the gravity of a poor patient satisfaction report for their health-care system. Applying critical thinking, important conversations are needed with the whole team, including the analysts, to find out much more. For example, find out more about the items on the surveys, response rates to the specific items, the sample and the target population, response rate, and missingness of data.

In the practice of health-care management, there is an abundance of data. The challenge is identifying salient existing data that can captured, exported, and transformed for meaning for various purposes. This may often entail linking data from various sources. Sources of data may include administrative data, health records, Joint Accreditation Commission of Healthcare Organization (JCAHO) regulatory surveys, and required surveillance data. The explosion of health-care technology allows even

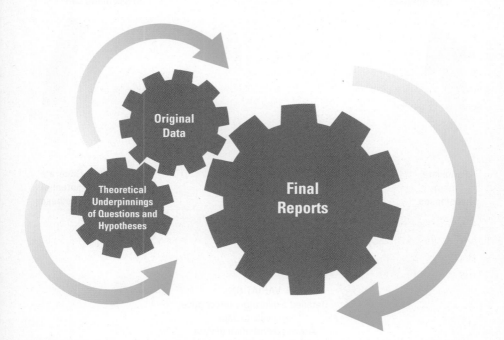

FIGURE 2.3. Making sense of data-driven reports begins with knowing theoretical underpinnings applied and quality of the original data.

more sophisticated uses of all the existing data. Applying statistical thinking to the big questions and all possible data that can be used to answer these questions would be quite productive.

Statistical thinking is an iterative process that begins with fully understanding what the big picture is. A key premise of statistical thinking is that scrutiny of the data should be applied in anywhere in the cycle where data is used to represent meaning of phenomenon. Special attention in statistical thinking is given to variation in processes and how the variation is quantified and explained (Chance, 2002). The steps of the process of statistical thinking can be systematically learned. Figure 2.4 attempts to illustrate the cyclic nature of the analytical processes once data are obtained. This iterative process can be applied to existing health-care data in everyday health-care and nursing practices. This process can begin either with scrutinizing the original data or the big picture that the data represent. Questions to ask of data are listed in Table 2.5.

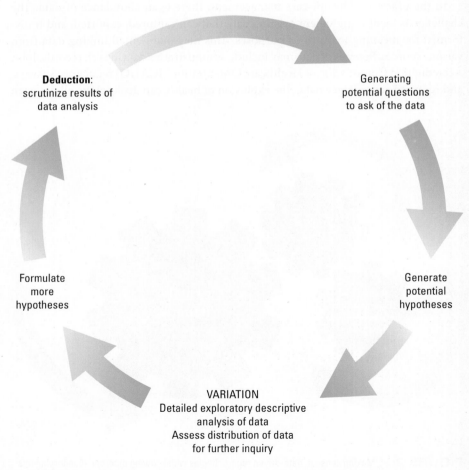

Deduction: scrutinize results of data analysis

Generating potential questions to ask of the data

Formulate more hypotheses

Generate potential hypotheses

VARIATION
Detailed exploratory descriptive analysis of data
Assess distribution of data
for further inquiry

FIGURE 2.4. Statistical thinking applies cyclic and iterative processes to data.

TABLE 2.5. Statistical Thinking Questions to Ask of Data and Data-Driven Reports

Big Picture Questions	What is the big picture about the structure, processes, and outcomes of care that we are concerned about?
	What data is available about these structure, processes, and outcomes?
Data Scrutiny Questions	What does the original data represent?
	Where does it come from?
	Who collects it and how is it managed? What measures to ensure reliability?
	Are other data collected concurrently? Are other data available but not used? Why?
	Are the data pulled from electronic databases? Depending on the implications of these data, scrutinize the electronic databases for variables, defaults, user ease, etc.

SUMMARY AND CONCLUDING REMARKS: EDUCATING THE NURSE EXECUTIVE DNP STUDENT

In summary, the DNP academic degree offers great hope and promise for nursing executives and the profession of nursing. Realizing these promises entails thinking outside of the box—perhaps to places where both DNP faculty and DNP students have never been before. The AACN essentials sets the stage, now the rest is up to those involved to maximize unique learning experiences for our most esteemed nursing leaders seeking their most advanced and terminal nursing practice doctoral degree. DNP faculty must be courageous to relinquish their traditional ways they approached doctoral students; otherwise, they may hinder potential innovation that will evolve. These nurse executive DNP students bring their exemplar professional health-care administrative experiences to academia to a curriculum that emphasizes methods, applications, and applied research. Visibility of nursing processes and their contribution to overall patient outcomes of health-care use is growing because of significant advances in nursing science that have moved forward conceptualizing and validating important nurse-sensitive outcomes (Doran, 2011). The DNP graduate will continue these links of theory to practice. With enhanced statistical thinking approaches to data, DNP nursing scholarship of translating data-driven knowledge to practice has great promise. Bridging nursing leaders together in nursing academia and practice creates infrastructure, like never before, to collaborate and create think tanks to solve significant nursing and health-care issues using innovative methods and new knowledge to effect the kind of real change in their own organizations and practices that can improve outcomes for patients.

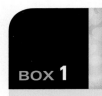

Bloch's Story to Academia and Bias about the DNP Academic Degree: Thrilled and Honored to Be Involved in Educating Nurse Executive DNP Students

BOX 1

I have been a faculty member in Drexel University's Doctor of Nursing Practice program since 2006. Yet, the journey that got me to this point began over 30 years ago when I was hired in my first clinical administrative/practitioner role after graduating with a Master of Science in Nursing (MSN) from the University of Pennsylvania in 1981. I was hired to reestablish inpatient and outpatient OB/GYN services in a hospital that served a socioeconomically disadvantaged Philadelphia neighborhood. Infant mortality rates and the rates of pregnant women who had inadequate prenatal care were especially high after the OB/GYN department closed 5 years prior.

Essentially in this role, I was a pioneer women's health nurse practitioner (WHNP) in the city of Philadelphia and then in Connecticut when I was hired first at the University of Connecticut and then at Kaiser Permanente. Those of us, who were nurse practitioners (NPs) back then, can remember the confusion and bitter battles over what our name should be and what educational pathway was sufficient. The system was broken and needed to be fixed. Despite the controversies within the nursing profession, the role of the NP emerged and evolved into a credible and well-respected role. Vulnerable, marginalized populations benefited greatly from increased access to care. Does not this seem similar to where we find ourselves today?

So, as my story continued, standing on the shoulders of giant leaders in the WHNP movement, Miriam Manisoff, BSN, MA, and Sandy Worthington, BSN, CNM, I was greatly inspired by them. Miriam Manisoff had the vision of developing the NP role in women's health. She wrote the first grant that secured federal funding for a curriculum she developed in collaboration with medical experts. Receiving federal funding through Planned Parenthood Federation of America, she and Ms. Worthington led the WHNP movement for decades in developing and implementing the high standards of WHNP education and practice as we know it today. Privileged to work closely with them in educating WHNPs and planning postgraduate educational seminars, my admiration for the profession of nursing just grew because of the impact that these two nurses had. Therefore, I was most proud to continue forward in my nursing journey by enrolling in a nursing doctoral program at the University of Pennsylvania. Honestly, I had no idea what a PhD was, but it was the most advanced degree in my profession, so I went for it. The DNP had not yet been developed.

Knowing that data drives policy but knowing my disciplinary home was nursing, I strategically designed my doctoral journey to know how this is really done. Enjoying the challenge of pushing my quantitative acumen to places that others in health-care service research go, I pushed my doctoral education not only inside the profession of nursing but also outside the profession to the business school (Wharton) to learn how others are taught in a */ continues*

/ *continued*   PhD-level health economics course and regression modeling in business and epidemiology in the School of Medicine. I tailored my PhD journey to learn how to conduct health outcomes research. Culminating my journey in doctoral education, I was awarded a post-doctoral research fellowship in Dr. Linda Aiken's Health Policy and Health Outcomes Research Center.

Unbeknown to me when I started my doctoral journey is that I would not return to a leadership practice role. Somewhere along my journey, I found my professional home in academia honing my research skills and knowledge as a perinatal health disparities researcher. Although my love of practicing nursing is strong and I am able to carve out a 4-hour a week practice caring for pregnant women, I am acutely aware that I have little time to develop, implement, and lead changes in the real world of health practice. The best I can do is to generate new knowledge (and data) for my practice colleagues to use as evidence to justify developing innovative approaches to nursing and health-care practices. In essence, my work means nothing unless I can partner with leaders in nursing practice so the plethora of health disparities research can be translated into practice to improve health care and health outcomes for all. After all, nurses are the largest workforce caring for those populations most burdened with health disparities.

To these ends, I bring a strong bias that strong DNP–PhD alliances must occur. During these tumultuous times of a heavily regulated health-care system undergoing tumultuous changes, I appreciate the stressors of nurse executive DNP students who are at the front lines. With tremendous responsibilities, I am in awe with deep respect for the nurse executives who choose to embark on their doctoral educational journey. Looking at the current context and reflecting back to when the new role of the NP emerged, I have fond memories of pride and empowerment, recognizing our collective ability to think outside of the box and create incredible programs of care for individuals and their families.

Thus, I have great expectations that nurse executive DNP graduates will apply their "higher level of education" to help fix some of the systems in disarray, such as practice, education, and/or policy. At this time, in an ever-changing world, we need, as a profession, to join together with wisdom to advance the discipline of nursing in both academia and practice. With exemplar collaboration, inside and outside professional boundaries, we can build strong bridges in which *all* stakeholders benefit.

REFERENCES

American Association of Colleges of Nursing. (2006). *The essentials of doctoral education for advanced nursing practice.* Retrieved from http://www.aacn.nche.edu/publications/position /DNPEssentials.pdf

American Nurses Credentialing Center. (2014a). *Announcing a new model for ANCC's Magnet Recognition Program©.* Retrieved from http://www.nursecredentialing.org/MagnetModel

American Nurses Credentialing Center. (2014b). *ANCC National Magnet Conference®.* Retrieved from http://www.nursecredentialing.org/conferences#magconf

Bloch, J. R., Dawley, K., & Suplee, P. D. (2009). Application of the Kessner and Kotelchuck prenatal care adequacy indices in a preterm birth population. *Public Health Nursing, 26*(5), 449–459.

Buchholz, S. W., Budd, G. M., Courtney, M. R., Neiheisel, M. B., Hammersla, M., & Carlson, E. D. (2013). Preparing practice scholars: Teaching knowledge application in the Doctor of Nursing Practice curriculum. *Journal of the American Association of Nurse Practitioners, 25*(9), 473–480.

Chance, B. L. (2002). Components of statistical thinking and implications for instruction and assessment. *Journal of Statistics Education, 10*(3). Retrieved from www.amstat.org /publications/jse/v10n3/chance.html

Conn, V. S. (2012). Unpacking the black box: Countering the problem of inadequate intervention descriptions in research reports. *Western Journal of Nursing Research, 34*(4), 427–433.

Donabedian, A. (1981). Criteria, norms and standards of quality: What do they mean? *American Journal of Public Health, 71*, 409–412.

Donabedian, A. (1984). Quality, cost, and cost containment: The health care professions. *Nursing Outlook, 32*(3), 142–145.

Donabedian, A. (1986). Criteria and standards for quality assessment and monitoring. *QRB: Quality Review Bulletin, 12*(3), 99–100.

Doran, D. M. (2011). *Nursing outcomes: The state of the science* (2nd ed.). Sudbury, MA: Jones and Bartlett Learning.

Fawcett, J. (2005). *Contemporary nursing knowledge: Analysis and evaluation of nursing models and theories* (2nd ed.). Philadelphia, PA: F. A. Davis.

Glazer, G., & Fitzpatrick, J. J. (2013). *Nursing leadership: From the outside in.* New York, NY: Springer.

Goodson, P. (2010). *Theory in health promotion research and practice.* Sudbury, MA: Jones and Bartlett.

Gopee, N. (2002). Human and social capital as facilitators of lifelong learning in nursing. *Nurse Education Today, 22*(8), 608–616.

Heckman, J. J. (2000). Policies to foster human capital. *Research in Health Economics, 54*, 3–56.

Institute of Medicine. (2011). *The future of nursing: Leading change, advancing health.* Washington DC: Author.

Institute of Medicine. (2013). *U.S. health in international perspective: Shorter lives, poorer health.* Washington, DC: Author.

Ketefian, S. (2013). Is the DNP fulfilling its promise? *Dean's Notes, 35*(2), 1–2.

Kirkpatrick, J. M., & Weaver, T. (2013). The Doctor of Nursing Practice capstone project: Consensus or confusion? *Journal of Nursing Education, 52*(8), 435–441.

Kupperschmidt, B. (2013). The Executive Leader Doctor of Nursing Practice (EL DNP): The rest of the story. *Oklahoma Nurse, 58*(2), 8.

Melnyk, B. M. (2013). Distinguishing the preparation and roles of Doctor of Philosophy and Doctor of Nursing Practice graduates: National implications for academic curricula and health care systems. *Journal of Nursing Education, 52*(8), 442–448.

Merrill, J. A., Yoon, S., Larson, E., Honig, J., & Reame, N. (2013). Using social network analysis to examine collaborative relationships among PhD and DNP students and faculty in a research-intensive university school of nursing. *Nursing Outlook, 61*(2), 109–116.

National Organization of Nurse Practitioner Faculties. (2010). *Clinical education issues in preparing nurse practitioner students for independent practice: An ongoing series of papers.* Retrieved from http://c.ymcdn.com/sites/www.nonpf.org/resource/resmgr/imported/clinicaleducationissues pprfinalapril2010.pdf

National Organization of Nurse Practitioner Faculties. (2013). *Titling of the Doctor of Nursing Practice project*. Retrieved from http://c.ymcdn.com/sites/www.nonpf.org/resource/resmgr /dnp/dnpprojectstitlingpaperjune2.pdf

Nelson, J. M., Cook, P. F., & Raterink, G. (2013). The evolution of a doctor of nursing practice capstone process: Programmatic revisions to improve the quality of student projects. *Journal of Professional Nursing, 29*(6), 370–380.

Sebastian, J. G., & White Delaney, C. (2013). Doctor of Nursing Practice programs: Opportunities for faculty development. *Journal of Nursing Education, 52*(8), 453–461.

Sonson, S. L. (2013). DNP-prepared APRNs: Leading the Magnet® charge. *Nursing Management, 44*(7), 49–52.

Swanson, M. L., & Stanton, M. P. (2013). Chief nursing officers' perceptions of the Doctorate of Nursing Practice degree. *Nursing Forum, 48*(1), 35–44.

Sylvia, M., & Terhaar, M. (2014). An approach to clinical data management for the doctor of nursing practice curriculum. *Journal of Professional Nursing, 30*(1), 56–62.

Szanton, S. L., Taylor, H. A., & Terhaar, M. (2013). Development of an institutional review board preapproval process for Doctor of Nursing Practice students: Process and outcome. *Journal of Nursing Education, 52*(1), 51–55.

Wiggins, G., & McTighe, J. (2005) .*Understanding by design* (2nd ed.). Upper Saddle River, NJ: Pearson Merrill Prentice Hall.

3

The Health-Care Environment

Diane F. Hunker

Defining the current health-care environment is kind of like being asked to predict the future. It is easy to describe the structure that has been in place for the last 30 years, but it is a bit more challenging to describe the health-care environment as it will look in the next 30 years. With the aging of society (there are 77 million baby boomers reaching retirement age of 65 years in 2011 [American Association of Retired Persons, 2011]), the enhanced management of chronic conditions, the advancements in technology, the changes in reimbursement, emphasis on safety, quality and value, the looming health-care reform, and a projected labor shortage, the health-care environment of the future most likely will look vastly different than it does today. Although challenging given all of the other responsibilities, a nurse executive must remain abreast of these changes and advancements in order to be able to fully examine, understand, and project environment shifts in the future.

So what is the health-care environment? The health-care environment encompasses the health-care system itself and is complicated by a myriad of services including acute care, rehabilitative care, palliative care, outpatient care, home care, and long-term care. In addition to the health-care systems that include our traditional hospital settings, health-care environments also include the consumers of the systems. These are the patients who use the services. Some authors describe the health-care environment as a partnership between those who give care and those who receive care; however, there are many more sectors involved. The health-care environment also includes the suppliers, the regulators, and the payers.

The United States currently has a pluralistic health system. This includes a mix of insured and uninsured, U.S. citizens and foreign residents, government and nongovernment providers, and government- and nongovernment-funding streams (Penner,

2004). Other countries use a universal coverage system, which includes differing ratios of government involvement. Although the cost of the U.S. health-care system currently far exceeds any other health-care system in the world while still having a large uninsured population with inconsistent patient outcomes, countries with universal coverage experience health-care rationing and longer wait times for care (Agency for Healthcare Research and Quality, 2011).

PROVIDERS OF HEALTH CARE

The providers in the health-care environment include all of the physical settings as well as the staff who work in them. Nurses make up the largest group of providers (Almanac of Policy Issues, 2011). Most nurses work in hospitals and, with the exception of managers and some advanced practice nurses, are hourly wage employees. Nursing remains an attractive field to many adults due to the wide variety of settings and specialties that may be experienced. Nursing shortages have been a hot topic in the media for the past 30 years due to a multitude of reasons, including shortage of nursing faculty, aging of the profession, declining interest by the younger generations, increased need for care providers due to aging of society and increase in chronic conditions, and perceived salary caps (American Association of Colleges of Nursing, 2011). Public debate ensues regularly regarding the scope of nursing practice and the variability advanced practice nurses have across the United States in terms of the need for physician supervision and practice autonomy. This issue will become an even more important topic as the need for more primary care providers potentially increases exponentially over the next decade. Another popular issue for the nursing profession that has spurred much debate involves the recommended pre-licensure education structure. Currently, the possible entries to practice include the hospital diploma program, associate's degree program, or baccalaureate degree program, all associated with varying pros and cons for consumers, providers, and potential students.

Physicians are another large group of providers and are often considered to have the most influential voice in the health-care industry (Finkler, Kovner, & Jones, 2007). Physicians provide care in various settings and can either be an employee or guest of the health system they work in or an owner of their own practice. In most cases, physicians are guests of the hospital they work in and can have privileges in multiple hospitals (Finkler et al., 2007). Hospitals are incented to recruit and adhere to physicians' requests because physicians play a vital role in sending patients to a particular hospital, thus providing revenue streams and ensuring market share.

Hospitals are traditionally thought of as a source of all care outside of the home or physician office setting. Hospitals can also be designated by specialty (e.g., pediatric, psychiatric) and types of care (acute, tertiary, and rehabilitative). Hospitals house expensive, sophisticated technology and employ staff. Hospitals typically provide both emergent care and 24-hour care.

The federal U.S. government is also considered a key provider because it operates hospitals that provide services to the active military, the veterans, and the federal prisoners. State and local governments can also function as a provider by offering services for mental health, state prison systems, outpatient's facilities and clinics, and care for the aging.

There are other key providers that make up the health-care environment. These include other types of health professionals, such as physical therapists and pharmacists, as well as other types of physical settings such as home care agencies, nursing homes, and community centers. The health system as a business entity may own various entities and employ various health professionals. Other professionals and entities may function independently, completely independent of the government or a larger health-care system. Health-care organizations can be for-profit, meaning that the profits that the organization makes go to stakeholders, or not-for-profit, meaning that the profits that the organization makes go back into the system for development. Nonprofit entities can either be a voluntary or a government-run entity.

Providers of the future may include new and innovative care models that focus on performance and outcomes. Such facilities will have a focus on primary care and seamless transition of care and will need to demonstrate a lower cost of operating than the traditional health-care systems. There are several new models of care being tested and discussed in order to produce savings, increase value, improve transition of care, manage chronic diseases, and promote community-based care and overall wellness (Fairman, Rowe, Hassmiller, & Shalala, 2011). Some of these new models include medical homes, enhanced home health models, transitional care service models, nurse-managed clinics, and pay-for-performance models. Similar to the medical home model, accountable care organizations, whose charter is to improve quality and reduce costs, will present another model in the health-care environment in which nurse executives will need to function and impact change. The accountable care organization model emphasizes collaboration between participating health-care providers, hospitals, and health plans to improve care and service to patients. It requires that all health-care providers share responsibility for the wellness of patients as well as associated financial payments.

Urgent care centers or walk-in clinics have already become a convenient, often cheaper alternative to the traditional care setting of a private physician office or emergency department. Urgent care centers will continue to play a key role in the health-care environment as cost shifting occurs as a result of health-care reform, changes to the payer mix, increase in the number of insured, and shortage of primary care physician offices.

CONSUMERS OF HEALTH CARE

The participants of the health-care environment include those who receive care and their families. Historically considered to have a quiet voice, the consumers of today tend to be more health literate and more technologically savvy (MedlinePlus, 2011).

Consumer awareness of services and resources have resulted in a higher demand for discussion, satisfaction, and improved outcomes. In addition to the necessary inter-professional collaboration already required, nurse executives often need to practice collaboration, tolerance, and understanding of the more demanding voice of today's consumer.

Presently, there are millions of uninsured individuals living in the United States. These individuals include all socioeconomic statuses as well as U.S. citizens, foreign guests, and immigrants, both legal and illegal, who are using the U.S. health-care resources. In March 2010, Congress passed and the president signed into law the Affordable Care Act. The Affordable Care Act mandates comprehensive health insurance reforms that will hold insurance companies more accountable, lower health-care costs, provide more health-care choices, and enhance the quality of health care for consumers. The Affordable Care Act is projected to reduce premium costs for millions of families and small business owners who cannot afford coverage today. This could help as many as 32 million Americans who have no health care today receive coverage (HealthCare.gov, 2011).

PAYERS OF HEALTH CARE

A view of the American consumers of health care leads to a natural discussion of who pays for their health care. In some cases, the consumers are considered "the payer." These consumers are termed *self-pay consumers*. Rates for care are usually higher than those with either government-negotiated or private insurer-contracted rates. Self-payers typically represent the upper and lower classes of society (Finkler et al., 2007). Oftentimes, health-care bills from self-pay consumers never get paid, resulting in cases of bankruptcy for the patient and lost revenue for the provider. Every 30 seconds in the United States, someone claims bankruptcy following a serious illness as a result of unpaid medical bills (Warren, 2005).

Outside of the patient, and the cost of care incurred by the provider itself, other payers for care are called *third-party payers*. Private insurance companies are one of the most common third-party payers. Insurance companies collect money from individuals and employers, pool the resources, negotiate competitive rates from the health-care systems, and then pay the providers for their participants' care. Insurance companies are able to secure discounted rates, referred to as *contractual allowances*, through a formal, complex contract drawn up between the health-care provider and the insurance company. Over the years, private insurance companies have been able to increase enrollment, increase revenues, and maximize profits by offering varying types of managed care coverage options, such as the preferred physician organization (PPO), health maintenance organization (HMO), and point of service (POS) plans. With an HMO, the consumers must see a primary care physician within the care network that has been defined and use that primary care physician to coordinate all of their care. In a PPO, the consumers' paid coverage depends on if they go in or out of the prescribed care network for their care. Either way, the consumers receive coverage, but they get more coverage if they remain in the company's network. In a POS, the consumers are permitted to choose in or out of network each time they need care. Insurance companies usually require a co-payment, co-insurance, out-of-pocket expenses, or deductible as part of the consumer's plan. The thought behind this process is not only about sharing in the cost of care but also assumes that risky behavior potentially is minimized if the consumer has to share in the costs.

The government is thought to be the largest payer of patient care. Governed by the Centers for Medicare and Medicaid Services (CMS), Medicare is afforded to those individuals age 65 years and older and individuals with certain disabilities and illness younger than age 65. Medicare is divided into three parts: (1) hospital and other care settings, (2) physician fees and outpatient services, and (3) prescription drug coverage. The Medicaid program, funded and run jointly by state and federal government, is primarily available to low-income families and individuals with physical and mental disabilities. Since their inception in 1966, it has been suggested that Medicare and Medicaid have had the most dramatic effect by far over any other factor on the rising costs of health care (Kim, Majka, & Sussman, 2011). Finally, other payers of health care include employers and philanthropic charities. Employers, especially larger ones, include health-care benefits and pay a portion of the insurance premium for their employees. Unfortunately with the rising costs of health care, this practice has jeopardized smaller businesses to remain profitable and still practice this employee benefit. Employers are able to negotiate discounted rates for their business with private insurance companies. As the unemployment rates increase, naturally so does the rate of the uninsured. Charitable contributions for health-care costs unfortunately have also declined over the years. As the rates of health care increase, and the government role increases, so does the ability for philanthropic charities to make a dent in the high cost of care today (Finkler et al., 2007).

SUPPLIERS OF HEALTH CARE

Hospitals and physician offices would not be able to operate without the suppliers. Suppliers include manufacturers and distributors of all pharmaceuticals, medical supplies, medical equipment, and health information technology (HIT). HIT refers to hardware, software, integrated technologies or related licenses, intellectual property, upgrades, and information technology (IT) support for health-care entities in order to access or exchange health information (Baker & Baker, 2011).

Health-care suppliers are for-profit companies that usually remain profitable, even in times of economic downturns. They also have contributed to the high cost of health care and have direct contact with the hospitals, physicians, consumers, and government. Their role in developing new innovations for care and quality is pivotal as the focus in the 21st century moves away from treating a certain volume of patients to improving patient outcomes and increasing quality.

REGULATORS OF HEALTH CARE

The goal of the regulatory bodies at the federal, state, and local level is to ensure the health and physical well-being of the consumers of health care. Typically not laws, regulations often add to the already complex structure of the health-care environment. Regulations are in place that govern the rules and actions of the provider, the payer, and the consumer. Regulations vary widely from state. For example, licensure is an example of regulation that varies between states. Regulations may be mandatory or voluntary. As both a provider and a payer of health care, the government is often subject to its own regulations and requirements.

IMPLICATIONS FOR NURSE EXECUTIVES: LOOKING INTO THE FUTURE HEALTH-CARE ENVIRONMENT

In the past, the health-care environment was one driven by a volume-driven model of economics (Kim et al., 2011). Decisions were based on census, utilization, space, and service needs despite the skyrocketing costs to support the volume-based model (Kim et al., 2011). Today, the focus for health-care executives appears to be on value, safety, improved patient outcomes, and improved accessibility to health care. The proposed health-care reform will obviously accelerate the process of facilitating this change. In addition to understanding the pieces and parts of the health-care system and the payer mix, nurse executives must also understand important questions and issues surrounding increased competition for new innovative health-care delivery models, complex information systems, and evidence-based practice.

New models of care and changing relationships will necessitate the optimal functioning of the interdisciplinary team. Historically, nurses have been an integral participant in health-care teams and have been collaborating with other members of the health-care team for decades. Nurse executives, in particular, are well versed and knowledgeable on the other roles that are performed in various health-care settings.

With the passing of the Affordable Care Act, the number of insured individuals will increase dramatically over the next decade, eliciting the need for more available health-care providers, particularly at the outpatient setting. Both government and private insurance companies will participate in this massive growth, thereby necessitating communication and collaboration on both fronts by health system executives. With the need for more outpatient settings, also comes the need for more primary care providers. The need for additional primary care providers presents an opportunity for advanced practice nurses functioning as a nurse practitioner to alleviate that deficit. The Doctor of Nursing Practice (DNP)–prepared nurse executive is positioned best to oversee and coordinate those efforts and staff and lead nurse practitioners as future primary care providers.

At the same time the demand for primary care explodes, hospital admissions may shift significantly due to an increase in elective procedures requested by the newly insured, or maybe even a decrease in requested services as a result of increased consumer financial responsibility put forth by the private insurers. As safety practices, renewed focus on health outcomes, and consumer health literacy improve, hospital admissions may also be affected negatively by these changes as well. These potential shifts in utilization require the nurse executive to be proficient in staffing, forecasting, and budgeting.

Financial implications of the changes in payer mix and costs will also mandate nurse executives to think innovatively and proactively about the future. Changes in payer mix and costs have been estimated to impact health system operating costs by 10% to 15% (Kaufman, 2011). Changes to Medicare and Medicaid payment rates as a result of changes in reimbursement and an increase in insured individuals will result in a strategic financial plan that incorporates these changes. Contract negotiations with private, commercial payers will also be transformed in light of the potential changes in requested services, increased focus on primary care, and possible shifts in hospital admissions. Capital expenditures will also need to be reexamined as well as careful consideration for any risk-based decision making. Because patients are required to pay more of their own health-care costs, the amount of bad debt incurred by the health systems will also increase. With the potential for drastic shifts in financial metrics, nurse executives will need to be able to identify and react quickly to changing financial conditions.

Nurses have firsthand experience identifying and treating the needs of the consumer, their families, and their communities as it has been a foundation of nursing education for the past 50 years. Nurses are employed as providers in a wide variety of settings in the community. In addition to providing leadership to all of these nurses, nurse executives working in a particular community are aware of the specific care needs of the people in that community and are best positioned to provide insight and knowledge for those people. Providing leadership to the largest group of providers of care in the health-care environment, nurse executives will be uniquely positioned to drive the change in their communities.

There could not be a more exciting time for nurse executives to contribute to the decision making and health-care environment design of the future. The time for the DNP-prepared nurse executive is evident because the need for advanced practice nurses enriched with knowledge of leadership and evidence-based practice is vital. A nurse executive well versed in both the clinical aspect of patient care as well as the changing health-care environment and associated financial changes is best prepared to meet the needs of the future health-care environment. It is imperative that nurse executives keep abreast of their knowledge of the environment in which providers and payers function.

To meet the challenges of the 21st century, nurse executives will need leadership skills that encompass various competencies. Obtaining a DNP degree is a first step in developing those competencies. By further understanding the complex health-care environment as it exists today and how it may look in the future, nurse executives will best be able to provide strategic planning and decision making for the future while being a high-performing leader.

General City Health System

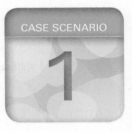

CASE SCENARIO

General City Health System (GCHS) offers comprehensive health services. It is located in the town of General City. General City is the 22nd largest urban area in the United States. The estimated population of the city in 2010 was 315,000. The population was 64.0% White, 26% Black or African American, and 10% Other. The median income for a household in the city was $28,500, and the median income for a family was $38,800. Thirty-five percent of the citizens are of German and Irish descent.

GCHS is a nonprofit organization. GCHS is the area's largest employer, with almost 25,000 employees, and ranks as the number two employer in the state. GCHS has deployed an electronic health record across its hospitals and outpatient centers. GCHS operates 12 academic, community, and specialty hospitals and 150 outpatient sites; employs more than 1,200 physicians; and offers an array of rehabilitation and long-term care facilities. GCHS has created an integrated health delivery system with centers of excellence in transplantation, cancer, neurosurgery, psychiatry, rehabilitation, geriatrics, and women's health.

▌ Discussion Questions

1. What potential additional services could GCHS open that would serve as a revenue stream for the health-care system?
2. How might the addition of these services at GCHS might be affected by the potential changes to the payer mix and cost shifting predicted for the next decade?
3. What shifts in personnel should be predicted at GCHS for next 5 years?
4. How might changes in the health-care environment in the future affect the total nursing work force?
5. How might nurse-driven evidence-based practice affect GCHS?
6. Why might GCHS want to start their own private commercial insurance company?
7. How is the current electronic health record in place at GCHS an asset to the health-care system as it exists today, and how the health-care system might look in 5 years?
8. What does it mean for consumers to be health literate? Why is this shift in literacy occurring?
9. How might the predicted changes in payer mix affect inpatient and outpatient utilization at GCHS?
10. Search and explore examples of nurse-driven innovative health-care delivery models. How could these be implemented at GCHS?
11. Describe the Affordable Care Act of 2010. How might this affect GCHS?
12. Discuss the benefits of an accountable care organization. How might GCHS go about incorporating this model in their health-care system?
13. Give examples of how suppliers may have added to the cost of health care at GCHS.

14. Give examples of how suppliers may have improved the health of General City's community.

15. How might the chief nurse executive at GCHS prepare for her role in the health-care system of the future?

REFERENCES

Agency for Healthcare Research and Quality. (2011). *The high concentration of U.S. health care expenditures*. Retrieved from http://www.ahrq.gov/research/ria19/expendria.htm

Almanac of Policy Issues. (2011). *Nursing shortages: A growing concern*. Retrieved from http://www.policyalmanac.org/health/archive/nursing_shortages.shtml

American Association of Colleges of Nursing. (2011). *Nursing shortage*. Retrieved from http://www.aacn.nche.edu/media/factsheets/nursingshortage.htm

American Association of Retired Persons. (2011). *AARP search*. Retrieved from http://www.aarp.org/applications/search/search.action?q=baby%20boomers

Baker, J. J., & Baker, R. W. (2011). *Healthcare finance: Basic tools for non-financial managers*. Sudbury, MA: Jones and Bartlett.

Fairman, J. A., Rowe, J. W., Hassmiller, S., & Shalala, D. E. (2011). Broadening the scope of nursing practice. *The New England Journal of Medicine, 364*(3),193–196.

Finkler, S. A., Kovner, C. T., & Jones, C. B. (2007). *Financial management for nurse managers and executives*. St. Louis, MO: Saunders Elsevier.

HealthCare.gov. (2011). *About the law*. Retrieved from http://www.healthcare.gov/law/about/index.html

Kaufman, N. S. (2011). Changing economics in an era of healthcare reform. *Journal of Healthcare Management, 56*(1), 9–13.

Kim, C., Majka, D., & Sussman, J. H. (2011). Modeling the impact of healthcare reform. *Healthcare Financial Management, 65*, 50–60.

MedlinePlus. (2011). *Managed care*. Retrieved from http://www.nlm.nih.gov/medlineplus/managedcare.html

Penner, S. J. (2004). *Introduction to health care economics and financial management*. Philadelphia, PA: Lippincott Williams & Wilkins.

Warren, E. (2005, February 9). Sick and broke. *The Washington Post*, A23.

Professional Practice Environments

Al Rundio

Creating the best practice environment is an essential function of nurses who function in executive roles. Such environments will vary based on the practice experience of the nurse executive as well as the educational level of this executive. The mentorship that they had received while in practice will also shape the nurse executives creation of an excellent practice environment.

The Magnet Recognition Program by American Nurses Credentialing Center (ANCC) is an excellent model to implement in any practice setting whether or not the organization has the intent to pursue Magnet status.

Magnet organizations will serve as the fount of knowledge and expertise for the delivery of nursing care globally. They will be solidly grounded in core Magnet principles, flexible and constantly striving for discovery and innovation (American Nurses Credentialing Center [ANCC], 2008a).

They will lead the reformation of health care; the discipline of nursing; and care of the patient, family, and community (ANCC, 2008a).

ANCC Magnet designation is recognition for nursing excellence and identifies health-care organizations that epitomize outstanding quality and professionalism.

Designation can be achieved by a health-care organization regardless of its size, setting, or location (ANCC, 2008b).

A BRIEF HISTORY OF MAGNET HOSPITALS

The history of Magnet organizations really began with a nurse researcher named Dr. Marlene Kramer. The initial Magnet study that she conducted was completed in the early 1980s. One of the questions centered on what attracted a registered nurse to a hospital and kept him or her in place like a magnet. In the initial study, there were two hospitals in New Jersey that this author is familiar with. The two hospitals in New Jersey were Morristown Memorial Hospital and Union Hospital. Both hospitals were located in the northern part of the state. As a new nurse executive at the time, the author had the opportunity to network with the nursing leaders at these hospitals. These leaders were very progressive. For example, in 1970, the nurse executive at Morristown Memorial Hospital had implemented a clinical ladder program (some now refer to this as a clinical advancement program). Such programs reward nurses at the bedside monetarily for criteria such as the achievement of certification and advanced degrees. This was a very forward-looking nursing executive because many hospitals to this day do not have such innovative programs. It was very clear from the initial Magnet hospital study that excellent nursing leadership was critical to attracting and retaining registered nurses at the bedside. These leaders had strong advocacy for registered nurses and nursing. These were stable leaders, who had been at their respective organizations for some time. These leaders embraced a transformational style of leadership.

The Magnet hospital study was replicated in the late 1980s, and the ANCC developed the Magnet Program in the 1990s. This program has now been expanded from hospitals to all types of health-care organizations. The program has grown beyond the borders of the United States and is now an international recognition program for nursing.

The initial Magnet program focused primarily on structure and process indicators. Today, the program focuses on outcomes. Excellent nursing practice and care should achieve excellent patient outcomes.

> **Structure**—defined as the characteristics of the organization and the health-care system, including leadership, availability of resources, and professional practice models (ANCC, 2008b, p. 3).
>
> **Process**—defined as the actions involving the delivery of nursing and health-care services to patients, including practices that are safe and ethical, autonomous, and evidence-based, with efforts focused on quality improvement (ANCC, 2008b, p. 3).
>
> **Outcome**—defined as the quantitative and qualitative evidence related to the impact of structure and process on the patient, nursing workforce, organization and consumer. These outcomes are dynamic and measurable and may be reported at an individual unit, department, population, or organizational level (ANCC, 2008b, p. 4).

When the ANCC implemented the Magnet Recognition Program, the focus was primarily on structure and process. Today, the focus has shifted to outcome.

TABLE 4.1 The Five Major Forces of Magnetism

Forces of Magnetism	Empirical Domains of Evidence	Magnet Model Components
Quality of nursing leadership	Leadership	Transformational leadership
Organizational structure	Resource utilization and development	Structural empowerment
Professional models of care	Professional practice model	Exemplary professional practice
Quality of care: research and evidence-based practice; quality improvement	Research	New knowledge; innovation and improvements
Quality of care	Outcomes	Empirical quality outcomes

Let us review in detail the 5 major forces now apparent in the Magnet model (Table 4.1). The 5 new forces have the original 14 forces embedded within them. The first force is the quality of nursing leadership. Excellent nursing leadership is essential to the creation of a Magnet organization. Transformational leadership is critical to this process. Let us describe what a transformational leader is. A transformational leader is concerned with meeting the goals and objectives of the organization; however, the transformational leader is also concerned about staff having self-esteem and reaching their full potential. The transformational leader raises the bar higher so that staff achieves excellence. This is the leader who motivates staff to achieve certification, advanced education, continuing education, and other factors that advance one's profession. This leader is not a laissez-faire leader. This leader has his or her finger on the pulse of the organization. This leader encourages one to take risk. If the individual fails at the risk-taking strategy, this leader does not reprimand but rather applaud the individual for taking a risk. This leader recognizes that in order to achieve higher goals and aspirations, one must take a risk. This leader recognizes that risk also involves failures at time. Without taking a risk, nothing would be achieved. If a risk-taking strategy should fail, one still learns by such failure and will usually do better the next time. Dr. Timothy Porter O'Grady is a noted nursing leader who has written about transformational leadership. One may want to explore some of Dr. O'Grady's work.

To summarize this section on transformational leadership, the transformational leader is one who then transforms the entire organization with their leadership style. Such transformation involves changing the entire culture of the organization. This can be a process that takes some time. Thus, even though the crown of Magnet is quite an accomplishment, the most important aspect of Magnet is the journey. Every organization can and should embark on such a journey because that will truly improve nursing practice and the ultimate care to the patient.

Force 2 centers on the organizational structure. This force describes the structural pieces of the organization that must be in place. Nursing needs to be involved in personnel policies, procedures, and programs that affect nursing. Nursing must have strong influence within the health-care organization in the community that it serves. The image of nursing is crucial. Nursing must be respected in the organization, and other departments must recognize this. The organizational structure must provide for the professional development of nurses. Such development includes ongoing education both formally and in a continuing education format, the encouragement of certification in one's specialty field of practice, and other factors that contribute to one's professional development.

Force 3 centers on the professional model of care. A nursing organization should evaluate and select a model of care for nursing practice that improves patient care. There are several models available. For example, the author is familiar with a hospital that recently selected relationship-based care as their nursing model. The nursing practice counsel at this organization evaluated and selected this model. The nursing practice counsel developed a logo for the organization that incorporates the elements of this model. Another example of a nursing model would be family-centered care where the family as well as the patient is at the center of care delivery by the nurse.

Other factors contained within the professional model of care are inclusive of the following: Nurses consult other experts in their organization, for example, the use of advanced practice nurses for consultation to other nurses in order to improve care to the patient. In the professional model of care, nurses are also teachers. Nurses teach patients, family members, other nurses, and other individuals within the organization. The quality of the education must be evaluated, and the educational material must be written at an appropriate age level for all patients. Health literacy must be evaluated in the respective organization. Professional practice models also include interdisciplinary relationships. Nursing does not function as an island within the organization but rather practices collaboratively with other departments and individuals within the organization because the primary purpose of every department is to improve the care to the patient. Professional practice models should also include ethical standards and guidelines as well as patient safety. The provision of quality care is inherent within such professional practice models. Quality improvement is a vital force contained within such models. Professional practice models should incorporate the concepts of decentralization and autonomous practice. Nurses, who practice within the professional practice model, must be able to be autonomous clinicians who can make instantaneous decisions about patient care. A decentralized practice model encourages and supports decision making at the point of service. Thus, in the case of nursing, we are talking about decisions that are made at the point care. It is also understood that such decisions will involve other clinicians and other bargains in interdisciplinary fashion.

To summarize this force, the goal of the professional practice model is exemplary professional nursing practice focused on excellent quality outcomes for the patient.

Force 4 centers on quality care that results from research and the implementation of evidence-based practice. Quality care results from interventions that are based on current evidence. Today, many interventions are still based on ritual rather than current evidence. There is a move in health care to incorporate current evidence into practice so that the best patient outcomes are achieved. When evidence does not exist, then a primary research study is warranted in order to develop new knowledge to answer a question about practice. The professional practice environment must be an environment that encourages research and the use of best evidence in the care of patients.

Force 5 centers on the quality of care rendered to the patient. Patient outcomes must be measured. Empirical quality outcomes include both quantitative and qualitative evaluations. Patient satisfaction surveys are critical.

The characteristics of nursing in a Magnet health-care environment include the following: high-quality nursing care, clinical autonomy, shared decision making, strong nursing leadership, excellent communication, community involvement, an opportunity and encouragement for professional development, and the use and implementation of evidence-based practice to improve patient care.

THE 14 FORCES OF MAGNETISM

This section of the chapter will discuss the 14 forces of Magnetism.

Force 1: There is congruence between mission, vision, values, philosophy, and strategic plan of nursing that relates to scholarly practice for the patient. Nurse leaders seek input from nurses at every level through decision-making bodies in the organization as well as other mechanisms.

Force 2 relates to the organizational structure: The organizational structure is dynamic and responsive to change. Strong nursing representation is apparent throughout the organizational committee structure.

The chief nursing officer typically reports directly to the chief executive officer in the organization. This creates a stronger powerbase for the nurse executive. The nurse executive makes certain that the nursing organization has a functioning and productive system of shared participatory decision making.

Force 3 relates to management style: Nurse leaders use a participatory management style that empowers all nurses at all levels of the organization. Feedback of staff is encouraged, supported, and valued. Nurses, who serve in leadership positions, are visible, accessible, and committed to communicating effectively with staff. A leader who is not visible is a non-leader. Thus, visibility of the leader is critical to the creation of a Magnet environment.

Force 4 relates to personnel policies and programs: Personnel policies and programs are created with involvement of nurses at every level. Such policies and programs support professional nursing practice, balance in the nurse's work and life, career development, and the ultimate delivery of quality patient care. Creative and flexible staffing models are used that support a safe and healthy work environment. The nurse's salaries and benefits are competitive with both unionized and nonunionized health-care organizations.

Force 5 relates to the professional model of care: A professional practice model describes how nurses practice, collaborate, communicate, and develop professionally to provide the highest quality of care for those served by the organization. Such service is rendered to patients, families, and the community.

Force 6 relates to the quality of care: Nurses serving in leadership positions are ultimately responsible for providing an environment that positively influences patient outcomes. There is a pervasive perception among nurses that they provide high-quality care to the patients that they serve.

Force 7 relates to quality improvement: The organization has structures and processes for measuring and improving the quality of care. There is involvement of nurses at every level of the organization related to quality improvement. The nurse executive has a role in the selection of the type of quality improvement system that is used in the organization. Research and evidence-based practice are conscientiously integrated into the clinical and operational processes of the organization consistent with the institutional and community resources.

Patient outcomes include the following: risk adjusted mortality index; nosocomial infections; falls and injuries associated with falls; hospital-acquired pressure ulcer occurrence and prevalence, in particular, stage III and stage IV pressure ulcers; ventilator-associated pneumonia; overall patient satisfaction; and patient satisfaction with nursing care.

There is ongoing monitoring, evaluation, and improvement of nurse-sensitive outcomes appropriate to the clinical setting. These outcomes are benchmarked with external entities. Such outcomes include and are not limited to the following: level of nurse engagement, level of nurse satisfaction, perception of nurse autonomy, turn-over and vacancy rates, percentage of direct care registered nurses who have achieved certification in their specialty, percentage of nurse leaders and administrators who have achieved certification in their specialty, educational preparation of staff, rates and types of staff injuries, staff perception of a safe culture and work environment, and staff perception of orientation and/or effectiveness of continuing education programs.

Force 8 relates to consultation and resources: The health-care organization provides adequate resources, support, and opportunities for the use of experts, in particular, advanced practice nurses. Advanced practice nurses are inclusive of the following: nurse practitioners, clinical nurse specialists, nurse midwives, and certified registered nurse anesthetists. In addition, the organization promotes involvement of nurses in professional organizations and among peers in their community. For example, nurses are encouraged and supported in joining the American Nurses Association, their respective state nurses associations, and their specialty organizations.

Force 9 relates to autonomy: Autonomy in nursing is the ability of the nurse to assess and perform nursing actions for patient care based on competence, professional expertise, and the nurse's knowledge. Common sense and critical thinking are encouraged and implemented. The nurse is expected to practice autonomously, exercising independent judgment within the context of interdisciplinary, cross-disciplinary, and multidisciplinary approaches to patient care.

Force 10 relates to the community and the hospital: Relationships are established within and among all types of health-care organizations and other organizations in order to develop strong partnerships that support improved patient outcomes and the health of the communities that they serve.

Force 11 relates to nurses as teachers: Professional nurses are involved in educational activities within the organization and the community. Nurses include teaching in all aspects of their practice. There is a development and mentoring program for staff preceptors for every level of student, inclusive of undergraduates, new graduates, and experience nurses. There is a patient and family education program that meets the diverse needs of patients in all of the health-care settings of the organization. Health literacy is assessed and educational materials are developed based on the health literacy of the population served.

Force 12 relates to the image of nursing: The services provided by professional nurses are characterized as essential by other members of the health-care team. Nurses effectively influence system-wide processes and are viewed as integral to the health-care organizations ability to provide care.

Force 13 relates to interdisciplinary relationships: Collegial working relationships within and among the disciplines are valued by the organization and the employees within the organization. Mutual respect is based on the premise that all members of the health-care team make essential and meaningful contributions to the achievement of clinical outcomes in patients.

Force 14 relates to professional development: The health-care organization values and supports the personal and professional development of their staff; a continuous learning environment is evident. Programs that promote formal education, professional certification, and career development are evident. For example, one hospital worked collaboratively with a local university to provide the registered nurse to Bachelor of Science in Nursing (BSN) program at the health-care organization. The health-care organization paid for professional nurses to get their BSN. This same health-care organization paid a higher salary for those nurses who achieved professional certification. Competency-based clinical and leadership/management development is promoted. Adequate human and fiscal resources for all professional development programs are provided by the health-care organization.

REFERENCES

American Nurses Credentialing Center. (2008a). *The commission on Magnet recognition.* Retrieved from http://www.nursecredentialing.org/magnet/programoverview
American Nurses Credentialing Center. (2008b). *Magnet Recognition Program.* Retrieved from http://www.nursecredentialing.org/Magnet/International/MagnetProgOverview

5

Ritual to Relevance: Changing the Paradigm to Evidence-Based Practice

Al Rundio

This chapter focuses on evidence-based practice in nursing. Research and evidence-based practice are critical to the creation of a professional practice environment.

When we explore research, the philosophy of science must be considered. If we look at the history of research, logical positivism was the nature of research. Research centered on exclusive experimental designs. It was reductionistic in nature. The researcher was an observer. It involved in pure gold testing in the form of an experiment. The primary purpose of research was to demonstrate cause and effect. Understanding this is important as we move more from primary research and as we incorporate different types of research as well as integrate evidence from the research into practice.

Everything that we do in this world and in nature is really evolutionary. If we look at nursing and go back several years, nursing was very task-oriented and very ritualistic in nature. Then in the 1980s, the push was for theory-based nursing practice. Some of the broad conceptual models for nursing as well as the series for nursing, primarily the grand theories, were implemented in practice. Nursing was trying to define itself through theory-based practice. It must be noted, however, that grand theories and conceptual models are difficult to implement and test in practice. Thus, this did not work well with staff who was engaged in practice every day. The good news is that nursing then began to be involved in research. The creation of the National

Institute for Nursing Research (NINR) was a pivotal moment for nursing. In the late 1980s and since the 1990s: Nursing has become more and more involved with the research process. In the late 1990s and now in this millennium: Not only has primary research been important, but evidence-based practice has become critical. By conducting research and by implementing evidence-based practice, nursing has placed itself in the limelight with other research professions.

Thomas Kuhn defined the structure of scientific revolutions in 1970 (Kuhn, 1996). He describes normal science as that which involves continuing research that concerns a particular field of study. Thomas Kuhn is the one who incorporated the paradigm as a working model. He states that scientific revolutions results when there is a major paradigm shift. Certainly, the incorporation of research and evidence-based practice into nursing is one of those major paradigm shifts.

A wonderful example of a scientific revolution and a new paradigm is chaos theory. This theory refutes classical physics theory, where regularity and predictability abounded. Chaos was a new paradigm where randomness, irregularity, and unpredictability are the norm.

It must be noted that the paradigm continuously changes in the human and social sciences. Culture and time are the major separating factors. For example, viewing through the spectacles of the Greeks, such as Aristotle and Plato, versus our own spectacles is quite different. Objects will change secondary to time and culture, and the one uniting force is the discovery for new knowledge and learning.

In this postmodern era of science, research has changed were applied research is the norm. The researcher is no longer an observer but an active participant in the research process. There is repetitious cycling. There are new paradigms for the research process. There is acceptance for qualitative research designs, and there are many mixed methods and varied types of research methodologies.

One must question himself or herself, what is so magical about research and evidence-based practice? Is research a myth or reality? Is research doable in practice? Why should one engage in the research process? What is in it for me?

The difference between primary research and evidence-based practice are the following: In primary research, a question is posed. A search of the literature is conducted. The question may be further refined. The methodology, in particular in experimental designs, incorporates the use of theory. The methodology is defined. In quantitative studies, numbers and statistics are used. In qualitative studies, words are used. The purpose of primary research is to generate new knowledge to change the world around us. Evidence-based practice, on the other hand, poses a clinically relevant question. The database search is conducted, often times, reviewing meta-analyses and meta-syntheses to see if the question has been answered. The evidence is critically evaluated and appraised using an appraisal tool. If the evidence demonstrates that a practice change should be made, then the evidence is translated into practice. The outcomes of this translation are then measured to see if patient care has improved.

Although Magnet status mandates research, the translation of evidence-based knowledge into practice is not the primary reason why we should do it. If nursing is really an art and a science, then the practice needs to be rooted in research. The art and the science both need exploration, validation, and testing. If evidence demonstrates that patient care can be improved by evidence-based interventions, then the reason to do such is to provide the patients with the best outcome.

The following provides some examples of changing the paradigm. For example, once upon a time, when one went on to the postpartum unit, one had to be appropriately dressed in a cover gown, shoe booties, and a surgical cap. The reason for this was to prevent infection. Research conducted in newborn nurseries (the most vulnerable population) found that cover gowns were not necessary. Rush, Fiorino-Chiovitti, Kaufman, and Mitchell (1990) demonstrated that there were no differences in infection rates of newborns whether a cover gown by staff and visitors was worn or not worn. Thus, the practice has changed. Another example is presurgical shave preparations. In the past, the patient's surgical site and all surrounding areas would be shaved preoperatively. Research demonstrated that more postoperative infections developed from the presurgical shave preparations. This practice has changed. In the past, families were not permitted at resuscitation events. That practice has now changed. It has been demonstrated that underweight infants can be cared for at home with visits by an advanced practice nurse as well as the patient can be cared for in the hospital. Look at how critical pathways and the measurement of variance in patient populations has improved care and decreased hospitals length of stay.

Evidence-based practice incorporates a systematic search of the clinical question. The evidence is critically appraised in an attempt to answer the burning clinical question. A clinician's clinical expertise as well as patient's preferences and values are considered and will serve as lower forms of evidence. The five steps of evidence-based practice are described as the following: the need for information that is placed into a clinically relevant, answerable question; a systematic retrieval of best evidence that is available; a critical appraisal of the evidence for validity and clinical relevance; translation and application of the critically appraised evidence into clinical practice; and evaluation of outcomes.

Evidence-based practice involves clinical judgment. Decision making and problem solving incorporate the skills of engaged practical reasoning so that patterns may be recognized. Clinical judgment involves understanding about a patient's needs, concerns, or health problems, followed by the decision to act or not to act, and to use or modify standard approaches as deemed appropriate by the patient's response. Clinical reasoning incorporates the thinking process by which clinicians make their judgments, and this includes processes of generating alternatives, weighing the risk against the evidence, and choosing the right course of action.

Most facilities use an evidence-based practice model as a framework for evaluating and implementing evidence into practice. When evaluating and appraising the evidence, one model levels the evidence in the following manner: level I evidence, which is strong evidence, includes experimental designs and meta-analyses of rigorous controlled clinical trials; level II evidence includes quasi-experimental designs; and level III evidence, the lowest form of evidence in this model, includes qualitative studies and meta-syntheses.

When an evidence-based practice project is completed and the results demonstrate an improvement in patient care, the evidence must then be disseminated. Dissemination of evidence can take many forms. Some examples are the following: a poster presentation at a conference, a journal article, the podium presentation at a conference, a speaking engagement, a chapter in a book, and presentations in classrooms to students. The following section provides two exemplars of evidence-based practice.

The first exemplar describes the American Heart Association (AHA) emergency cardiac care guidelines for resuscitation. In 2005, the AHA defined the importance of maximizing cardiopulmonary resuscitation (CPR), decreasing the amount of ventilation, the importance of early fibrillation to those patients requiring such, and minimizing the time to shock if needed. The research evidence at this time demonstrated the importance of increasing the coronary perfusion pressure and decreasing the mean intrathoracic pressure in the chest. The importance of priming the pump by good quality chest compressions and decreased ventilations was inherent. Quality chest oppressions are critical to achieving return of spontaneous circulation. Chest compressions must be done hard and fast with complete recoil of the chest so that the heart is adequately primed. The 2010 AHA emergency cardiac care guidelines for resuscitation further supports the importance of high-quality CPR. Now, when the victim of cardiac arrest is identified, chest compressions are started for ventilations. This again reinforces quality chest compressions.

The second exemplar describes evidence-based interventions to reduce medication errors in the acute care hospital environment. The Institute of Medicine (IOM) in 1999, 2003, and 2007 reported nearly 100,000 iatrogenic events that occur in healthcare facilities on an annual basis. Since 2003, the goal of the IOM is to decrease these iatrogenic events, with a resultant increase of the quality of care provided to patients.

Medication errors are estimated to account for more than 7,000 deaths annually (Institute of Medicine [IOM], 2007). When analyzed, there are multifactorial reasons why medication errors occur. Studies document those interruptions both in the preparation and administration of medications as a major factor. Noise is one of these factors that contribute to medication errors. The purpose of this project was to determine if implementing evidence-based interventions would decrease the number of interruptions incurred by nurses during the medication administration process within outcome of decreased medication errors. Many evidence-based practice models use the "PIC OT" format. The "P" is the patient population; in this study, the target population with a diverse sample of registered nurses into acute care hospital settings who administer medications on medical-surgical nursing units. The "I" stands for the intervention. The intervention in this study was the development of a "quiet" zone for registered nurses by having them wear an armband with the word *quiet* written on the armband. The intervention also incorporated having the charge nurse and the unit secretary manage phone calls for the nurse who was administering medications. A quiet area was also developed for medication preparation. In addition, health-care team members were educated on the negative impact that interrupting the nurse during medication administration would have on patient safety. The "C" stands for the comparative group or intervention. In this study, medication events would be totaled for the same time period in 2010 (study period) compared to 2009 on the pilot units in order to assess if medication errors increased or decreased during the study time period. The "O" stands for outcome. In this study, a decrease in the number of medication error events, which ultimately prevents adverse medication reactions and results in improved quality of care provided to the patient would hopefully be the outcome. The "T" stands for time. This study was conducted from August of 2010 through November of 2010, thus the time of study was for 3 months.

The results: One of the medical-surgical units had zero medications during the study time. During the same time, the year prior to the study, there were a total of seven medication error events. The other medical-surgical unit had one medication error during the study time period. This same unit had six medication error events occur during the same time the previous year. The conclusions were that creating a quiet zone significantly decreased medication error events. The plan is to repeat the same study the following year on to other nursing units. Should that study demonstrate the same results, then a quiet zone will be implemented on all nursing units throughout both hospitals.

To summarize, then, evidence-based practice is crucial to the provision of quality patient care. There are many evidence-based practice projects that can be initiated through any health-care system. This chapter describes two examples. The question that one must raise is the following: Is this evidence-based practice for you? The question is not a pro or con, but the real question is when.

REFERENCES

American Heart Association. (2005). *2005 American Heart Association Guidelines for CPR and ECC*. Dallas, TX: Author.

American Heart Association. (2010). *2010 American Heart Association Guidelines for CPR and ECC*. Dallas, TX: Author.

Institute of Medicine. (1999). *To err is human: Building a safer health system*. Washington, DC: National Academies Press.

Institute of Medicine. (2003). *Crossing the quality chasm. A new health system for the 21st century*. Washington, DC: National Academies Press.

Institute of Medicine. (2007). *Preventing medication errors*. Washington, DC: National Academies Press.

Kuhn, T. S. (1996). *The structure of scientific revolutions* (3rd ed.). Chicago, IL: University of Chicago Press.

Rush, J., Fiorino-Chiovitti, R., Kaufman, K., & Mitchell, A. (1990). A randomized control trial of a nursing ritual: Wearing cover gowns to care for healthy newborns. *Birth, 17*(1), 25–30.

Continuous Organizational Improvement: DNP Leadership Promoting High-Reliability Organizations

Carol Patton

Health-care delivery organizations are chaotic and frenetic with everyone claiming their health-care system is all about quality and safety to enhance patient outcomes. The reality of the matter is health-care delivery organizations are chaotic, complex systems of constant change, and the organization must continually focus on organizational improvement continuously no matter how good one believes their organization is. Health-care organizations that survive and surpass all others in the 21st century are indeed going to be those that create and sustain an organizational mission and philosophy of quality and safety. For example, the costs associated with creating an organizational culture of quality and safety are much less than offering poor quality. In July 2005, the Patient Safety and Quality Improvement Act was enacted to foster and promote a national initiative to have a national reporting system that signifies the federal government's commitment to fostering a culture of patient safety (Key, 2005).

Continuous health-care organizational improvement certainly is linked to continuous assessment and evaluation. In many health-care organizations, continuous assessment and evaluation may be centralized or decentralized functions. Continuous assessment and evaluation of health-care organizations may fall under the concept of continuous quality improvement (CQI), but CQI is only one important element in

59

creating a culture of continuous health-care organizational improvement. In addition to CQI, other health-care organizations may focus on risk management. It is relevant to note that risk management is a concept that evolved from insurance industry programs (Napier & Youngberg, 2011).

CREATING A CULTURE AND INFRASTRUCTURE TO SUPPORT CONTINUOUS HEALTH-CARE ORGANIZATIONAL IMPROVEMENT

Another major issue to keep in mind is that continuous health-care organizational improvement is a culture and not a single event, process, or outcome when something does not go according to plan. For many health-care organizations, creating a culture of continuous health-care organizational improvement involves a major organizational paradigm shift with administrative support, resource allocation, and stakeholder buy-in to create the systems and supports necessary to foster and promote a culture of continuous health-care organizational improvement.

No matter how one organizationally structures continuous assessment and evaluation, there is a clear and compelling need to make certain continuous assessment and evaluation is not complex and everyone is involved in the process and secondly that everyone from the macrosystem to the microsystem level is engaged in continuous organizational improvement initiatives. There are many reasons for continuous assessment and evaluation of every aspect of organizational operations at the macro-, micro-, and mesosystems levels because these initiatives are imperatives in contemporary health-care delivery systems. For example, continuous health-care improvement is not only needed to enhance patient quality and safety, but health-care organizations must also focus on quality and safety initiatives for other reasons including health-care worker retention, consumer satisfaction, employer satisfaction, and ultimately having a health-care organization that works and is responsive to challenges when and if they occur. The focus of this chapter is to examine what is driving health-care organizational improvement, why organizational improvement is relevant and timely, and the nurse executive role of the Doctor of Nursing Practice (DNP) in fostering and promoting continuous organizational improvement through a culture of quality and safety.

DRIVERS OF CONTINUOUS HEALTH-CARE ORGANIZATIONAL IMPROVEMENT

Developing continuous health-care organization improvement means creating a culture of change and support for all health-care professionals and staff. The ultimate goal of continuous health-care organization improvement is to create a resilient organization that is able to move and navigate with continuously changing internal and external stimuli like governmental change. There must be a rapidly responsive system in place if an organization is to be truly transformational when it comes to creating a culture of continuous health-care organization improvement. For example, creating a culture of continuous health-care organization improvement means never facing a challenge but seeing change as an opportunity for growth and meeting continuously changing demands at the macro-, micro-, and mesosystems levels of the health-care organization.

CLINICAL MICROSYSTEM LEVELS IN HEALTH-CARE ORGANIZATIONS

Continuous health-care organization improvement must be grounded in a firm organizational commitment at the clinical systems level, and it cannot be by doing some things right some of the time and being lucky or unlucky the rest of the time. For example, continuous health-care organization improvement results when organizations are highly functioning and at peak performance 10% of the time. This is certainly a tall order, but those health-care organizations that can and make this level of commitment to their key stakeholders are those that will excel in the 21st century. It is this level of commitment that builds and purposefully designs health-care organization systems that provide the right care, in the right way, at the right time, for the right patient, every time.

CLINICAL MICROSYSTEM AS A MODEL FOR CONTINUOUS HEALTH-CARE ORGANIZATION IMPROVEMENT

Systems are a network of independent components working together (Deming, 1986). Health-care systems are also independent components working together to accomplish the organizational mission and philosophy. In health-care organizations, there are many independent and yet interconnected departments or units with strong linkages between and among the various departments or units. Without a culture of support for the frontline staff and health-care personnel at the point of care, there will be many challenges for fostering and promoting continuous health-care organization improvement. The key message is that the managers and leaders cannot do this important work without direct buy-in and support from all health-care professionals and staff in the health-care system.

Although DNPs may be in various clinical leadership roles, they are in positions to create positive change and cultures of quality and safety at the clinical micro-, macro-, and mesosystems levels. Some literature refers to patient care at the microsystem level as the "sharp end of care" (Batalden, Nelson, Gardent, & Godfrey, 2007). The *sharp end of care* is defined as the point at which the patient interacts and comes into contact with the health-care system (Batalden et al., 2007, p. 74). The "blunt end of care" is at the clinical macrosystem level at the highest level of the health-care delivery (Batalden et al., 2007, p. 74). The DNP is in a prime role to increase interprofessional team collaboration and build capacity by assisting other health-care providers at the clinical microsystem level to understand the complexity and interrelationships that are essential to have a highly reliable health-care team with quality outcomes. For example, the DNP is in a prime role to create a culture at the sharp end of care and also to apply skills and competencies to shape policy and create change at the highest level of the organization, the macrosystem level. The DNP is in a unique role to facilitate and oversee clinical care that results in high performance and is disseminated and spread throughout the entire organization to macro- and mesosystems levels.

Although a health-care organization may profess to create a culture of continuous health-care organization improvement, there may be very different models for accomplishing this major goal. It really does not matter what kind of model is used to foster and promote continuous health-care organization improvement, but what does matter is that a model is subscribed to providing guidance and direction for cost-effective and efficient patient-driven outcomes. For example, some of the models that may work well in health-care organizations are the American Nurses Credentialing Center Magnet Recognition Program and The Pathway to Excellence Program (American Nurses Credentialing Center, n.d.a, n.d.b) (Table 6.1).

IMPETUS FOR CONTINUOUS HEALTH-CARE ORGANIZATION IMPROVEMENT

Nursing as a profession is focused on patient quality and outcomes even from the early days of Florence Nightingale (Nightingale, 1860). Nurses may choose different models to implement patient care that is linked to continuous health-care organization improvement, but regardless of the model of care, nurses are patient advocates for continuous health-care organization improvement. One of the major challenges for nurses, both nurse leaders and followers, is the ability to garner necessary human and financial support for initiatives related to continuous health-care organization improvement. For example, it is not uncommon in many health-care organizations that if a nursing activity is not directly related to patient care, then the initiative is not supported with adequate human and financial resources.

In the 21st century, there have been some major initiatives driving continuous health-care organization improvement, and nurses who understand these major initiatives can see them as opportunities to lead and support continuous health-care organization improvement. Some of the major drivers of change in health-care organizations are certainly consumerism, governmental regulations, and key stakeholders who are demanding high reliability and cost control in addition to quality and safety in all health-care organizations.

TABLE 6.1. Overview of the American Nurses Credentialing Center Magnet Recognition Program and The Pathway to Excellence Program

Magnet Recognition Program	The Magnet Recognition Program recognizes health-care organizations for quality patient care, nursing excellence, and innovations in professional nursing practice. Consumers rely on Magnet designation as the ultimate credential for high-quality nursing. Developed by the American Nurses Credentialing Center, Magnet is the leading source of successful nursing practices and strategies worldwide.	Benefits of Magnet Designation • Attract and retain top talent • Improve patient care, safety, and satisfaction • Foster a collaborative culture • Advance nursing standards and practice • Grow your business and financial success
The Pathway to Excellence Program	The Pathway to Excellence Program recognizes health-care organizations for positive practice environments where nurses excel. Any size or type of health-care group where nurses care for patients may apply. A dedicated application and review process exists for long-term care institutions. To qualify, organizations meet 12 practice standards essential to an ideal nursing practice environment. Applicants conduct a review process to fully document the integration of those standards in the organization's practices, policies, and culture. Pathway designation can only be achieved if an organization's nurses validate the data and other evidence submitted, via an independent, confidential survey. This critical element exemplifies the theme of empowering and giving nurses a voice. Nurses trust that Pathway-designated organizations, respect nursing contributions, support professional development, and nurture optimal practice environments. Communities want satisfied nurses because they are better equipped to deliver higher quality care. Organizations may hold Pathway and Magnet designations simultaneously.	Benefits of Pathway to Excellence Designation • Improve nurse satisfaction • Retain choice nursing staff and leaders • Cultivate interprofessional teamwork • Champion high-quality nursing practice • Support business growth

A major impetus for continuous health-care organization improvement is supported by several major organizations and think tanks advocating the need for examination and change in health-care organizations particularly related to health-care quality and safety. For example, there are numerous references attesting to the need for quality and safety in health care and need for paradigm change in approaches to quality and safety, and these initiatives are not new by any means, but the time has certainly come for continuous health-care organization improvement (Donaldson & Mohr, 2000; Institute for Healthcare Improvement, 2012; Institute of Medicine, 2001; Nelson et al., 1995; Quinn, 1992).

HEALTH CARE AS A HIGH-RISK INDUSTRY

There is much to be learned about the nature and sources of risk in health-care organizations from non-health-care organizations. There has clearly been an impact in health-care quality and safety initiatives largely due to the way health care has handled safety issues in a personal and punitive manner when an error has occurred. A "high-hazard industry" is one that "involves potent activities that have the potential to kill or maim" (Youngberg, 2011, p. 294). The characteristic of a high-hazard organization is that the organization is prone to error and injury while operating effectively and consistently despite potential for system failure and catastrophic outcomes (Youngberg, 2011, p. 295). Although health-care organizations are high-hazard industries, they still have great potential to embrace models with potential for a radical paradigm shift that creates a culture of safety and quality. Although organizational infrastructure may or may not be required for this paradigm shift, there must be integration of safety and quality with every member of the interprofessional health-care team despite the great potential of a hazardous event with catastrophic outcomes.

WHAT IS A HIGH-RELIABILITY ORGANIZATION AND WHY THIS CONCEPT MATTERS?

Reliability is defined as a "defect-free" operation (Reinertsen & Clancy, 2006). With this definition, one can readily envision the challenges with creating a culture within a health-care organization that could claim "a defect-free care policy." Although this may appear as a lofty goal for health-care organizations, it is the culture that will truly set one health-care organization apart from others in the 21st century, and creating a culture of reliability is very appealing to all major stakeholders. A high-reliability organization is one that will not be replicable and sets health-care organizations apart from their counterparts through creating and sustaining a competitive edge. High-reliability organization is one that provides more than quality improvement or risk management but that engages in continuous efforts to provide patient-centered, relationship-based care that is always safe and minimizes error as well as make certain each patient received the right care, at the right time, in the right way, every time.

One of the major challenges in 21st century health-care organizations is maintaining a competitive edge in the health-care marketplace. It is often said that competition is good, and in health care as with all organizations and businesses, there will be leaders and there will be followers of the leaders trying to mimic the product or deliverables. For example, it is a challenge in health care to create a "look-alike or knockoff" of quality health care and that is quite a bit different than a purse manufacturer creating a look-alike or knockoff purse. The DNP has an opportunity in health-care organizations at the micro-, macro-, and mesosystems levels to create a competitive advantage for the health-care organization by creating a competitive edge in the health-care market by providing health care that is not easily replicated and is unique in service and delivery.

To move toward creation of a health-care competitive edge, the DNP has skills and competencies to apply concepts and models of care that are genuine, timely, relevant, and provide care by high-quality interprofessional teams and care that is focused on quality outcomes with each patient encounter. For example, the DNP has the requisite skills and competencies to create a paradigm shift that provides and supports foundational change and movement away from an industrial model that has been so common in health-care organizations for decades. Health-care changes and models must reflect public opinion and the opinion and preferences of many stakeholders who shape health-care services. There is nothing stagnant in health-care organizations, and DNPs have to read widely and be knowledgeable of shifting sands and times with numerous stakeholders. Table 6.2 provides an overview of major key stakeholders and foci of their vested interests in health-care delivery.

TABLE 6.2. Major Key Stakeholders and Foci of Their Vested Interest in Health-Care Delivery

Major Key Stakeholder	Vested Interest in Health-Care Delivery
Government	Dominant authorities in health-care services and payment of services as major payers of health-care services through Medicare and Medicaid
Health-care organizations	Shape the care and services provided and models of care for services including acute care, specialty care, long-term care, home health, palliative care, community-based care, outpatient services, hospice, and public health
Health-care providers	Members of the interprofessional health-care team who provide services to patients and carry out the care and comprise the major cost of health-care delivery but without whom care cannot be provided
Health-care insurers	Those whose companies cover health-care costs and benefits for individuals or groups of individuals and who determine the cost of reimbursement and co-pays or deductibles for health-care services and contracts
Public	People who are recipients of all health care across the life span in all types of health-care delivery settings regardless of whether or not they have health-care insurance
Employers	Pay for much of the health-care costs through employee benefits and who also shape and form partnerships with health-care organizations based on services provided and costs of those services

High-reliability theory is a strength in health-care organizations to focus on patient-centered, relationship-based care. According to Riley (2009, p. 239), "reliability principles include methods of evaluating, calculating, and improving overall operating performance of complex systems." High-reliability organizations can only be so if there is an overall organizational commitment and creation of culture to safety and quality. These concepts cannot be mere rhetoric, and there must be organizational support from every level to truly make this kind of organizational commitment. For example, there must be ongoing education and support for every member of interprofessional health-care teams to truly embrace a culture of safety and quality. The DNP is in a capacity to be a leader and mentor with respect to high-reliability organizations particularly looking at organizational safety and quality failures as systems issues and not individual personnel issues.

Creation of capacity in interprofessional health-care teams, and according to Riley (2009, p. 241), there are key characteristics of effective teams that must be embraced in order to enhance interprofessional communication and team functioning. The DNP is in an excellent position to foster and promote team knowledge, skills, and attitudes (KSAs) in team leadership, backup behavior, mutual performance monitoring, communication adaptability, and mutual trust/team orientation. Interprofessional health-care teams must become high-reliability teams and not just groups of expert health-care providers carrying out their unique professional roles. To be a high-reliability team, the sum of an interprofessional health-care team must be greater than the sum of its parts. "The team is the primary vehicle through which problems are analyzed, solutions are generated, and change is evaluated" (Fried & Carpenter, 2013, p. 117).

ROLE OF THE DNP IN A HIGH-RELIABILITY ORGANIZATION

The DNP plays a major role in ensuring that patients consistently receive high-quality care at the sharp end of care or the patient impact level when the patient has contact with the health-care organization. This role provides an excellent opportunity for the DNP to apply all the American Association of Colleges of Nursing (AACN) DNP Essentials to shape and reform health-care delivery amidst complexity and challenges that are ever-changing and dynamic. The DNP is in a key capacity to work from a model of high-reliability theory to shape the quality of health care within each clinical microsystem and between clinical microsystems. For example, who is better than the DNP to facilitate health outcomes in diverse populations, shape, or reform policy for patient handoffs and communication between and among clinical microsystems? The DNP applies strategies integrating professional presence and behavior to make these needed changes and reformations through communication and leadership styles that empower nurses at the sharp end of care to embrace their key roles in shaping the "front lines" of health-care delivery.

CONCLUSION

Perhaps the greatest benefit of the skills and competencies of the DNP is to shape, form, and reform health-care organizations into high-reliability organizations. There is a clear and compelling need for leadership to provide 21st century health care that is patient-centered and relationship-based so care is provided in the right way, at the right time, every time. DNPs are leaders in clinical excellence and perhaps it may be that other nurses have been functioning at higher levels until the advent of the DNP. That said, the DNP plays a major role to be empowered and to empower others in advancing professional nursing and accountability elevating the role of the nurse to where it should be in contemporary 21st century health-care organizations. There is a clarion call for DNPs to be leaders and shapers of health-care organizational cultures that are calling for radical paradigm shift with respect to administrative support, resource allocation, and stakeholder buy-in to create the systems and supports necessary to foster and promote a culture of continuous health-care organizational improvement at the micro-, macro-, and mesosystems levels. To negate this role or do otherwise is failing the nursing profession and society.

REFERENCES

American Nurses Credentialing Center. (n.d.a). *Magnet Recognition Program® overview.* Retrieved from http://www.nursecredentialing.org/Magnet/ProgramOverview.aspx

American Nurses Credentialing Center. (n.d.b). *Pathway program overview.* Retrieved from http://www.nursecredentialing.org/Pathway/AboutPathway.aspx

Batalden, P. B., Nelson, E. C., Gardent, P. B., & Godfrey, M. M. (2007). Chapter 4 Leading microsystems and mesosystems for microsystem peak performance. In E. G. Nelson, P. B. Batalden, & M. M. Godfrey (Eds.), *Quality by design: A clinical microsystems approach* (pp. 69–105). San Francisco, CA: John Wiley & Sons.

Deming, W. E. (1986). *Out of the crisis.* Cambridge, MA: MIT Center for Advanced Engineering Study.

Donaldson, M. S., & Mohr, J. J. (2000). *Exploring innovation and quality improvement in health care microsystems: A cross-case analysis.* Washington, DC: Institute of Medicine.

Fried, B., & Carpenter, W. R. (2013). Understanding and improving team effectiveness in quality improvement. In W. A. Sollecito & J. K. Johnson (Eds.), *McLaughlin and Kaluzny's continuous quality improvement in healthcare* (4th ed., pp. 117–153). Burlington, MA: Jones & Bartlett.

Institute for Healthcare Improvement. (2012). *How to improve.* Retrieved from http://www.ihi.org/knowledge/Pages/HowtoImprove/default.aspx

Institute of Medicine. (2001). *Crossing the quality chasm: A new health system for the 21st century.* Washington, DC: National Academies Press.

Key, C. M. (2005). A review of the Patient Safety and Quality Improvement Act of 2005. *Health Law, 18*(18), 1–20.

Napier, J., & Youngberg, B. J. (2011). Risk management and patient safety: The synergy and the tension. In B. J. Youngberg (Ed.), *Principles of risk management and patient safety* (pp. 1–22). Sudbury, MA: Jones & Bartlett.

Nelson, E. C., Greenfield, S., Hays, R. D., Larkin, C., Leopold, B., & Batalden, P. B. (1995). Comparing outcomes and charges for patients with acute myocardial infarction in three community hospitals: An approach for assessing "value." *International Journal for Quality in Health Care, 7*(2), 243–258.

Nightingale, F. (1860). *Notes on nursing: What it is, and what it is not.* Retrieved from http://digital.library.upenn.edu/women/nightingale/nursing/nursing.html

Quinn, J. B. (1992). *Intelligent enterprise: A knowledge and service based paradigm for industry.* New York, NY: Free Press.

Reinertsen, J. L., & Clancy, C. (2006). Keeping our promises: Research, practice, and policy issues in healthcare reliability. A special issue of health services research [Foreword]. *Health Services Research, 41*(4), 1535–1538.

Riley, W. (2009). High reliability and implications for nursing leaders. *Journal of Nursing Management, 17*(2), 238–246. doi:10.1111/j.1365-2834.2009.00971.x

Youngberg, B. J. (2011). Chapter 22 Creating systematic mindfulness: Anticipating, assessing, and reducing risks of health care. In B. J. Youngberg (Ed.), *Principles of risk management and patient safety* (pp. 293–303). Sudbury, MA: Jones & Bartlett.

The Chief Nurse Executive as an Organizational Leader and Its Moral Compass: Should a Doctorate in Nursing Practice Be a Requirement?

Jean Barry

Today's chief nurse executives (CNEs) work within a health-care industry which is rapidly changing, highly complex, and technologically driven (Rundio & Scott, 2011). Health-care organizations in which CNEs practice are considered complex adaptive systems (CASs). CASs are hallmarked by dynamic human and technologic interdependencies distinguished by multiple interrelated components and pathways interacting nonlinearly (Fairchild, 2010). One of the major challenges of working within a CAS is that it is fundamentally unpredictable and, thus, to a great degree, unknowable (Anderson & McDaniel, 2000). Escalating levels of decisional ambiguity in resolving complex patient care issues and the varying perceptual lens through which multiple team members view and experience these situations create the potential for significant value conflicts.

Yet, these complex environments must be continuously transformed to create climates where patient outcomes are outstanding, interdisciplinary collaboration is the norm, nursing flourishes, and frontline decision making thrives. Organizational culture is often referred to as the personality or the "social glue" of the organization (Kane-Urrabazo, 2006). Arising from multiple and multilevel interactions among employees, shared perceptions emerge which influence employee attitudes and behaviors (Olson, 1998). *Ethical climate* (EC), a critical aspect of organizational culture, is defined as the collective perception and knowledge of principles that guide moral decision making in the care of patients (Rathert & Fleming, 2008). EC is part of a complex, adaptive system in which multiple disciplines must interact in patient-related situations that can be marked by great uncertainty, moral ambiguity, and potential moral discord (Badger & O'Connor, 2006; Robichaux & Parsons, 2009).

The CNE plays a vital role in the transformation of organizational cultures so that a robust EC is created and sustained (Kane-Urrabazo, 2006). CNE expertise in sense making in the context of complexity and unpredictability, sophisticated relationship building, scientific analysis of issues, framing and asking the next best questions in ambiguous situations, adroit and innovative improvisation when needed, and the empowerment of frontline teams to make and execute clinical decision-making based on the best available evidence are all essential (Anderson & McDaniel, 2000; Porter-O'Grady, 2009; Talbert & Dennison, 2011). In addition, CNEs must be a highly expert in the redesign of systems, based on the theory and science of administrative practice, sophisticated systems thinking, robust evidence-based strategies, and fully functioning stakeholder partnerships (Porter-O'Grady & Malloch, 2011).

Excellence and innovation require CNEs who are highly educated at the graduate level. The fundamental premise of the author is that this advanced education should be at the doctoral level and that Doctor in Nursing Practice (DNP) programs that provide a specialty track in nursing administration can best meet the needs of practicing CNEs.

In this chapter, the necessity of organizational transformation to ensure optimal ECs will be discussed. Salient research supporting this necessity will be synthesized, and common sources of organizational ethical challenges will be identified. The relevance and necessity of doctoral preparation for CNEs to successfully enact their role in creating and sustaining an optimal ethical milieu will be elucidated through a discussion of relevant DNP outcomes and the Essentials as promulgated by the American Association of Colleges of Nursing (AACN) (Zaccagnini & White, 2011).

EVIDENCE FOR SIGNIFICANCE OF ETHICAL CLIMATES

Achieving ethical environments where nurses can practice in harmony with the nursing profession's code of ethics has been described as one of the "most difficult challenges CNEs face" (Storch, Rodney, Pauly, Brown, & Starzomski, 2002). Political, financial, and organizational ideologies often serve as potent barriers to the ethical practice of nursing. Indeed, the institutional resistance and barriers to nursing's involvement in decision making can be staggering when nurses attempt to enact their patient advocacy role (Nathaniel, 2006).

Most health-care organizations are traditional bureaucratic power structures in which nurses are in subordinate positions to administration and medical dominance and physician sovereignty are hallmarks (Corley, 1995, 2002; Kennard, Speroff, & Puopolo, 1996). Nurses are often not free to operate as moral agents because of these institutional constraints, especially in the acute care setting (Storch et al., 2002). Indeed, hospital environments have been found to mitigate against nurses' involvement in ethical decision making (Corley, Minick, Elswick, & Jacobs, 2005). Within hospitals, physicians and administrative leaders have passively and, at times, actively excluded nurses from involvement in the resolution of ethical conflicts (Dodd, Jansson, Brown-Saltzman, Shirk, & Wunch, 2004).

Despite the challenges in achieving an optimal EC, which is harmonious with nursing values and ethics, research suggests that this type of climate is essential for staff nurse retention. Studies have indicated that the quality of the hospital EC is a strong factor influencing nurses' decisions to leave their positions or the profession (Hart, 2005; Uhrich et al., 2007). Hospital EC focused on doing the right thing and has also been shown to be associated with positive perceptions of teamwork; hierarchical regression analysis further indicated that a leadership style focused on continuous quality improvement significantly influenced the relationship between EC and teamwork (Rathert & Fleming, 2008).

Other research suggests that as gaps in compliance with professional ethical codes increase, nurses experienced increased role conflict and decreased job satisfaction (Biton & Tabak, 2003). In other words, the CNE must demonstrate commitment to the organizational mission and values, which espouse an EC, both in words and action. She must "walk the talk," which at times may require great moral courage given the organizational challenges described earlier (LaSala & Bjarnason, 2010).

When nurses know what the right moral action to take on behalf of the patient and are prevented from doing so, they may experience the phenomenon of moral distress. *Moral distress* is defined as a phenomenon in which nurses are aware of the morally appropriate action to take on behalf of a patient but are thwarted by either internal (e.g., fear of confrontation or low self-esteem) or external obstacles (e.g., lack of collaborative relations with medical staff, restrictive hospital policies) (Fogel, 2007; Hanna, 2004; Nathaniel, 2006). Although the bulk of the research has had acute care as the site of study, moral distress has also been found to occur in palliative care (Weissman, 2009), public health (Oberle & Tenove, 2000), and long-term care (Green & Jeffers, 2006).

This phenomenon has been associated with nurses leaving a job or, indeed, the profession as well as distancing themselves from patients and families. Moral distress has been recognized as a response to an ethical environment that is lacking in structures and processes that support nurses in their ethical comportment. Studies suggest that ECs can moderate the effect of moral distress and intent to leave (Fogel, 2007) and also predict the degree of moral distress intensity (Corley et al., 2005). Moral distress has been found to be associated with emotional exhaustion, distressful and painful feelings, and work disengagement (Corley et al., 2005; Hamric & Blackhall, 2007; Hanna, 2004; Meltzer & Huckabay, 2004; Wilkenson, 1987; Zuzelo, 2007).

In addition, perceptions of powerlessness when nurses attempt to engage in ethical decision making can contribute to a toxic work environment in which nurses experience high levels of moral distress (Erlen & Frost, 1991; Erlen & Sereika, 1997), nurses are reluctant to communicate key patient issues to medical staff (VitalSmarts, 2005), patient safety is compromised (Wlody, 2007), and staff nurse suffering often exists (Jezuit, 2004).

The state of the science as it pertains to the importance of EC for the nursing profession and the phenomenon of moral distress is scant. It is predominated by primary studies that are descriptive in design, have small sample sizes, and usually use single sites. However, what evidence there is suggests that the existence of an optimal EC is associated with work satisfaction and retention of nursing staff. Also, findings from several studies suggest that moral distress has been found to contribute to unsafe practices and negative staff nurse mood states.

ORGANIZATIONAL AND CLINICAL CHALLENGES

The following section identifies five of the most common ethical challenges facing CNEs. It is not meant to be comprehensive but rather to provide examples that illustrate the complexity and rigor required on the part of the CNE to address ethical issues. As previously mentioned, most health-care organizations are traditional bureaucratic power structures hallmarked by administrative and medical dominance and in which nurses are in subordinate positions.

The authority gradient between nurses and physicians has been noted as a major issue in terms of resolving ethical issues and the experience of moral distress (Corley et al., 2005; Edmundson, 2010; Kirchhoff & Beckstrand, 2000; Redman & Fry, 2000; Storch et al., 2002). Status differentials among members can have a profound impact on the behavior of individuals within teams. Individuals lower in status more often accept the opinions and ideas of the higher status members and frequently do not offer nor are asked for relevant information only they might have (Thomas, Sexton, & Helmreich, 2003). Because nurses are viewed by medical staff as not being equal to them in hierarchical status, valuable nursing information is not sought by physicians and, often, not offered by nurses (Baggs, Norton, Schmitt, & Sellers, 2004).

When nurses do not believe that medical staff will be receptive to their input or perceive that their CNE is unsupportive of them, these nurses may become reluctant to advocate for their patients due to fear of retribution or ridicule from medical staff or because of the lack of confidence in their knowledge and their expertise (Curtis, 2004). An authentic CNE leadership style accompanied by CNE role modeling has been shown to increase the likelihood that nurses will actively speak up during difficult ethical situations (LaSala & Bjarnason, 2010; Wong, Laschinger, & Cummings, 2010).

CNEs are in a unique position when compared to other members of the administrative team in that they must fluidly move between clinical and administrative domains, balancing the needs of patients and families, clinical staff, providers, and the organization (Edmundson, 2010; Talbert & Dennison, 2011). Marginalization is always a risk for CNEs given this dual role. Pressure to adopt the values and standards of the administrative and medical power structures with the possible exclusion of what is in the best interests of nursing could lead to this marginalization (Shirey, 2005).

As the hospital industry aggressively moves to increase the safety of patients, new ethical issues have arisen related to patient safety policy and practice initiatives. Administrators espouse the notion of nonpunitive identification and reporting of errors and the view that errors arise from flawed systems rather than unsafe practitioners. However, changing the ethical culture so that these beliefs are embedded in the fabric of the organization can be challenging (Johnstone, 2007).The CNE must take a critical leadership role in shifting the culture but may come up against considerable resistance when dealing with individual patient safety errors with pronounced negative patient outcomes.

Related to the patient safety, the overall approach to registered nurse staffing can be fraught with ethical challenges in today's financially constrained environment. In a study by Cooper and associates, out of 20 challenges, nursing administrators ranked intense market competition and the necessity for the administrative team to be focused on the bottom line and less on ethics as the two top rated ones (Cooper, Frank, Gouty, & Hansen, 2003). The third and fourth highest rated challenges involved conflicting loyalties and accountabilities between duty to the CNEs' employers and their duty to employees and customers. This is one of the most difficult challenges with pressures from chief executives officers to contain staffing costs and from the nursing staff to provide safe patient care consistent with nursing's values. Again, it takes advanced knowledge in ethics, finance, and interdisciplinary team building to approach workable resolutions that are responsive in the long run to needs of organizational stakeholders. One of the most common sources of moral distress reported by researchers is related to staff nurse perceptions of inadequate staffing levels (Corley et al., 2005; Zuzelo, 2007).

With aging baby boomers, end-of-life issues will become increasingly prevalent in the health-care industry. Models of care delivery, which support the provision of comfort care, are critical in the 21st century. Organizational structures in the form of policies and high-functioning interdisciplinary teams including medical staff are essential to ensure that dying patients' wishes are met (Badger & O'Connor, 2006; Corley, 2002; Kirchhoff & Beckstrand, 2000). Yet, end-of-life care in the United States remains highly aggressive and invasive with concerns about futile care proliferating (Guitierrez, 2005; Hamric & Blackhall, 2007; Hanna, 2004). The most common source of the moral distress cited in the research is nursing's perception that they are causing unnecessary suffering for terminal patients due to the provision of futile care (Guitierrez, 2005; Hamric & Blackhall, 2007; Kirchhoff & Beckstrand, 2000).

THE NEED FOR CNE DOCTORAL PREPARATION

In 2004, in their DNP position statement, the AACN called for a transformational change in the educational preparation of nurses practicing in the most advanced level of professional nursing roles; AACN endorsed the need for advanced education for nurses engaged in advanced practice nursing, including the specialty focus of aggregate, systems, and organizational nursing practice (American Association of Colleges of Nursing [AACN], 2004). The demands of a rapidly changing and complex health-care industry require that nurses engaged in advanced levels of clinical or administrative specialty practice and must have in-depth scientific knowledge and expertise in the practice setting. Research has supported the notion that there is a link between higher levels of education and better patient outcomes (Aiken, Clarke, Cheung, Sloane, & Silber, 2003; Kutney-Lee & Aiken, 2009).

Although most nurses are aware that a Doctor of Philosophy (PhD) degree prepares one for a research career and for academia, many are still unaware of the national movement toward the DNP degree. DNP programs are rapidly proliferating across the United States with 241 schools across 49 states having DNP programs in place. Over 100 additional schools of nursing are considering starting programs (AACN, 2014). This rapid proliferation of programs is in response to many factors impinging on the health-care industry.

These factors include national concerns about the quality and safety of the care provided to patients and major policy developmental needs at the state and national level to ensure adequate provision of care to America's vulnerable populations. Major shortages of nursing faculty prepared with doctoral degrees and the continued increase in educational expectations for the preparation of other health professionals (e.g., doctor of pharmacy, doctor of physical therapy) contribute to this movement toward the DNP educational credential (Barry, 2009; Brown-Benedict, 2008; Royeen & Lavin, 2007).

Following the 2004 position paper, the AACN conducted a 2-year national consensus process. Eight core essential competencies, which formed a common framework for the design of DNP programs, were approved by the AACN Board of Directors (Table 7.1). Although these core essentials listed in Table 7.1 apply to any type of advanced nursing practice, brief descriptions that illustrate application to the CNEs work in designing ECs are also provided in Table 7.1 (AACN, 2006).

Although all DNP graduates must demonstrate the competencies of essentials 1 through 8, further DNP preparation falls into two general categories of specializations: nurses who specialize in the clinical care of individuals and who plan to function as nurse practitioners and nurses who specialize in care at an aggregate or systems or the organizational level. Those DNP programs with nursing administration and/or health service leadership tracks must also provide course work and practicum, which prepare students to assume the multifaceted role of a CNE in today's health-care industry with all its complexity and confounding problems.

TABLE 7.1. The Eight AACN Essentials for DNP Education

Essentials	DNP Graduate Competencies for CNEs
1. Scientific underpinnings for practice	1. CNEs will have the ability to translate a wide array of knowledge gleaned from the sciences to quickly and effectively improve systems of care and enact an advanced leadership role.
2. Organizational and systems leadership for quality improvement and systems thinking	2. CNEs will be prepared to use principles from multiple sciences and practices to create effective strategies for the management of ethical dilemmas at individual and the complex systems level. In addition, they will be able to use advanced communication methods to ensure stakeholder partnerships.
3. Clinical scholarship and analytic methods for evidence-based practice (EBP)	3. CNEs will have in-depth, scientific knowledge to use analytic methods to critique existing evidence for relevance and to design EBP interventions to transform and sustain ECs.
4. Information systems/ technology and patient care technology for the improvement and transformation of health care	4. CNEs will have advanced knowledge and abilities to use information systems and technology to improve patient care and systems, enhance communication, and to evaluate care at the individual and systems level. He or she will also be prepared to address the ethical and legal implications of using such technology.
5. Health-care policy for advocacy in health care	5. CNEs will be prepared to design, influence, and put into action health-care policies to address ethical issues at the organizational level to design and implement ethical environments. They will also have the knowledge and skills to improve ethical care of multiple patient populations at the community, state, and national levels.
6. Interprofessional collaboration for improving patient and population health outcomes	6. CNEs will have advanced preparation both in theory and practicum to design effective interdisciplinary team structures and processes to ensure that a strong and effective EC is a hallmark of the organizational culture. Advanced preparation in the areas of change and conflict negotiation will also be part of the DNP graduate's repertoire.
7. Clinical prevention and population health for improving the nation's health	7. The foundation provided by this essential will enable CNEs to analyze epidemiological, occupational, and environmental data to work with community stakeholders to improve the health of the citizens.
8. Advanced practice nursing	8. This essential refers to the foundational knowledge needed in order to ensure competence in highly complex areas of specialization, in this case nursing administration. CNEs will demonstrate advanced levels of judgment, systems thinking, and accountability in the design of organizations that have a robust EC.

AACN, American Association of Colleges of Nursing; CNE, chief nurse executive; DNP, Doctor of Nursing Practice; EC, ethical climate.

From American Association of Colleges of Nursing. (2006). *The essentials of doctoral education for advanced nursing practice*. Retrieved from http://www.aacn.nche.edu/dnp/pdf/Essentials.pdf

The DNP program culminates with a scholarly project, which differs from the type of dissertation associated with a PhD degree. The PhD dissertation requires the generation of new knowledge through the conduct of original research. The DNP scholarly project is focused on the application or translation of knowledge from original research studies and other forms of evidence into the clinical arena. The knowledge and skill to take an evidence-based project from the problem identification phase through a robust evaluation requires expert knowledge and skill in all domains articulated in the Core Essentials document (AACN, 2006).

Nurses interested in the field of nursing administration can still obtain a master's degree in this field. However, nursing administration experts are now beginning to question whether the curricula in nursing administration master's programs are sufficiently robust to prepare the CNEs of the 21st century to assume the top nursing executive roles in the health-care industry (Rundio & Scott, 2011; Talbert & Dennison, 2011).

It is important to note that these Core Essentials were not created in a vacuum. The AACN convened a task force of multiple constituencies across the United States. In addition, 2 years of consensus building occurred in multiple locales at multiple times during the construction of the Essentials document (AACN, 2006). Additionally, various professional organizations have identified key competencies for nurse executives. Although the American Organization of Nurse Executives (AONE) has not at this time endorsed the DNP degree as a requirement, they do believe that there are five key competencies which nurse executives must master. These include communication and relationship building, knowledge of the health-care environment, leadership, professionalism, and business skills (American Organization of Nurse Executives [AONE], 2005). These core competencies are aligned with the AACN Core Essentials. Although AONE still believes that nursing administration master's degree programs should remain intact, this organization does view nursing executive practice as a subspecialty which requires advanced executive knowledge (Talbert & Dennison, 2011).

The American Nurses Association (ANA) Nursing Administration: Scope and Standards of Practice is also an important source for the identification of nurse executive practices and behaviors and are aligned with the AACN Core Essentials (American Nurses Association [ANA], 2009). Finally, the American College of Healthcare Executives (ACHE) Code of Ethics supports the importance of providing a work environment that supports the free expression of ethical concerns and mechanism to address these concerns (American College of Healthcare Executive [ACHE], 2007). This Code also calls for the creation of an organizational culture in which adverse errors are minimized and that supports the reporting and remediation of these errors.

The prior sections of this chapter described the challenges faced by CNEs in the highly complex environment in which health care is provided and the difficult and arduous process of creating and sustaining optimal ethical work environments.

"Nurses in the role of clinical executive are no longer invited to the table solely based on their clinical insight but more so for their ability and capacity to lead organizations based on their leadership [knowledge and] competencies" (Talbert & Dennison, 2011, p. 151). Thus, in reviewing and reflecting on the DNP Essentials promulgated by the AACN (2006) and in light of the current and future challenges in the healthcare industry, it is becoming increasingly clear that doctoral level education in the form of a DNP program best prepares CNEs to lead their organizations and their communities.

REFERENCES

Aiken, L., Clarke, S., Cheung, R., Sloane, D., & Silber, J. (2003). Educational levels of hospital nurses and surgical patient mortality. *Journal of the American Medical Association, 290*(12), 1617–1623.

American Association of Colleges of Nursing. (2004). *AACN position statement on the practice doctorate in nursing.* Retrieved from http://www.aacn.nche.edu/DNP/DNPPositionStatement.htm

American Association of Colleges of Nursing. (2006). *The essentials of doctoral education for advanced nursing practice.* Retrieved from http://www.aacn.nche.edu/dnp/pdf/Essentials.pdf

American Association of Colleges of Nursing. (2014). *DNP fact sheet.* Retrieved from http://www.aacn.nche.edu/media-relations/fact-sheets/dnp

American College of Healthcare Executive. (2007). *American College of Healthcare Executives code of ethics.* Retrieved from http://www.ache.org/ABT_ACHE/code.cfm

American Nurses Association. (2009). *Nursing administration: Scope and standards of practice.* Washington, DC: Author.

American Organization of Nurse Executives. (2005, February). AONE nurse executive competencies. *Nurse Leader,* 50–56.

Anderson, R., & McDaniel, R. (2000). Managing health care organizations: Where professionalism meets complexity science. *Health Care Management Review, 25*(1), 83–92.

Badger, J., & O'Connor, B. (2006). Moral discord, cognitive strategies, and medical intensive care unit nurses. *Critical Care Nursing Quarterly, 29*(2), 147–151.

Baggs, J., Norton, S., Schmitt, M., & Sellers, C. (2004). The dying patient in the ICU: The role of the interdisciplinary team. *Critical Care Clinics, 20,* 525–540.

Barry, J. (2009). To use or not to use: The clinical use of the title "doctor" by DNP graduates. *Journal of Nursing Administration, 39*(3), 99–102.

Biton, V., & Tabak, N. (2003). The relationship between the application of the nursing ethical code and nurses' work satisfaction. *International Journal of Nursing Practice, 9,* 140–157.

Brown-Benedict, D. (2008). The doctor of nursing practice degree: Lessons from the history of the professional doctorate in other health disciplines. *Journal of Nursing Education, 47*(10), 448–577.

Cooper, R., Frank, G., Gouty, C., & Hansen, M. (2003). Ethical helps and challenges faced by nurse leaders in the healthcare industry. *Journal of Nursing Administration, 33*(1), 17–23.

Corley, M. C. (1995). Moral distress of critical care nurses. *American Journal of Critical Care, 4*(4), 280–285.

Corley, M. C. (2002). Nurse moral distress: A proposed theory and research agenda. *Nursing Ethics, 9*(6), 636–650.

Corley, M. C., Minick, P., Elswick, R., & Jacobs, M. (2005). Nurse moral distress and ethical work environment. *Nursing Ethics, 12*(4), 381–390.

Curtis, J. (2004). Communicating about end-of-life care with patients and families in the intensive care unit. *Critical Care Clinics*, *20*, 363–380.

Dodd, S., Jansson, B., Brown-Saltzman, K., Shirk, M., & Wunch, K. (2004). Expanding nurses' participation in ethics: An empirical examination of technical activism and ethical assertiveness. *Nursing Ethics*, *11*(1), 15–27.

Edmundson, C. (2010). Moral courage and the nurse leader. *Online Journal of Issues in Nursing*, *15*(3).

Erlen, J., & Frost, B. (1991). Nurses' perception of powerlessness influencing ethical decisions. *Western Journal of Nursing Research*, *13*(3), 397–407.

Erlen, J., & Sereika, S. (1997). Critical nurses, ethical decision-making, and stress. *Journal of Advanced Nursing*, *26*, 953–961.

Fairchild, R. (2010). Practical ethical theory for nurses responding to complexity of care. *Nursing Ethics*, *17*(3), 353–362.

Fogel, K. (2007). *The relationship of moral distress, ethical climate, and intent to turnover* (Unpublished dissertation). Loyola University Chicago, IL.

Green, A., & Jeffers, B. (2006). Exploring moral distress in the long-term care setting. *Perspectives*, *30*(4), 5–9.

Guitierrez, K. (2005). Critical care nurses' perceptions of and responses to moral distress. *Dimensions in Critical Care Nursing*, *24*(5), 229–241.

Hamric, A., & Blackhall, L. (2007). Nurse-physician perspectives of the care of dying patients in the intensive care units: Collaboration, moral distress, and ethical climate. *Critical Care Medicine*, *35*(2), 422–429.

Hanna, D. (2004). Moral distress: The state of the science. *Research and Theory for Nursing Practice: An International Journal*, *18*(1), 79–83.

Hart, S. (2005). Hospital ethical climates and registered nurses' turnover intentions. *Journal of Nursing Scholarship*, *37*(2), 173–177.

Jezuit, D. (2004). Suffering of critical care nurses with end-of-life decisions. *MedSurg Nursing*, *9*(3), 145–152.

Johnstone, M. (2007). Patient safety ethics and human error management in ED contexts. Part II: Accountability and challenge to change. *Australasian Emergency Nursing Journal*, *10*, 80–85.

Kane-Urrabazo, C. (2006). Management's role in shaping organizational culture. *Journal of Nursing Management*, *14*, 188–194.

Kennard, M., Speroff, T., & Puopolo, A. (1996). Participation of nurses in decision-making for seriously ill adults. *Clinical Nursing Research*, *5*, 199–219.

Kirchhoff, K., & Beckstrand, R. (2000). Critical care nurses' perceptions of obstacles and helpful behaviors in providing end-of-life care to dying patients. *American Journal of Critical Care*, *9*(2), 96–105.

Kutney-Lee, A., & Aiken, L. (2009). Effect of nurse staffing and eduction on the outcomes of surgical patients with co-morbid serious mental illness. *Psychiatric Services*, *59*(12), 1466–1469.

LaSala, C., & Bjarnason, D. (2010). Creating workplace environments that support moral courage. *Online Journal of Issues in Nursing*, *15*(3).

Meltzer, L., & Huckabay, L. (2004). Critical care nurses' perceptions of futile care and its effects of burnout. *American Journal of Critical Care*, *13*(3), 202–208.

Nathaniel, A. (2006). Moral reckoning in nursing. *Western Journal of Nursing Research*, *24*(4), 419–438.

Oberle, K., & Tenove, S. (2000). Ethical issues in public health nursing. *Nursing Ethics*, *7*(5), 425–438.

Olson, L. (1998). Hospital nurses' perceptions of the ethical climate of their work setting. *Image: Journal of Nursing Scholarship*, *30*(4), 345–349.

Porter-O'Grady, T. (2009). Creating a context for excellence and innovation. *Nursing Administrative Quarterly, 33*(3), 198–204.

Porter-O'Grady, T., & Malloch, K. (2011). *Quantum leadership: A resource for health care innovation* (3rd ed.). Boston, MA: Jones & Bartlett.

Rathert, C., & Fleming, D. (2008). Hospital ethical climate and teamwork in acute care: The moderating role of leaders. *Health Care Management Review, 33*(4), 323–331.

Redman, B., & Fry, S. (2000). Nurses' ethical conflicts: What is really known about them? *Nursing Ethics, 7*, 360–366.

Robichaux, C., & Parsons, M. (2009). An ethical framework for developing and sustaining a healthy workplace. *Critical Care Nursing Quarterly, 32*(3), 199–207.

Royeen, C., & Lavin, M. (2007). A contextual and logical analysis of the clinical doctorate for health practitioners. *Journal of Allied Health, 36*(2), 101–106.

Rundio, A., & Scott, L. (2011). Leadership and the DNP-educated nurse executive. In H. M. Dreher & M. Glasgow (Eds.), *Role development for doctoral advanced nursing practice* (pp. 245–256). New York, NY: Springer.

Shirey, M. (2005). Ethical climate in nursing practice: The leader's role. *JONA's Healthcare, Law, Ethics, and Regulation, 7*(2), 59–67.

Storch, J., Rodney, P., Pauly, B., Brown, H., & Starzomski, R. (2002). Listening to nurses' moral voices: Building a quality health care environment. *Canadian Journal of Nursing Leadership, 15*(4), 7–16.

Talbert, T., & Dennison, R. (2011). The role of the clinical executive. In H. M. Dreher & M. Glasgow (Eds.), *Role development for doctoral advanced nursing practice* (pp. 141–156). New York, NY: Springer.

Thomas, E., Sexton, J., & Helmreich, R. (2003). Discrepant attitudes about teamwork among critical care nurses and physicians. *Critical Care Medicine, 31*(3), 956–959.

Uhrich, C., O'Donnell, P., Taylor, C., Farrar, A., Danis, M., & Grady, C. (2007). Ethical climate, ethical stress, and the job satisfaction of nurses and social workers in the United States. *Social Science & Medicine, 65*, 1708–1719.

VitalSmarts. (2005). *Silence kills: The seven crucial conversations for healthcare.* Retrieved from http://www.silencekills.com

Weissman, D. (2009). Moral distress in palliative care. *Journal of Palliative Care, 12*(10), 865–866.

Wilkenson, J. (1987). Moral distress in nursing practice: Experience and effect. *Nursing Forum, 23*(1), 16–29.

Wlody, G. (2007). Nursing management and organizational ethics in the intensive care unit. *Critical Care Medicine, 35*(2), S29–S35.

Wong, C., Laschinger, H., & Cummings, G. (2010). Authentic leadership and nurses' voice behaviour and perceptions of care quality. *Journal of Nursing Management, 18*, 889–900.

Zaccagnini, M., & White, K. (2011). *The doctor of nursing practice essentials: A new model for advanced practice nursing.* Sudbury, MA: Jones & Bartlett.

Zuzelo, P. (2007). Exploring moral distress of registered nurses. *Nursing Ethics, 14*(3), 344–359.

8

Delegation Dilemmas

Al Rundio

PART 1: THE ART OF DELEGATION

Why Delegate?

The Doctor of Nursing Practice at the executive level is in a pivotal position to foster growth in the management and nursing staffs by having them educated and embracing the concept of delegation. This will become more important as health care and nursing address increased costs, quality patient outcomes, and staff satisfaction.

Delegation was an art and skill that I learned on the job (OTJ). No one ever taught me how to delegate effectively. No one educated me in nursing school to be a good delegator. It was more a process of osmosis and trial and error. How did I learn to delegate? For me, the answer is easy. I moved up the management ranks; as my responsibilities increased, I quickly learned that I could not do it all and, hence, began to delegate. What I have learned over the years is that delegation is an art and science, and probably, a little more art than science. I have also learned that delegation can be taught and that all nurses should be taught this skill. In addition, I have also learned that the practice of delegation is what most dramatically improves the skill. Do not be afraid to take the steps to delegation. Learn from your mistakes and move on. So, what follows is information that should help you learn the *art of delegation* and become a more effective delegator.

Delegation is an essential element of any manager's or nurse's job (after all, we manage patient care) if he or she is going to be effective in his or her role. Benefits can be realized by employees when managers and nurses delegate effectively. Oftentimes, the best possible results can be achieved when skillful delegation is employed.

Managed care and the nursing shortage have warranted changes in care delivery. Registered nurses (RNs) at the bedside have to learn how to render care differently. A nurse can no longer be the be-all and the end-all to the patient. Nurses have had to learn how to function interdependently with other caregivers. As many health-care delivery systems have incorporated unlicensed assistive personnel in the practice setting, nurses must learn the art of delegation. According to Parsons and Ward (2000), the use of unlicensed assistive personnel is the single most prevalent factor for patient care management redesigned care delivery models.

As nursing is a practice discipline, RNs are in a role where they directly supervise caregivers with less qualifications even though the RN may not be in a management role per se. In order for quality patient care to occur, it is then necessary for RNs to employ the art of delegation.

One of the major problems that affects why RNs do not delegate care and other tasks is that they have not been educated to do so. Parsons and Ward (2000) further notes that most nurses lack the expertise that is needed to direct a multi-skilled workforce.

What can be delegated by nurses? Basically, everyday small tasks to major leadership initiatives can be delegated. Some examples of delegation include a certain project such as the time schedule to specific patient care tasks such as the taking and the recording of vital signs.

According to Heller (1998), "delegation involves entrusting another person with a task for which the delegator remains ultimately responsible." Several state boards of nursing clearly specify that the RN cannot delegate a task that he or she is only licensed to perform. For example, the RN can certainly delegate vital signs because nursing assistants are permitted to be educated in the taking and recording of vital signs. The RN could not delegate the starting of an intravenous line to the nursing assistant because the nurse practice act in the vast majority of states state that only an RN can start an intravenous line. Many state boards of nursing have also developed and implemented delegatory clauses that specify what and what not RNs can delegate. The basic premise of these delegatory clauses centers on the issue of licensure and what one can perform and not perform legally from a licensure standpoint.

As RNs hold a license from an individual state, it is recommended that nurses contact their respective state board of nursing and ascertain if they have a delegatory clause or if a statement exists on delegation in their nurse practice act.

So, then, what actually is delegation and how does one go about it?

Delegation is allowing your "delegates" to think and decide for themselves in your absence. Delegation encourages subordinates to make decisions in certain situations that you would usually make. Delegation empowers someone else to act on your behalf within a specified scope of practice or work.

You can see that delegation encourages empowerment and autonomy, which are two key concepts that most nurses want. Certain studies have demonstrated that these two concepts, that is, empowerment and autonomy, when employed properly, contribute to nursing retention.

There are some things to consider when exploring delegation. Delegation is not just giving away tasks randomly. Some individuals do not want to have anything delegated to them. Some individuals do not have the proper training or education for certain delegated tasks. Some individuals do not possess the proper credentials or licensure for delegated tasks.

Delegation is not abdicating decision making and is not replicating you in your absence.

In addition, delegation involves you being there for support and monitoring. Many individuals have the notion that delegation is simply delegating the task and forgetting about it. In other words, one has passed the "buck" so to speak and now, it is the other person's responsibility. This is not delegation. *When one delegates a specific task, that person is still accountable for the outcome.* For example, if I delegate the task of vital signs to a nursing assistant, I am responsible to make certain that the nursing assistant has taken the vital signs. I am also responsible to make certain that the vital signs are taken according to nursing standards and are documented correctly. In lieu of the nursing shortage today, many nurses are willing to delegate tasks, but then, they do not follow up to see that the task has been done according to practice standards.

Although the tasks that one delegates in nursing are tasks that a lower level care provider can render, for example, vital signs, bed baths, and transportation of patients in a health-care facility, running errands, etc., these tasks all center on the fact that the individual to whom the task is delegated must be competent to do the task. Let us look at the example of taking vital signs. A nursing assistant, who is delegated the task of taking and recording vital signs, must be competent to perform this delegated task. This nursing assistant should have had an educational program on how to take vital signs, and, most importantly, this nursing assistant should have periodic reassessment of this skill in order to assure competency. Looking at this example further, let us say that a nursing assistant was delegated the task of taking vital signs and this nursing assistant is incompetent to do so. This nursing assistant records a blood pressure of 120/80 mm Hg on a patient who was admitted with signs and symptoms of a transient ischemic attack. This nursing assistant continues to record a blood pressure in the 120/80 mm Hg range for a couple of days on this patient. The patient suddenly, one morning, suffers a massive ischemic stroke. One of the staff RNs assigned to this nursing unit takes the patient's vital signs while the patient is in the process of having the stroke. The RN records a blood pressure of 260/140 mm Hg. The RN who delegated the task of taking and recording vital signs to the nursing assistant would be held accountable if it is discovered that the nursing assistant was not competent to take and record vital signs. Such competency of delegated tasks can only be assured through continued competency assessment, evaluation, and direct observation of the skill.

Table 8.1 lists some questions you should ask yourself prior to delegating any task.

TABLE 8.1. Questions for Your Consideration Prior to Delegating a Task

- What work should you delegate?
- What authority and limits are you delegating?
- Have I ensured that the delegate is adequately educated to perform the task at hand?
- Am I able to delegate the task according to my respective state's nurse practice act?
- Is the delegate looking at the task with a fresh eye?
- Are too many steps involved in the process of the delegated task?
- Is the delegate able to complete the task in a timely and competent manner?
- What support and feedback will your delegate need/require?
- How clear is the "delegate" on the scope of authority and decision making?
- Is an ongoing assessment system in place to identify any issues/problems with the delegated task?
- What improvement in care will result by delegation of this task?
- What cost savings can be realized by delegation of this task?
- Is a continuous quality improvement process in place so that delegation continues to improve?

Barriers to Delegation

When delegating any task, one must realize that there are certain barriers to the delegation process. Barriers will exist on both the person who delegates the task as well as the person to whom the task is being delegated. Some barriers may be minor and not create an issue on either side of the delegation process. Other barriers will impede the success of delegation. It is important that both the delegator and the delegate realize that barriers do exist, and these barriers should be discussed with the goal of eliminating as many as possible prior to the delegation process being implemented.

Table 8.2 lists some barriers to delegation.

Some Other Thoughts on Delegation

It is always best to approach any situation that one is going to delegate in a professional, adult-to-adult manner. What am I referring to? Adults at times are in a

TABLE 8.2. Barriers to the Delegation Process

- Doing it yourself—only I can do it right
- Overburdening staff
- Being inexperienced as a delegator
- Losing control of tasks
- Staff not being competent to perform task
- I may not want to delegate a certain task that would make me look good in front of my superior as I am up for a promotion at any time now
- Not having the right equipment for a delegated task thus the task is not delegated
- Dealing with fear
- Feeling insecure
- Being suspicious
- Lacking trust
- Being too busy
- Human diversity
- Gender issues

child-to-child mode. I am not saying that this is a bad thing. It is good at times when one gets in touch with his or her inner child. However, delegation is not one of those times. The interpersonal process of delegation is greatly enhanced if relationships are conducted in an honest and open adult-to-adult way.

The United States is a country of diversity. A wonderful example on diversity was provided to me when I was making home visits to elderly bound patients. I took my grandson on one of those visits. A very bright 91-year-old woman, who had more than her full mental capacity, questioned me about what nationality my grandson was. I advised her that he was Italian, English, German, French, American, Czechoslovakian, and an entire side to him that we did not even know. Her response was, "Boy, this country is just like minestrone soup, isn't it?" It is one of the best analogies that I have heard about cultural diversity, and it is true. It is one of those unique attributes that make America so great. Diversity exists in all aspects of our lives. One will see it at work, at school, at stores, at church, etc. Such diversity needs to be considered when delegating tasks. Not every culture believes and trusts what American medicine and nursing does.

Religious beliefs and the value system of the delegate also have to be taken into consideration when delegating certain tasks. Nurses in the United States today have to always recognize and accommodate the various cultures and the human diversity that exists in our society.

One should use delegation to benefit you, your staff, and your organization. One of the key goals of delegation is to empower and encourage the growth and development of others as well as allow you time to do others things. One of the overriding goals is organizational improvement for your place of work.

After a task has been delegated, one should always be positive when reviewing progress—expect to hear good news. One should show faith in your chosen delegate, even if others have reservation. Remember, you should not have randomly selected the delegate. Your selection is largely based on the fact that the individual is competent and able to perform the delegated task. A delegator should also have the right experience in order to coach others. Coaching is an artful skill that involves confrontation and feedback. Coaching done in a positive manner is one of management's most effective tools.

For delegation to be successful, it is vital to have an effective and responsive system for controls. Use such systems to monitor delegates and the progress of assignments.

A good monitoring system consists of a light rein and a tight hand. You can always exercise more control if you feel that it is necessary, but you should do so with tact and sensitivity. This is especially the case if your delegate is inexperienced. You will score far more points in the delegation process if you approach your delegate in a positive manner even when you have to correct something in order to get the process back on the right track.

And, finally, if delegation is not working, one needs to ask himself or herself: "What I am doing incorrectly? Where have I gone wrong?" The art of delegation is most incumbent on the person doing the delegating.

PART 2: EXEMPLAR: AN EDUCATIONAL MODULE TO EDUCATE CLINICAL NURSING LEADERS AT THE BEDSIDE

This exemplar describes a new nursing care delivery model and an educational module to educate clinical nurse leaders at the bedside. A six-module educational program was designed to educate nurses into the clinical nurse leader role. This educational program can be used in various ways. The most commonly used educational methods include (1) totally online, (2) traditional in-classroom, or (3) a blended methodology that incorporates both traditional in-classroom presentation as well as online learning. This educational program consists of six core modules. The focus of module 4 is issues in delegation. Case studies and stories on delegation dilemmas are highlighted.

Health care in acute care hospitals and other settings has changed dramatically over the years. Secondary to diagnosis-related groups (DRGs), managed care, utilization management, case management, and other systems that drive the cost of care, patients are generally more ill when they present for inpatient services. Parsons (1999) concluded that changing care delivery models secondary to managed care have significantly changed the RNs role on the health-care team. Nursing shortages tend to be cyclical in nature. The current shortage that began in the mid-1990s is projected to last for an indefinite time into the future. This is secondary to an aging population, the baby boomer generation at or near retirement age, and the number of retirees eventually exceeding the number of persons working and the changes in health-care reimbursement.

As a result of the nursing shortage, RNs at the bedside have to learn how to render care differently. A nurse can no longer be the be-all and the end-all to the patient. Nurses have had to learn how to function interdependently with other caregivers. As many health-care delivery systems have incorporated unlicensed assistive personnel in the practice setting, nurses must learn the art of delegation. According to Parsons and Ward (2000), the use of unlicensed assistive personnel is the single most prevalent factor for patient care management redesigned care delivery models. They further state that most nurses lack the expertise that is needed to direct a multi-skilled workforce.

This chapter addresses a timely issue and focuses on the development of an educational program that incorporates a delegation educational module to educate nurses on delegation skills.

Review of the Literature

The reality of the workplace is that nurses have to delegate an increasing number of nursing tasks to other care providers. Thomas and Hume (1998) explored how recently graduated baccalaureate prepared nurses felt about the delegation experience as practicing nurses. A focus group methodology was used for this research project. Responses from participants in the focus group demonstrated that delegation skills are learned by trial and error in the workplace rather than by a planned educational program. These graduates further reported that less than 1 hour of theory was dedicated to the specific topic of delegation. The topic of delegation was discussed in the fourth-year leadership course, and no simulated delegation situations or scenarios were used as part of the educational experience. Strong communication skills were also essential for these graduates to delegate effectively. The authors concluded that a varied educational approach was required to teach nurses and nursing students about delegation. Examples are inclusive of seminars, situational case studies, clinical learning experiences, and use of a nursing decision grid for teaching decision making in delegation. The authors also stated that nursing practice acts had to be analyzed.

Parsons (1999) studied the effects of a structured teaching intervention for delegation decision making and its effect on RNs' confidence and delegation knowledge. This study was an experimental study that was an intervention study. A convenience sample of 90 RNs from varied medical-surgical nursing units employed at a 282-bed tertiary suburban hospital in Central Alabama was the study participants. These nurses with varied educational backgrounds were assigned to an experimental or a control group. RNs in the experimental group were taught specific information contained in a delegation decision-grid model. RNs in the control group were not provided with specific information on how to make delegation decisions based on the delegation decision-grid model. The study author concluded that use of the delegation decision-making model with selected medical-surgical case studies created a greater awareness of the laws that govern the practice of nursing. She further concluded that hospitals and other health-care institutions should offer staff development sessions and continuing education programs on delegation for practicing RNs.

Anthony, Standing, and Hertz (2000) discussed a national survey of licensed nurses concerning patient outcomes when nursing activities were delegated to unlicensed assistive personnel. Experience of both the licensed nurses as well as the unlicensed assistive personnel in the current work setting were correlated with more positive outcomes and events. Routine observation of the delegated activity also contributed to more positive outcomes and events. More negative events were associated with a lack of direct supervision by the licensed nurse to the unlicensed assistive personnel. The authors concluded that the recognition of the importance of the supervisory process has implications for educational activities that focus on improving nurses' delegation competencies.

Anthony, Standing, and Hertz (2001) studied nurses' beliefs about their abilities to delegate and supervise direct nursing activities. Differences in beliefs based on professional and job-related factors were explored. A national sample of 148 licensed nurses working in three different practice settings was surveyed. The nurses reported a high level of comfort, frequency, preparedness, confidence, competence, and control. Differences in beliefs were attributed to education, practice setting, and the type of work and responsibilities associated with their work.

Thomas, Barter, and McLaughlin (2000) conducted a study that examined United States and territorial boards of nursing approaches to the use and regulation of unlicensed assistive personnel in acute care hospitals. This study also examined state and jurisdictional authority, oversight, and disciplinary action related to RN delegation, supervision, and assignment. Educational preparation for unlicensed assistive personnel and future projections for their use was also examined. An exploratory design that incorporated the use of a survey instrument was used. The survey was administered to 53 state and territorial boards of nursing in 1998. Results demonstrated that most states reported that they had regulations and guidelines for RNs who supervised unlicensed assistive personnel. Regulations also existed that protected the use of the RN title. Most boards of nursing formulated their own definitions for delegation rather than use other agency definitions. Most state boards of nursing also reported that no standardized curriculum were in place for the education of unlicensed assistive personnel who are employed in acute care hospitals. More than half of these states also reported that no plans were in the process for the development of such a curriculum.

A Case Study in Delegation

Review of the literature clearly demonstrates that delegation is a learned skill and that a formal curriculum that incorporates a case study methodology appropriate for the practice setting of the RN assists in nurses learning the art of delegation.

A large, for-profit, acute care hospital system in the United States decided that clinical nursing needed to be enhanced at the bedside in order to improve the quality of patient care. The chief nursing officer at a for-profit health system in the United States in collaboration with her executive council decided to embark on a new patient care delivery model that would enhance clinical nursing leadership skills. The model became known as *high-impact nursing*. The title of "high-impact nursing" was selected because this particular model of care delivery incorporated a "caring moment" based on Watson's (2012) work on caring. After a pilot test of the model at one of the hospitals in the system, it was decided that an educational component was needed to further educate nurses on clinical leadership skills. This pilot study also verified the need for delegation to be a key component of the educational program. The health system collaborated with a well-respected university to develop the educational component for the new care delivery model. The following describes key components of the care delivery model and the educational program that was developed.

Program Description

The key aspect of high-impact nursing incorporates the concept of team nursing. This has been conceptualized in this care model as nurses working together cohesively, not the old concept of team nursing. One of the other key components of the care delivery model is that of the caring moment. The caring moment is based on Watson's work on caring. The RN is expected to take a minimum of 5 minutes or so with each patient daily. The purpose of this caring moment is for the nurse to address patient needs proactively with the patient; for example, the nurse may discuss lab results with the patient prior to the patient inquiring about the results. Monitoring outcomes, a significant decrease in patients ringing their call bell was noted once the caring moment was implemented.

The team in this care delivery model consists of the RN, patient care assistants, and a unit coordinator. Generally, there are two RNs and two patient care assistants for every 12 patients. Some of the system's hospitals are considering utilization of one RN and one licensed practical nurse as the licensed personnel in the care delivery model. The unit coordinator is for the entire complement of patients, that is, a 36-bed nursing unit would have one unit coordinator.

The following describes the educational program.

Educational Program

The university was responsible for development of the educational component. The project team consisted of the dean of the college of nursing and health professions; two faculty members, who were former vice presidents of nursing in acute care community hospitals; and a current chief nursing officer from one of the large tertiary acute care hospitals.

The educational program incorporates a flexible program design in order to meet the needs of various users. This educational program can be used in various ways. The most commonly used educational methods include (1) totally online, (2) traditional in-classroom, or (3) a blended methodology that incorporates both traditional in-classroom presentation as well as online learning.

The educational program consists of six-course modules that focus on leadership and management issues. The six-course modules are the following:

1. Nurses transforming nursing
2. Clinical nursing leadership
3. Communication and team building
4. Issues in delegation
5. Time management
6. Putting it all together

It is recommended that all course modules be used in order to maximize learning; however, select modules may be used. It is recommended that the modules be used in the outlined sequence; however, the user may elect to use certain elements from each module for presentation.

The following describes the various types of products that are incorporated into the design of the educational program:

1. Each module begins with an introduction. This section of the module introduces the user to the course content contained within that module.

2. PowerPoint slide presentation. Many useful PowerPoint slide presentations have been developed. Participants may access these by clicking on the appropriate icon. You must either have the PowerPoint program software or have downloaded the PowerPoint reader to view the slide presentations. These slides contain valuable information on topics discussed in the course.

3. Discussion boards. The educational program has incorporated the use of discussion boards. These discussion boards are strategically placed throughout each module. The purpose of the discussion board is to allow participants to interact with the course facilitator and other participants by engaging in a threaded discussion centered around a topic of interest or a question posed by the course facilitator. The user needs to "click" the discussion board topic. Here they will find that they can read each other's responses as well as respond to individual responses. The format of the discussion board is totally asynchronous, meaning that anyone enrolled in the program can access and respond to the discussion board at any time.

4. Case studies/stories. The educational program includes a variety of different cases/stories on the related course material. Each module contains case studies/stories. The vast majority of these case studies/stories are events that actually have occurred in practice. Nurses and other health professionals seem to learn quite well from the case study/story methodology. Case studies/stories can be used in various ways. Participants can certainly read and problem-solve the case studies/stories. Questions are posed at the end of the case study/story in an effort to stimulate discussion. The case studies/stories can also be used for role-playing scenarios. Many of these case studies/stories lend themselves well to a role-play. It is recommended that role-playing events be planned. Educators may want to ask for volunteers from the audience prior to conducting the role-play. Educators should allow the volunteers ample time to practice the role-play scenario should they feel that this is warranted. Spontaneity also occurs, and at times, a role-play evolves naturally just from the interaction of the participants discussing the case study/story. Some case studies/stories contain decision trees. These have been placed deliberately to assist the clinical nursing leader with critical thinking. The case studies/stories are one of the most valuable pieces of information contained within this program.

5. Text documents. Several text documents were created for the different modules. The text documents further describe and enhance learning material. Some text documents may be forms and checklists as examples of tools used in clinical practice. Facilitators can have participants review and discuss the text documents were deemed appropriate.
6. External links. Links to various websites with appropriate information that is module-specific are incorporated into some of the modules. The purpose of the external links is so that students can further explore information related to module-specific material on their own.

Issues in Delegation

Issues in delegation is the fourth module that was developed. This module incorporates an introduction to the module, PowerPoint slide presentations on delegation, discussion board topics on delegation issues, specific case studies and stories on delegation issues with decision trees for problem-solving activities, and text documents; for example, the module was pilot-tested with a large group of nurse managers at a university tertiary teaching hospital in New Jersey. Data from participants on delegation issues are highlighted in a text document in this module. The module also incorporates external links to websites to boards of nursing's legislation on delegation and other sites on delegation issues.

Appendix A and B are examples of real cases on delegation that have been incorporated into module 4. Appendix C and D are examples of practical delegation checklists for the staff member and for the registered nurse that also have been incorporated into module 4.

SUMMARY

Nursing organizations continually evaluate and revisit care delivery models in an effort to improve nursing practice and the care to the patients that are served. This exemplar has provided an overview to an educational program with a specific focus on one of the course modules that focuses on delegation. This program was developed for a large tertiary health system's new nursing care delivery model by well-respected university. A specific focus on module 4, issues in delegation, has been provided.

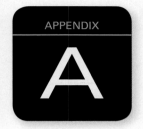

APPENDIX

A

CASE STUDY An Example of an Incompetent Staff Member

Diane S. has just assumed the nurse manager position on a busy oncology unit in a community acute care hospital.

Diane S. has always been a stickler for detail. She would always uphold the highest of nursing standards and care. That was one of the main reasons why she was selected for this position.

Diane S. is a no nonsense type of person. You know the type. Do what you are supposed to do and you will never hear from Diane S. Should one not adhere to standards of care or should one consistently call out when they are scheduled, well, then you will definitely hear from Diane S.

Diane S. is noted for consistency with management. She treats everyone the same. She has no favorites and that is what the staff really likes about her. She is also always willing to "pitch in" when times are tough and the unit is short-staffed.

The previous unit manager had hired a new nursing assistant. One of the job functions of nursing assistants at this hospital was the taking of all routine vital signs.

One day, when Diane S. was reviewing patient records, she noticed that there was an unusually high number of patients who all had the same blood pressure reading of 130/80 mm Hg. At first, she thought that this was just a coincidence. She began checking the patient vital sign records weekly and noted similar patterns of blood pressure recordings on subsequent chart audits. Diane S. began to question the accuracy of the blood pressures that were being taken and recorded by the nursing assistant.

Mr. J. had terminal cancer and had been dying for some time. One bright spring day, it happened that Mr. J. left the good planet earth. The nursing assistant was making her rounds that day and was taking and documenting the patient's vital signs. She went to Mr. J's room and recorded a BP of 130/80, a HR of 76, and a RR of 18 on Mr. J.

Please consider the issues that this case encompasses. Record your thoughts and ideas and then proceed to the second item in this folder for some issues that the author has identified.

1. Competency of the nursing assistant
2. Education and training of the nursing assistant
3. Preceptor program for educating and training the nursing assistant
4. Regulations/credentialing of nursing assistants
5. Management issues, such as a corrective action plan, hiring, disciplinary action, firing of incompetent employees
6. What about all of the other patients who had erroneous vital signs recorded?

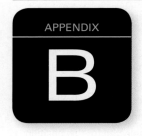

APPENDIX

B

CASE STUDY When a Staff Member Refuses to Do a Patient Assignment

A good friend of mine shared this story with me.

She was in her 20s and had just graduated from a diploma nursing school. It was the mid-1970s. She had just accepted a charge nurse position on a medical-surgical unit in a tertiary care hospital in Philadelphia.

Lorraine G. had been a stellar nursing student. She was an "A"-driven student and an "A"-driven nurse who always put patient care above everything else.

Dolly P. was a nursing assistant who had been employed on 5 South (Lorraine G.'s unit) for 20 years now.

Patients, who were going to have surgical interventions done back in the 1970s, always had extensive shave preps done the night prior to surgery. For example, if someone was having a hernia repair, the shave prep was from the nipple line to midthigh. The shave prep also included all pubic hair, and one had to be shaved to the bedside as well. As one surgeon taught me back then, "You have to shave the patient so their skin is like a newborn baby."

It was an extremely hectic evening on 5 South. There was a minimum of 15 patients going to surgery the next day. Lorraine G. requested Dolly P. to do a shave prep on Mr. J. who was going to have a cholecystectomy the following day. When asked, Dolly P. responded, "I do not know how to do shave preps." Lorraine G. found this statement daunting as it was the role of the nursing assistant to do the shave preps the evening prior to surgery and Dolly P. had been employed on that unit for 20 years now.

Lorraine G. decided that she could not let this go, so she went and spoke with the evening supervisor. She advised her of what the nursing assistant had told her about shave preps. The nursing supervisor responded, "Of course, Dolly P. knows how to do shave preps. She has been there for 20 years now. She is just trying to see how much she can pull over you." The nursing supervisor advised Lorraine G. to go back to Dolly P. and request her again to do the shave prep and add in a reminder on how to do the prep and the statement that she (Lorraine G.) would be available should she need her. Lorraine G. approached the nursing assistant in this manner and Dolly P. agreed to do the shave prep.

On a piece of paper, list some major issues surrounding this case.

▶ **Issues Identified by the Author**

1. The task delegated is refused by the person assigned to the task.
2. The importance of following a chain of command, that is, going to the immediate supervisor to discuss the issue at hand
3. Motivation
4. Trust—the nursing assistant had to develop a trust for this new charge nurse.
5. Competency of the nursing assistant

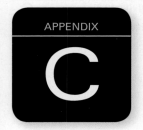

A Practical Delegation Checklist for the Staff Member/Delegate Who Has Been Delegated a Task

Staff Members Want to Make Certain That They Can Competently Perform Delegated Tasks

▶ **Checklist for the Staff Member/Delegate**

If you are a staff member who has been delegated a task, you need to check and recheck the following.

▶ **State Nurse Practice Act on Delegation**

For delegates who hold professional licensure in nursing:

Have I assessed my state's respective nurse practice act in order to ascertain if the task delegated to me meets regulatory compliance?	○
Do I have a copy of that law or web access to it?	○
After reviewing the practice act, is it clear to me what can be delegated to me and what cannot be delegated to me?	○

Hospital Policy and Procedure on Delegation

Does the hospital have policy and procedures related to what tasks and job functions I can safely perform as a delegate?	○
If I am a licensed person, are these policies consistent with the state nurse practice act?	○
As a staff member, whether a licensed or unlicensed staff member, am I familiar with the policies and procedures governing delegation in my institution?	○
As a licensed staff member, are there tasks in the nurse practice act prohibited for delegation?	○

Staff Competencies

Do I know my own capabilities and competencies for certain job functions?	○
Have my competencies been validated by my department manager?	○
If I am not certain of my specific competencies, do I check with my nurse manager or with staff development?	○
Am I thoroughly familiar with my position description?	○
Does my position description include what job functions I can safely perform?	○
Have I taken responsibility on my own to review delegation policies so that I am clear on reasons and rules guiding delegation practices?	○

Do I possess the right skills to perform the task that has been delegated to me? ○

Do I have enough time in my work schedule to perform the delegated tasks? ○

Do I have a problem saying "NO" to my manager when I know that I do not have enough time to complete the delegated task correctly? ○

Do I feel that I am the right person to do the delegated task, or should I recommend to my manager someone who I feel is a more competent person to complete the delegated task? ○

Patient Needs and Delegation

Have I sufficiently assessed the patients needing care so that priority setting and delegation are appropriate to the acuity level? ○

Do I take my own initiative in trying to handle the delegated task? ○

Are the tasks that I have been assigned appropriate to my skill level? ○

Am I afraid to ask for help from my manager with the task that has been delegated to me? ○

Am I willing to examine and revise my work process in handling the delegated task when necessary? ○

Do I consider all possibilities when handling a delegated task? ○

Do I allow enough time to complete the delegated task? ○

If patient acuity is high, have I considered advising my manager that I may need extra help with the delegated task? ○

Have I monitored the results of the task that was delegated to me and made corrections or improvements where necessary? ○

Communication and Delegation

Are my delegated assignments clear and unambiguous? ○

Do I clearly understand the tasks that have been delegated to me? ○

Do I confidently answer questions or concerns that my manager has about delegated assignments? ○

Do I request feedback from my manager on how I am handling the delegated task? ○

Do I revise my approach in handling the delegated task if questions or concerns from my manager warrant such action? ○

Am I open to learning from my mistakes in handling a delegated task? ○

Do I use any failures to learn valuable lessons for future tasks that may be delegated to me? ○

Do other staff members frequently challenge me for having tasks delegated to me? ○

If yes, have I consulted my manager on the best course of action? ○

Can I clearly communicate any problems or concerns to my manager? ○

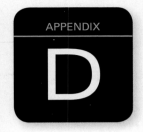

APPENDIX

D

A Practical Delegation Checklist for the Registered Nurse, Clinical Nurse Leader

Delegation is not merely the assignment of a task; it is the extension of your authority and expertise as a licensed registered nurse.

▶ Checklist for the Registered Nurse with Delegation Authority

If you are the RN delegating responsibilities to staff, you need to check and recheck the following.

State Nurse Practice Act on Delegation

Does the state nurse practice act have a delegation clause that specifies nursing functions that may or may not be delegated? ○

Do I have a copy of that law or web access to it? ○

After reviewing the practice act, it is clear to me what can be delegated and what cannot. ○

Hospital Policy and Procedure on Delegation

Does the hospital have policy and procedures related to delegating nursing care? ○

Are these policies consistent with the state nurse practice act? ○

Are all nursing staff, licensed and unlicensed, familiar with the policies and procedures governing delegation? ○

Are there tasks in the nurse practice act prohibited for delegation? ○

Staff Competencies

Do I know the capabilities and competencies of my staff? ○

Have staff competencies been validated in some formal way? ○

If I am not certain of specific staff competencies, do I check with the nurse manager or with staff development? ○

Am I thoroughly familiar with the position descriptions of staff to whom I delegate? ○

Have I reviewed delegation policies with staff so that they are clear on reasons and rules guiding delegation practices? ○

Do the staff members to whom I delegated responsibilities possess the required skills? ○

Will the staff member have time to complete all of the responsibilities that I have delegated? ○

Do I routinely select the appropriate staff member in my delegation activities or have I had poor outcomes with my delegation decisions? ○

Patient Needs and Delegation

Have I sufficiently assessed the patients needing care so that priority setting and delegation are appropriate to acuity level?	O
Are the tasks that I am assigning appropriate for routine delegation to an unlicensed staff member or to a licensed vocational nurse (LVN)?	O
If the task is not routine but can be delegated, does the unlicensed assistive personnel (UAP) or LVN require supervision and is the rationale for such supervision explicit and understood by all parties?	O
If patient acuity is high, have I considered that delegating "routine tasks" may require extra supervision?	O
Have I monitored the results of all care delegated and made corrections or improvements where necessary?	O

Communication and Delegation

Are my delegation assignments clear and unambiguous?	O
Have I considered how my directions/assignments were "heard" by others, that is, my tone, manner, and how I deliver the message?	O
Do I confidently answer questions or concerns from the staff about delegated assignments?	O
Do I revise assignments if questions or concerns from staff warrant such action?	O
Are my assignments frequently challenged by staff?	O
If yes, have I consulted my supervisor on the best course of action?	O

REFERENCES

Anthony, M. K., Standing, T., & Hertz, J. E. (2000). Factors influencing outcomes after delegation to unlicensed assistive personnel. *Journal of Nursing Administration, 30*(10), 474–481.

Anthony, M. K., Standing, T. S., & Hertz, J. E. (2001). Nurses' beliefs about their abilities to delegate within changing models of care. *Journal of Continuing Education in Nursing, 32*(5), 210–215.

Heller, R. (1998). *How to delegate.* London, England: Dorling Kindersley Limited.

Parsons, L. C. (1999). Building RN confidence for delegation decision-making skills in practice. *Journal of Nursing Staff Development, 15*(6), 263–269.

Parsons, L. C., & Ward, K. S. (2000). Delegation strategies for registered nurses practicing in turbulent health care arenas. *Scientific Nursing, 17*(2), 46–51.

Thomas, S. A., Barter, M., & McLaughlin, F. E. (2000). State and territorial boards of nursing approach to the use of unlicensed assistive personnel. *Journal of Nursing Administration, 2*(1), 13–21.

Thomas, S., & Hume, G. (1998). Delegation competencies: Beginning practitioner's reflections. *Nurse Educator, 23*(1), 38–41.

Watson, J. (2012). *Human caring science: A theory of nursing.* Sudbury, MA: Jones & Bartlett Learning.

Strategic Management for the Nurse Executive

Joseph Anton

INTRODUCTION

The U.S. health-care system is undergoing a fundamental transformation which will impact how care is accessed, delivered, and paid for. The Affordable Care Act (ACA) was signed into law by President Barack Obama on March 23, 2010. Together with the Health Care and Education Reconciliation Act, it represents the most significant regulatory overhaul of the U.S. health-care system since the passage of Medicare and Medicaid in 1965. The ACA was enacted with the goals of increasing the quality and affordability of health insurance, decreasing the uninsured rate by expanding public and private insurance coverage, and reducing the costs of health care for both individuals and the government. In addition to the passing of the ACA into law, there are several other societal drivers that are fueling the change to our health-care system in the United States:

1. Aging population. The nation's 65 years and older population is projected to reach 83.7 million in the year 2050, almost double in size from the 2012 level of 43.1 million, according to two reports released today from the U.S. Census Bureau. A large part of this growth is due to the aging of baby boomers (individuals born in the United States between mid-1946 and mid-1964), who began turning 65 years in 2011 and are now driving growth at the older ages of the population (U.S. Census Bureau, 2014).

2. Obesity. More than one-third of U.S. adults (34.9%) are obese. Obesity-related conditions include heart disease, stroke, type 2 diabetes, and certain types of cancer—some of the leading causes of preventable death. The estimated annual medical cost of obesity in the United States in 2008 was $147 billion; the medical costs for people who are obese were $1,429 higher than those of normal weight (Centers for Disease Control and Prevention, 2014).

3. Physician shortages. The Association of American Medical Colleges (AAMC) forecasts that in 15 years, the United States will face a deficit of up to 159,300 physicians. The AAMC projects that universal access to health care would increase the physician shortage by an additional 31,000 doctors. (Dill & Salsberg, 2008).

4. Emerging consumerism (patient management). The concept that an informed consumer will hold the system accountable for improved value and make more responsible choices regarding their own health and use of health-care services.

5. Advances in medical care. Advances in medical technology have contributed to rising overall U.S. health-care spending. Advances include the development of new treatments for previously untreatable terminal conditions and clinical progress, through major advances or by the cumulative effect of incremental improvements.

In order to achieve the necessary improvements in quality and cost reduction, we need to transform the full spectrum of care delivery. Hospitals, physicians, and payors need to collaborate and commit to an overarching vision with clear objectives to reduce cost, improve quality, ensure safety, and optimize the patient experience.

AN EMERGING CARE DELIVERY MODEL

Care Delivery, Payment Models, and Patient Engagement

Across the United States, systems of care are rapidly evolving and placing greater emphasis on well-coordinated, team-based care. Although the ACA is structured to make primary care more accessible, expansion of coverage will likely strain the current health-care infrastructure and may overload providers. There are several new models emerging in response to ACA and other societal drivers that are fueling change. The patient-centered medical home (PCMH) is leading the way in physician practices, whereas accountable care organizations (ACOs) and integrated health-care delivery systems (IDSs) are providing a larger framework that bridges delivery and payment challenges. Because clinical practice often follows payment, novel payment models hold the most potential for transforming our health-care systems. Many collaborative models are based on bundled case rates (fixed payments for a full episode of care) or global payments (single, risk-adjusted payments coupled with quality metrics). All payment schemes come with implications regarding how cost increases will be controlled, quality will be managed, and patients will be engaged. In the future, we are likely going to see increasingly sophisticated pricing methodologies deployed in health care. In addition, patients are expected to take a greater degree of ownership in their health to enable them to make more informed lifestyle and health-care utilization decisions. Many employer plans already use value-based benefit designs that motivate employees to make optimal choices in their consumption of care. Workplace incentives for programs such as smoking cessation and weight loss have existed for several years. Patient engagement will help hold the system accountable for improved value because increased transparency in cost and quality are demanded. Nurse executives are key stakeholders in the redesign of the payment and delivery systems because they are at the forefront of patient care and bring an extremely valuable perspective to the table.

Integrated Health-Care Delivery Systems

The U.S. health-care system has long been characterized as complex, fragmented, and costly, with significant variation in quality of care. Many health policy experts have called for the country to reorganize health-care providers and delivery systems through organizational or virtual integration called IDSs. An IDS is a formally organized network of providers that are clinically, financially, and administratively integrated to provide services to a defined population or community. The IDS concept is based on the fundamental belief that a higher level of integration will yield a more efficient health-care delivery system that produces higher quality, improves the patient experience, and reduces costs.

Accountable Care Organizations

An ACO is a coordinated network of provider partners, such as hospitals, primary care physicians, and specialists, who work together to improve care delivery, quality, and reduce costs. ACOs are expected to save Medicare up to $940 million in their first 4 years (U.S. Department of Health & Human Services, 2012). ACOs make providers jointly accountable for the health of their patients, giving them financial incentives to participate and reduce costs by avoiding unnecessary tests and procedures. The ACOs must meet a long list of quality measures to ensure they are not saving money by stinting on necessary care. Those that save money while also meeting quality targets would keep a portion of the savings. In a traditional fee-for-service system, physicians and hospitals typically are paid for each test and procedure. This model drives up costs by rewarding providers for doing more, even when it may not be needed. Although ACOs do not eliminate fee for service, they create an incentive to be more efficient by offering bonuses when providers keep costs down. Physicians and hospitals have to meet specific quality benchmarks, focusing on prevention and carefully managing patients with chronic diseases. Essentially, providers are incentivized to keep their patients healthy and out of the hospital. Physicians will likely refer patients to hospitals and specialists within the ACO network, but patients would still be free to see physicians of their choice outside the network without paying more. Insurers are essential to the success of an ACO because of their ability and access to track and collect the data on patients that allow systems to evaluate patient care and report their results. Some fear that the rush to form ACOs and the resulting hospital mergers and provider consolidation could have significant downside as the increase market share gives these health systems more leverage in negotiations with insurers, which could potentially lead to higher cost and few choices for patients. One key challenge for hospitals and physicians is that the incentives in ACOs are to reduce hospital stays, emergency room visits, and expensive specialist and testing services, which have historically been their major source of revenue. Nurse executives should be involved in the development of ACOs given the available evidence that links nursing to high-quality care (Institute of Medicine, 2011).

Patient-Centered Medical Home

The PCMH is a model in which primary care physicians manage all aspects of patient care. In the PCMH model, physicians serve as team leaders and care coordinators when patients require specialist services. They also work to engage patients as active participants in managing their health. The PCMH is a collaborative, team-based model that focuses on reducing hospitalization, emergency room visits, and readmissions. PCMH seeks to provide the right care, by the right provider, at the right time, in the right location, and at the right cost (Agency for Healthcare Research and Quality, n.d.). The PCMH has five primary attributes:

1. Comprehensive care. The PCMH is accountable for meeting most of each patient's physical and mental health-care needs, including prevention and wellness, acute care, and chronic care.
2. Patient-centered. The PCMH provides primary health care that is relationship-based with an orientation toward the whole person. Partnering with patients and their families requires understanding and respecting each patient's unique needs, culture, values, and preferences.
3. Coordinated care. The PCMH coordinates care across all elements of the broader health-care system, including specialty care, hospitals, home health care, and community services and supports.
4. Accessible services. The PCMH delivers accessible services with shorter waiting times for urgent needs, enhanced in-person hours, around-the-clock telephone, or electronic access to a member of the care team.
5. Quality and safety. The PCMH demonstrates a commitment to quality and quality improvement by ongoing engagement in activities such as using evidence-based medicine and clinical decision-support tools to guide shared decision making with patients and families, engaging in performance

measurement and improvement, measuring and responding to patient experiences and patient satisfaction, and practicing population health management (Agency for Healthcare Research and Quality, n.d.).

Value-Based Purchasing

Value-based purchasing (VBP) is a payment methodology that rewards quality of care through payment incentives and transparency. VBP has significant implications for providers and health-care organizations. In health care, value can be considered to be a function of quality, efficiency, safety, and cost. VBP holds providers accountable for the quality and cost of the health-care services they provided by a system of rewards and penalties, conditional upon achieving specific performance measures. Incentives are structured to discourage inappropriate, unnecessary, and costly care. VBP is a departure from the fee-for-service payment system, which rewards excessive, costly, and complex services, rather than quality, and contributes to the unsustainable costs of health care. VBP payment reform is expected to reduce Medicare spending by approximately $214 billion over the next 10 years and has significant implications for health-care organizations. The Centers for Medicare and Medicaid Services (CMS) began implementing VBP pilots in 2003. Since then, many commercial health plans have followed suit with versions of VBP that align consistently with Medicare goals for better care, lower costs, and improved efficiency. These CMS pilots may be grouped in three categories (Center for Medicare & Medicaid Services, n.d.):

1. Pay-for-reporting (P4R)—a provider is incentivized to report information for public consumption.
2. Pay-for-performance (P4P)—a provider is incentivized to achieve a targeted threshold of clinical performance.
3. Pay-for-value—providers are incentivized to achieve both quality and efficiency improvements.

Goals for CMS Value-Based Purchasing Initiatives

1. Improve clinical quality.
2. Address problems of underuse, overuse, and misuse of services.
3. Encourage patient-centered care.
4. Reduce adverse events and improve patient safety.
5. Avoid unnecessary costs in the delivery of care.
(Center for Medicare & Medicaid Services, n.d.)

VBP provisions are mandatory, challenging providers to reorganize and prepare or face the possibility of substantial short-term losses. The goal is to avoid hospital admissions and, in particular, readmissions. If not already participating in VBP, hospitals and providers should integrate quality measure collection into routine business practices to position themselves to be successful in VBP. In addition, patient experience is a key driver, and attention should be paid to optimize patient experience quality measures (Center for Medicare & Medicaid Services, n.d.).

TRANSFORMATIONAL LEADERSHIP: EMBRACING AND LEADING CHANGE

The changes under way in the U.S. health-care system require nurse executives who can create and transit to new business models while continuing to manage the delivery of quality services and value. Organizations will have to be structured in different ways, and nurse executives will need different competencies in order to be successful.

System Changes/Challenges for the Nurse Executive

- A shift from a volume-driven, fee-for-service system to an integrated, patient-centered approach that rewards efficiency and quality
- Accelerated consolidation and integration
- Use of data-based quality standards that will reduce variation in care
- Increased use of outsourcing as a means to reduce costs
- Risk-based, "bundled" or capitated payments that incent the transformation through more integrated, cost-effective care

The extent to which any given transformation is a success will depend largely on the quality and characteristics of the leadership team guiding the process. Organizations that invest in the right nurse executives and the infrastructure to support them will be poised to capitalize on the dramatic changes ahead and will position themselves to deliver improved care at a reduced and sustainable cost. Transformational leadership is a major component of the Magnet model developed by the American Nurses Credentialing Center. In today's health-care environment, the ability to be a transformational leader is essential. The transformational leadership model is described as a process in which followers trust, admire, and respect their leader, and are consequently motivated to adopt and embrace a new vision or goal. This concept was introduced by J. M. Burns in 1978 and enhanced by B. M. Bass in 1985. The four key components of transformational leadership are charisma, inspiration, individual consideration, and intellectual stimulation (Bass, 1985).

1. Charisma. Transformational leaders motivate workers to transcend their self-interest for the good of the organization. Workers must identify with their leader's values and vision of the future. Transformational leaders can change an organization by identifying the need for change, articulating a new vision, and generating commitment to the new vision. The leader that empowers, develops, and inspires followers will transform an organization.

2. Inspiration. Transformational leaders motivate workers to go beyond their self-interest. Leaders can manage the impression they make through their dress, speech, and appropriate connections with those they visibly interact. Inspirational leaders must develop a realistic vision of the future that will motivate workers and be able to communicate the vision in such a persuasive manner that others are willing to commit to it.

3. Individual considerations. Transformational leaders exhibit concern for the workers' development through assignments that provide opportunities for growth. Considerate leaders know the developmental needs of each worker and should know what motivates and interests the workers.

4. Intellectual stimulation. Transformative leaders encourage new ideas from their followers and never criticize them publicly for the mistakes committed by them (Bass, 1985).

Health-care organizations need nurse executives and other leaders who can both lead in this consolidated, complex model and who can help their institutions transition to a model that delivers quality health care at a lower cost while providing an optimal patient experience.

REFERENCES

Agency for Healthcare Research and Quality. (n.d.). *Patient-centered medical home resource center.* Retrieved from http://pcmh.ahrq.gov/

Bass, B. M. (1985). *Leadership and performance beyond expectations.* New York, NY: Free Press.

Centers for Disease Control and Prevention. (2014). *Adult obesity facts.* Retrieved from http://www.cdc.gov/obesity/data/adult.html

Center for Medicare & Medicaid Services. (n.d.) *Hospital value-based purchasing.* Retrieved from http://www.cms.gov/Medicare/Quality-Initiatives-Patient-Assessment-Instruments/hospital-value-based-purchasing/index.html?redirect=/Hospital-Value-Based-Purchasing.

Dill, M. J., & Salsberg, E. S. (2008). *The complexities of physician supply and demand: Projections through 2025.* Washington, DC: Association of American Medical Colleges.

Institute of Medicine. (2011). *The future of nursing: Leading change, advancing health.* Washington, DC: National Academies Press. Retrieved from http://www.thefutureofnursing.org/IOM-Report

U.S. Census Bureau. (2014). *Fueled by aging baby boomers, nation's older population to nearly double.* Retrieved form http://www.census.gov/newsroom/releases/archives/aging_population/cb14-84.html

U.S. Department of Health & Human Services. (2012). *HHS announces 89 new accountable care organizations.* Retrieved from http://www.hhs.gov/news/press/2012pres/07/20120709a.html

10

Defining and Developing Self-Awareness in the Nurse Leader

William J. Lorman

INTRODUCTION

"He that would govern others, first should be the master of himself."

—Philip Massinger (1583–1640)

The unfortunate reality is that nurse leaders are not readily recognized nor fully appreciated. In the 1960s and 1970s, nurses with a master's degree in nursing (MSN) were preferred and recruited to manage nursing departments, but they were, as a rule, never really taken seriously because they were "clinical" and really did not know anything about finance. So, as long as they kept the nurses in line and assured coverage on all shifts and on all units so the hospital could maintain an optimal census, the nurse "leader" is doing his or her job to the full extent expected. Unfortunately, during the late 1970s and 1980s, with the arrival of managed care, financial issues became the major focus, and hospitals wanted nurse leaders who could manage the financial side—increasing revenues and decreasing costs—in order to maintain profits. Thus, the arrival of the nurse with a master's degree in business administration (MBA) became the hot commodity. An administrator's dream was to have a nurse whose primary responsibility was to run the nursing operation side of the business by min-imizing costs and maximizing revenue. Interestingly enough, this coincided with the increasing problems with malpractice litigation, nurse shortages (although this has always been a cyclic problem and cannot be blamed entirely on these developments), and most importantly—and we can blame these developments—there became a growing dissatisfaction with the practice of nursing by nurses. In the 1990s, The Joint Commission (which has gone through several name changes over the years but is back to being known as TJC [The Joint Commission]) realized that the expectation for nurse leaders was to advocate for the patients and nurse employees by primarily improving quality of care and not having a primary (also known as *restricted*) interest in profit making, although the nurse leaders of the new millennium must be ever cognizant that every clinical/nursing decision has financial consequences and every financial decision has clinical/nursing consequences. Although we could next move into the role of the successful nurse leader as someone who is able to understand the science (new research) and apply it to the work setting (the role of the Doctor of Nursing Practice [DNP]), this will be covered elsewhere in this text. However, this chapter is concerned more with personal issues because this also has become a time in nurse leaders' development where nurses must take better care of themselves and their direct reports in addition to the patient populations they serve. This requires a major paradigm shift in how nurse leaders act. The starting point in the development of this new paradigm is by understanding how you perceive yourself, how you per-ceive the world, and ultimately, how you respond to those perceptions.

THE CONCEPT OF SELF-AWARENESS

Self-awareness embodies the willingness to challenge yourself. This essential attribute includes awareness not only of your needs and motivations but also of your personal conflicts and problems and the potential influence they have on those around you. This concept—also called *emotional intelligence*—has been identified as one of the most important factors correlating to success in leaders (Boyatzis, Goleman, & Rhee, 1999). In addition, it is a more powerful predictor of success in life than intelligence quotient (IQ) (Goleman, 1995). Erich Fromm, a psychiatrist and student of Sigmund Freud, was one of the first to observe the close connection between one's self-concept and one's feelings about others. He said, "Hatred against oneself is inseparable from hatred against others" (Fromm, 1939). And so, the knowledge you possess about yourself, which makes up your self-concept, is at the core of improving your man-agement skills. However, individuals frequently evade personal growth and new self-knowledge in order to protect their self-esteem. They worry that in acquiring new knowledge about themselves, there is always the possibility that it will be nega-tive or that it will lead to feelings of inferiority. Abraham Maslow (1962) wrote,

> *We tend to be afraid of any knowledge that would cause us to despise ourselves or to make us feel inferior, weak, worthless, evil, [or] shameful. We protect ourselves and our*

ideal image of ourselves by repression and similar defenses, which are essentially techniques by which we avoid becoming conscious of unpleasantness or dangerous truths.

Sigmund Freud (1956) believed that to be completely honest is the best effort an individual can make because complete honesty requires a continual search for more information about the self and a desire for self-improvement.

So why is it so difficult to continually focus on who we really are? There is a *psychic pain threshold* or *level of sensitivity* that is part of our being. It is that point at which we become defensive or protective when we encounter information about ourselves that is in conflict with and differs from our own self-concept. We are often exposed to information about ourselves that is marginally inconsistent. For instance, someone might say to you, "You look tired. Are you feeling alright?" If you feel fine, this information is in conflict with your self-awareness. However, because it is a relatively minor discordance, it would most likely not invoke a strong defensive reaction. But if a more dissident interaction occurred, you would cross the psychic pain threshold and need to defend yourself. For example, if a coworker expressed that you were a poor manager, and you believed you were a competent manager, you would feel a need to defend yourself in order to protect the image you hold of yourself. When the threshold is crossed, you become rigid emotionally and in your thinking, and you tend to minimize any risk-taking activities. A parallel system exists in the physical domain. When you are frightened or in danger of harm, your body becomes rigid in order to protect itself and your thoughts are focused only on the feared object. Now back to the coworker example. Your response is one of regression: You rely on first-learned behavior patterns and emotions. You deny the possible validity of the information and use other defense mechanisms to ensure your self-concept remains stable. So, crossing the threshold creates rigidity and self-preservation.

Then how can self-knowledge and personal change ever occur if we are constantly guarding against crossing the psychic pain threshold? Studies have shown that low self-disclosers are less healthy and more self-alienated than high self-disclosers (Kelly, 1998). By controlling when and what kind of information you receive about yourself by involving others during the process of self-disclosure will contribute to greater self-awareness without crossing the pain threshold. So, start out cautiously—ask your closest allies what they really think about you. Ask for and expect honesty. Ponder on what they have expressed to you. You are still free to accept or reject what they have told you. The point is, become more at ease expanding your network of acquaintances and others by requesting feedback on your actions, attitudes, and decisions.

Paradoxically, when you focus on self-awareness, you are better able to identify differences among others with whom you interact. The management literature refers to this as *managing diversity*. Being able to recognize, respect, and incorporate differences among others improves your effectiveness as a manager because it makes your interactions more effective and insightful. Most people, however, tend to interact with individuals who are like themselves and exclude others who seem to be different (Berscheid & Walster, 1978). The reason for this is that differences are usually interpreted as frightening or threatening. And it is "safer" to be surrounded by similar-thinking individuals; however, this ultimately reduces creativity and complex problem solving. A lack of diversity in the composition of key decision makers makes it difficult to perceive the need for change, and if change is indicated, to respond in new and novel ways (Cameron, Kim, & Whetten, 1987).

The capacity for self-awareness separates us from other animals and enables us to make free choices. And even though we are limited by internal (genetic) factors and external (sociocultural) factors, the greater our level of self-awareness, the greater our possibilities to make choices and recognize the responsibility associated with the freedom to choose and to act. Alternatively, we have the capacity to know that we are being victimized, which allows us to take a stand on this situation and act or not act (May, 1961). In other words, we can determine the direction of our own lives or allow other people and environmental forces to determine it for us, and we can choose to establish meaningful ties with others or choose to isolate ourselves. And ultimately, we can take risks and experience the anxiety of deciding for ourselves, or we can choose the security of dependence. The philosophy/theory of existentialism is grounded on these tenets.

AREAS OF SELF-AWARENESS

There are many aspects of self-awareness that have been studied along with how those aspects change with maturity. However, only a few factors that seem to best correlate with effective management practices will be described. Effective leaders have been found to be competent decision makers, highly creative team performers, skillful communicators, and proficient at self-empowerment (Allan & Waclawski, 1999; Sosik & Megerian, 1999). Understanding these factors and how they affect you and those around you will help you develop your skills as an effective leader. As you will see, there is a good deal of overlap here and efforts to separate them are merely a mechanical means for providing a more clear explanation.

Personality

Our personalities do not generally change, they remain stably pervasive. However, an understanding of our personalities will help us identify areas in which we will thrive and also help us avoid situations in which we will experience too much stress. For instance, highly introverted persons are more likely to experience more stress in a position where they are required to interact with people on a regular basis as compared to extroverted persons who enjoy the interactions and seem to become more energized in such an environment. Should the introverted person hold a position in which he or she must interact regularly with many people, he or she would either learn skills to cope with these situations or ultimately fail to maintain such an undertaking. Awareness of your own personality helps you analyze decisions and situations such as this.

Values

The first area important in development of self-awareness is one's values. It is believed that we probably possess only a relatively small number of values and we all possess the same values only in different degrees (Rokeach, 1973). It is from our values that our attitudes and personal preferences are formed. Not only do we have our own basic values, but there are also values that characterize ethnic and cultural groups, professional organizations, and even the workplace. Sometimes these various group values are in conflict, and sometimes there is congruence. Values exist on a continuum and have been described as having a dimensional character (Trompenaars & Hampton-Turner, 1998). In general, we "move" along the continuum in both directions depending on the issue at hand. Naturally, our heritage, upbringing, and cultural background infuse values into us, and we more or less carry them with us throughout our lives unless and until a need to change them becomes manifest in which case we learn to adapt in order to survive, that is, to be successful. Here are a few examples of values that might be considered more cultural than personal. For instance, do you place more importance on your own contributions (individualism) or on the team's contributions (collectivism)? Many organizations rate managers higher based on their ability to function within a team. Yet, there are many times when your singular abilities are required to complete a project or task based on your level of expertise. Successful leaders can move back and forth on this continuum and, most importantly, know when and how much movement is necessary. Another cultural value that is considered important is how you display feelings in public (or how you respond to your colleagues). Is the showing of emotions valued (affective orientation), or are unemotional responses expected (neutral orientation)? Displays of loud laughter, anger, and intense passion may be important elements of your personality or of others. Obviously, there would be a conflict if you followed an affective orientation and your workplace valued a neutral orientation. How would you respond to this (and still maintain a high level of satisfaction and success)? As another example, suppose someone at work offended you and you became very upset. How likely would you show your feelings openly?

Another cultural dimension relates to focus of control. There are many people who believe they control their destinies and what happens to them is the result of their own actions or inactions (internal focus). There are also those who believe that they are controlled by outside forces and because of others' actions or inactions they encounter the consequences (external focus). Where do you stand and how do you relate to those who are mainly guided by the opposite dimension? You should begin to raise your awareness of individual differences around you and determine whether there is congruence or conflict. And if conflict, how will you resolve it? By engaging in this practice, you will begin increasing your sensitivity to others' values and also increase your own self-awareness.

Now we will approach values that are more personal than cultural. Here, our individual life experiences help us define and develop them. Rokeach (1973) describes a paradigm for personal values. He identifies *instrumental values*, which are process-oriented, such as ambition, competence, and honesty, to name a few. He also identifies *terminal values*, which are outcome-oriented. Examples of terminal values are happiness, self-esteem, social recognition, and equality. He further subdivides the terminal values into personal and social values. Personal values are those that are related to the individual and his or her private concerns; social values are those related to one's environment and people outside one's immediate circle of concerns. Family security would be an example of a personal value, whereas national security would be a social value. Rokeach also observed that an individual's top priorities at any given time are either personal or social. Thus, if a person increases the priority of a personal value, other personal values become higher in priority and social values decrease in priority. Alternatively, if a social value increases in priority, other social values follow and personal values decrease in priority. So, for example, an ambitious person works hard to obtain a comfortable life with all the amenities and has everything he desires. This person is operating primarily on personal values, which are a high priority for him. But suppose, along the way, he becomes aware of the growing concerns of global warming, the ozone layer destruction, and other harsh realities. He now is focused on creating a world of beauty, working diligently on educating people about the effects of their overuse and abuse of natural resources. He is now using his instrumental value of ambition aimed no longer on his personal values of personal comfort and wealth but on the social values of world beauty and safety for all inhabitants. The hypothesis is understood as each individual, at any given time, is either self- or others-oriented. Using Rokeach's list of values, a study was conducted (Schmidt & Posner, 1982) whereby managers in the workplace were asked to prioritize the instrumental values in the order they believed to be the most important to the least important. The vast majority selected *responsible* and *honest* as the most desirable. Interestingly, the least important values were identified as *polite* and *forgiving*. One must wonder how workplace civility is affected by these values. Does honesty trump politeness? Should we be brutally frank with our peers and direct reports without consideration of the effect such frankness will have on the receiver of the message? In light of the fact that we are seeing much more horizontal and vertical incivility in the workplace, we must conclude that our values have shifted or we have become less aware of them. Contemporary managers and managers of the future will most likely need to balance personal and social values in order to be more successful.

A third model related to values is that of values development in the decision-making process. The best known model is Kohlberg's model (1981), which is composed of three distinct levels. The first level is referred to as the *preconventional level*. A person who uses this level follows a very self-centered approach: Decision making revolves around increasing rewards and decreasing negative consequences for the individual. Here, compliance rather than motivation is the major force at work. These individuals follow rules and regulations in order to avoid the consequences of breaking them. The second level is called the *conventional level*. A person who follows this level conforms because of duty and commitment to do what is right. Generally, these people act through motivation. Most adults have been identified as residing in the conventional level. The third level is referred to as the *postconventional level*. People in this level are principle-centered in their thinking and are considered highly motivated and values-oriented. Although rules and regulations are followed, if this person is faced with a rule that is in conflict with a principle, the principle is chosen over the rule. Obviously, as one progresses through the levels, one's values and morals develop more fully. Although not a part of this chapter's discussion, the reader should ponder how values development affects ethical decision making. Ethics refers to what is and is not acceptable behavior. Certainly, the individual operating at the preconventional level would probably determine what is ethical behavior quite differently from someone operating at the postconventional level.

Rest (1979) proposed that people vary in how they assess a social issue based on the level of values development they have achieved. The following case study and the questions that follow demonstrate this:

> A man has been sentenced to prison for 10 years. After 1 year, however, he escaped from prison, moved to a new area of the country, and took on the name of *Thompson*. For 8 years, he worked hard, and gradually, he saved enough money to buy his own business. He was fair to his customers, gave his employees top wages, and gave most of his own profits to charity. Then one day, Ms. Jones, an old neighbor, recognized him as the man who had escaped from prison 8 years before and for whom the police had been looking. In your opinion, if you were in Ms. Jones's position, should you report Mr. Thompson to the police and have him sent back to prison?

Here are some questions you might ask yourself based on your level of values maturity to help define your opinion. Which questions would you consider to be most important to answer before you can determine your position?

1. Has not Mr. Thompson been good enough for such a long time to prove he is not a bad person?
2. Every time someone escapes punishment for a crime, does not that just encourage more crime?
3. Has Mr. Thompson really paid his debt to society?
4. How could anyone be so cruel and heartless as to send Mr. Thompson to prison?
5. Would it be fair to all the prisoners who had to serve out their full sentences if Mr. Thompson was let off?
6. Was Ms. Jones a good friend of Mr. Thompson?
7. Would not it be a citizen's duty to report an escaped criminal, regardless of circumstances?

8. How would the will of the people and the public good best be served?
9. Would going to prison do any good for Mr. Thompson or protect anybody?

Only questions 8 and 9 are based on principle-centered values. The first seven are based on duty/commitment values orientation.

Here is another example:

> A woman was dying of incurable cancer and had only about 6 months to live. She decided to finish her days at home surrounded by her family. She was in terrible pain, but she was so weak that a large dose of a pain killer such as morphine would probably kill her. She was delirious with pain, and in her calm periods, she would ask the nurse caring her to give her enough morphine to kill her. She said she could not stand the pain and that she was going to die in a few months anyway. If you were this nurse, what would you do?

Again, here are some questions for you to consider. Which are the most important in helping you reach a determination?

1. Is the woman's family in favor of giving her the overdose?
2. Is the nurse obligated by the same laws as everybody else?
3. Should the doctor make the woman's death from a drug overdose appear to be an accident?
4. Does the state have the right to force continued existence on those who do not want to live?
5. Should the nurse have sympathy for the woman's suffering, or should she care more about what society might think?
6. Is helping to end another's life ever a responsible act of cooperation?
7. Can only God decide when a person's life should end?
8. What values has the nurse set for herself in her own personal code of behavior?
9. Can society afford to let people end their lives whenever they desire?
10. Can society allow suicide or mercy killing and still protect the lives of individuals who want to live?

Question 3 is based on a self-centered values orientation; questions 4, 6, 8, and 10 are from a principle-centered values orientation. Questions 1, 2, 5, and 9 are from a duty/commitment values orientation.

Here is a third case to ponder:

> One of your colleagues with whom you work is also a good friend of yours. In fact, you socialize frequently together. Although both your jobs take you to different parts of the hospital throughout the day, you are still required to stay on premises until the shift is over in case there is an emergency. You know that your friend quite frequently leaves early when his work is completed. On one such occasion, the staff were unable to locate your friend in an emergency situation because he had left earlier before the end of his shift. An investigation ensues and he asks you to state he was with you at the time of the emergency. Would you lie for him?

As you can see from the cases, our values play a major role in helping us in reaching opinions and determining outcomes. We take each situation and apply our values system (by asking ourselves level-based questions as discussed earlier) and then concluding the best alternative.

Change

Another factor involved in the self-awareness process is how you perceive change. The one constant in the world in general and particularly in management is change. If the past 50 years is any indication, change has been occurring at an increasing pace and breadth. Technology, which affects management more than anything, is changing from one moment to the next. But how does change—or more specifically, how you view change—affect self-awareness? One area described by Whetten & Cameron (2002) is *tolerance of ambiguity*. Change involves a transition from a previously known process to a new, probably unknown, process. In between, there is a "blob"— an unclear, vague state of transient nonstructure and unorganization. Often, many processes in the workplace are in a state of flux or change and can usually be found in this transitory blob. How well are you able to effect change? How well can you change the blob into a structured and organized process? Three traits have been correlated to your ability to be successful in effecting change. The first is *novelty*, which measures how well you can tolerate new, unfamiliar information or situations. Obviously, this requires practice because the "novelty" trait, left unfettered, results in impulsive decision making, extravagance in approach to reward cues, and quick loss of temper. As examples, your novelty tolerability would be high if you would embrace, without a second thought, living in a foreign country for a while. Your novelty tolerance would be low if you what you are used to is always preferable to what is unfamiliar. The second is *complexity*, indicating how well you are able to tolerate multiple, variable, or unrelated data. First applied as a factor in mental health, "complexity" was later expanded within organizational theory referring to the ability of a person to perceive and respond to variables based on prior experience and prior developed personal constructs. Your complexity tolerance would be high if you believed that people who fit their lives to a schedule probably miss most of the joy of living. It would be low if you followed the guideline that a good job is one in which what is to be done and how it is to be done are always clear. The third is *insolubility*, which looks at how well you can deal with problems that are difficult to solve either because solutions are not readily evident or different parts of the problem do not seem to be related. If you believe that there is really no such thing as a problem that cannot be solved, then you have a low tolerance for insolubility. An example of high-insolubility tolerance as a trait would be if you think that many of our most important decisions are based on insufficient information. The more you are able to tolerate novelty, complexity, and insolubility, the more you perceive situations as promising rather than threatening and the more successful you will be as a manager. For more information on these traits and rating scales which measure these traits, see Budner (1982).

Habits

Habits are the behaviors that are repeated routinely and often automatically. Although we would like to possess the habits that help us interact effectively with and manage others, we can probably all identify at least one of our habits that decreases our effectiveness. For example, if you are a manager who never consults your staff before making decisions, that habit may interfere with your ability to build the staff's commitment to the decisions and their decision-making skills as well. Alternatively, if you routinely seek input from staff before making decisions and you use this input in finalizing your decisions, then staff take ownership for the decision and they are motivated to follow it.

Interpersonal Interactions

A final factor that plays a significant part in self-awareness development is your interpersonal orientation—how you relate to others. Here, unlike the previous factors, you move from your own internal processing to interpersonal processing. Understanding how you relate to others will help you minimize your level of frustration and dissatisfaction and optimize successful interactions. Shutz (1992) proposed a model with the basic assumption that people need people because we are social beings and as a result, three interpersonal needs develop that must be satisfied in order to function effectively. They are *need for inclusion*, *need for control*, and *need for affection*. It is important to note that not only do you require these but so do the people you deal with.

The degree of need for inclusion is dependent on where one lies on the introversion–extroversion continuum. However, it does not matter if you are an obligatory introvert, an obligatory extrovert, or somewhere in the middle, the need for inclusion is always operating, and you should be sensitive to this need in yourself and in those around you. The second interpersonal need, the need for control, is a concept that is measured on the independent–dependent continuum. According to Shutz (1958), everyone needs to have control—and also be controlled—at different times and in different situations. You must also be sensitive to this need in yourself and in others. The third need, the need for affection, is a very interesting construct. Although it is more about the need to like and be liked, if unchecked, it is often a cause for ethical boundary violations, especially when working with special patient populations. Generally, however, this need is best observed in those who either require distance versus closeness to individuals or groups in the work environment. Keep in mind, you express behaviors toward others who exhibit these needs (you meet their needs) and/or you express behaviors that demonstrate your own desires to have these needs met. Understanding how you relate to others, specifically around the three needs just discussed, will enhance your interpersonal interactions and can be an important part of your managerial success.

CONCLUSION

By developing self-awareness skills, you not only gain insight into your own *modus operandi* but you also begin to become sensitized to the differences of those around you. Today's successful manager is surrounded by people of diverse backgrounds and makeup and, when working as a team, will bring unlimited creativity, growth, and success to the workplace. Surrounding yourself with people just like you will most certainly lead to stagnation. Learning to understand diversity through a process of self-awareness can only lead to success.

REFERENCES

Allan, H., & Waclawski, J. (1999). Influence behaviors and managerial effectiveness in lateral relations. *Human Resource Development Quarterly, 10*, 3–34.

Berscheid, E., & Walster, E. H. (1978). *Interpersonal attraction*. Reading, MA: Addison-Wesley.

Boyatzis, R. E., Goleman, D., & Rhee, K. (1999). Clustering competence in emotional intelligence: Insights from the emotional intelligence inventory. In R. Bar-On & J. D. A. Parker (Eds.), *Handbook of emotional intelligence* (pp. 343–362). San Francisco, CA: Jossey-Bass.

Budner, S. (1982). Intolerance of ambiguity as a personality variable. *Journal of Personality, 30*, 29–50.

Cameron, K. S., Kim, M. U., & Whetten, D. A. (1987). Organizational effects of decline and turbulence. *Administrative Science Quarterly, 32*, 222–240.

Freud, S. (1956). *Collected papers*. London, United Kingdom: Hogarth.

Fromm, E. (1939). Selfishness and self-love. *Psychiatry, 2*, 507–523.

Goleman, D. (1995). *Emotional intelligence*. New York, NY: Bantam.

Kelly, R. E. (1998). *How to be a star at work*. New York, NY: Times Books.

Kohlberg, L. (1981). *Essays in moral development* (Vol. 1). New York, NY: Harper & Row.

Maslow, A. H. (1962). *Toward a psychology of being*. Princeton, NJ: D. Von Nostrand.

May, R. (Ed.). (1961). *Existential psychology*. New York, NY: Random House.

Rest, J. R. (1979). *Revised manual for the defining issues test: An objective test of moral judgment development*. Minneapolis, MN: Minnesota Moral Research Projects.

Rokeach, M. (1973). *The nature of human values*. New York, NY: Free Press.

Schmidt, W. H., & Posner, B. Z. (1982). *Managerial values and expectations*. New York, NY: American Management Association.

Shutz, W. (1958). *FIRO: A three-dimensional theory of interpersonal behavior*. New York, NY: Holt, Rinehart & Winston.

Shutz, W. (1992). Beyond FIRO-B—Three new theory-derived measures: Element B (behavior), Element F (feelings), and Element S (self). *Psychological Reports, 70*, 915–937.

Sosik, J., & Megerian, L. E. (1999). Understanding leader emotional intelligence and performance: The role of self–other agreement on transformational leadership perceptions. *Group and Organization Management, 24*, 367–390.

Trompenaars, F., & Hampton-Turner, C. (1998). *Riding the waves of culture*. New York, NY: McGraw-Hill.

Whetten, D. A., & Cameron, K. S. (2002). *Developing management skills* (5th ed.). Saddle River, NJ: Pearson Education.

Future of the DNP Nurse Executive

Elizabeth A. Gazza

INTRODUCTION

Visionary nurse executives anticipate and plan for the future and lead others, as together, they make their vision a reality. Nurse executives who have earned the Doctor of Nursing Practice (DNP) degree have been prepared for this executive leadership role. They understand that quality care must be rooted in evidence, and they are prepared to ensure that a culture of evidence-based practice is established in health care.

This chapter includes details about the competencies that DNP-prepared nurse executives possess and that when practiced to the fullest extent, can shape the future of health care. The impact that visionary nurse executives can have on the future of nursing and nursing practice is demonstrated through two exemplars.

COMPETENCIES OF DNP-PREPARED NURSE EXECUTIVES

In order to understand the impact that DNP-prepared nurse executives can have on the future of health care, it is necessary to look at formal nursing education programs that offer the DNP degree program. The Accreditation Commission for Education in Nursing (ACEN) and the Commission on Collegiate Nursing Education (CCNE) are two organizations that accredit nursing education programs. Both organizations have established standards and criterion that address the competencies that must be displayed by graduates of a nursing education program that culminates in a clinical doctorate. Program outcomes, including the skills of graduates, must be congruent with established professional nursing standards, and the curriculum must be designed to prepare graduates to practice from an evidence-based research perspective (Commission on Collegiate Nursing Education [CCNE], 2013; National League for Nursing Accrediting Commission, 2008).

Professional nursing standards that serve as the basis for a clinical doctorate include *The Essentials of Doctoral Education for Advanced Nursing Practice* (American Association of Colleges of Nursing [AACN], 2006) as shown in Table 11.1, and the *Nursing Administration: Scope and Standards of Practice* (American Nurses Association [ANA], 2009) as shown in Table 11.2. A nurse who has earned a clinical doctorate through a program based on these, or similar professional standards, has the foundational skills needed to advance nursing practice in accordance with his or her vision.

In addition to earning a clinical doctorate degree, nurses can pursue specialty certification as a nurse executive. The American Organization of Nurse Executives (AONE) has identified competencies specific to the nurse executive role (American Organization of Nurse Executives [AONE], 2013). It is interesting that these executive competencies align with the competencies of doctoral education identified by AACN (2006). Table 11.3 reflects the clear alignment between these two sets of competencies. This indicates that there is congruency between organizations that prepare and certify nurse executives regarding the skills and competencies needed to be successful in leading the future of nursing. How these competencies can be used by DNP-prepared nurse executives to shape the future must now be explored.

TABLE 11.1. Synopsis of the American Association of Colleges of Nursing Doctoral Education Essentials for Advanced Nursing Practice

1. Scientific underpinnings for practice
2. Organizational and systems leadership for quality improvement and systems thinking
3. Clinical scholarship and analytical methods for evidence-based practice
4. Information systems/technology and patient care technology for the improvement and transformation of health care
5. Health-care policy for advocacy in health care
6. Interprofessional collaboration for improving patient and populations health outcomes
7. Clinical prevention and population health for improving the nation's health
8. Advanced nursing practice

From American Association of Colleges of Nursing. (2006). *The essentials of doctoral education for advanced nursing practice.* Washington, DC: Author.

TABLE 11.2. Synopsis of the American Nurses Association Standards of Nursing Administration Practice

Standards of Practice

Standard 1. Assessment
Standard 2. Identifies issues, problems, or trends
Standard 3. Outcomes identification
Standard 4. Planning
Standard 5. Implementation
Standard 5a. Coordination
Standard 5b. Health promotion, health teaching, and education
Standard 5c. Consultation
Standard 6. Evaluation

Standards of Professional Performance

Standard 7. Quality of practice
Standard 8. Education
Standard 9. Professional practice evaluation
Standard 10. Collegiality
Standard 11. Collaboration
Standard 12. Ethics
Standard 13. Research
Standard 14. Resource utilization
Standard 15. Leadership
Standard 16. Advocacy

From American Nurses Association. (2009). *Nursing administration: Standards and scope of practice* (3rd ed.). Silver Springs, MD: Author.

TABLE 11.3. Comparison of Nurse Executive Certification and Doctoral Education Competencies

American Organization of Nurse Executives (2013) Nurse Executive Certification Exam Competencies	American Association of Colleges of Nursing (2006) Essentials of Doctoral Education for Advanced Nursing Practice
Communication and relationship building	Interprofessional collaboration for improving patient and populations health outcomes
Knowledge of the health-care environment	Scientific underpinnings for practice Clinical scholarship and analytical methods for evidence-based practice Health-care policy for advocacy* Clinical prevention and population health for improving the nation's health
Leadership	Organizational and systems leadership for quality improvement and systems thinking
Professionalism	Advanced nursing practice
Business skills	Information systems/technology and patient care technology for the improvement and transformation of health care Health-care policy for advocacy

THE VISION OF DNP-PREPARED NURSE EXECUTIVES

In 1990, the American Nurses Association (ANA) established the Magnet Hospital Recognition Program for Excellence in Nursing Services as a mechanism for recognizing nursing excellence in health-care organizations (American Nurses Credentialing Center [ANCC], 2014). The program is based on five model components that serve as the framework for achieving superior performance as evidenced by outcomes (ANCC, 2013). Essentially, this represents a vision of what is possible in the provision excellence in nursing care. As such, nurse executives who identify this as part of their vision will lead their organizations through the process of achieving Magnet recognition. Again, it is necessary to consider the skills and competencies a nurse executive must have in order to make this vision a reality. Table 11.4 indicates that the DNP-prepared executive has the skills that align with the five model components of the Magnet Program and is therefore prepared to lead this major undertaking aimed at achieving nursing excellence.

Through the review of professional nursing standards that serve as the basis for formal nursing education programs that lead to a clinical doctorate, competencies that must be displayed by certified nurse executives, and how such abilities align with a major initiative such as Magnet Recognition, a primary component of the nurse executive skill base has been identified. It is a thread that runs through degrees, certifications, the Magnet program, and professional nursing practice in clinical and educational settings. That thread is evidence-based practice (EBP), including knowledge about EBP, and the ability to lead the transformation of health care to a new culture; a culture in which evidence is consistently used as the basis for practice.

TABLE 11.4. Comparison of DNP Competencies and Magnet Recognition Model

American Association of Colleges of Nursing (2006) Essentials of Doctoral Education for Advanced Nursing Practice	American Nurses Credentialing Center (2014) Magnet Recognition Model
Interprofessional collaboration for improving patient and populations health outcomes Advanced nursing practice Information systems/technology and patient care technology for the improvement and transformation of health care	Exemplary professional practice
Scientific underpinnings for practice Clinical scholarship and analytical methods for evidence-based practice Clinical prevention and population health for improving the nation's health	New knowledge, innovations, and improvements Empirical quality results
Organizational and systems leadership for quality improvement and systems thinking	Transformational leadership Empirical quality results
Health-care policy for advocacy	Structural empowerment

DNP-prepared nurse executives are qualified to make that vision a reality in health care and nursing education.

Many of the practices in health care and nursing education are historically based, performed in a certain manner because that is how it was always done. In today's rapidly changing health-care arena, this is not the milieu in which practice should be rooted. Although there has been a dramatic increase in the areas of science and technology, health care, including nursing, has experienced a delay in translating knowledge to practice. This was clearly identified by the Institute of Medicine (IOM, 2001) as a factor contributing to the divide that existed between what is and what should be in health care. The use of evidence as the basis of practice is one of six nursing competencies identified by the IOM (2003) and subsequently a competency addressed at all levels of nursing education by the Quality and Safety Education for Nurses (QSEN Institute, n.d.) initiative. The IOM (2003) stated, "All health professionals should be educated to deliver patient-centered care as members of an interdisciplinary team, emphasizing evidence-based practice, quality improvement approaches, and informatics" (p. 3). By virtue of their formal doctoral level education, DNP-prepared nurse executives are knowledgeable about EBP and how to use this important competency to advance nursing practice. However, this is only one of two components needed to infuse EBP into health care.

The second component needed to infuse EBP as the basis for nursing practice focuses on the creation of a culture of EBP. This cultural transformation must occur at the micro and macro levels. In some cases, changes made at one level can impact another level. For example, Peters (2002) stated, "Of all the steps in the policy-making process, problem recognition/issue identification is most crucial" (p. 2). This indicates that a macro level change, such as the generation of a policy, can begin at the micro level, with the identification of a problem in clinical or nursing education practice in a particular setting. Both of these, policy generation and initiation of a practice change specific to an identified problem, are within the realm of practice for the DNP-prepared nurse executive.

Leading a cultural transformation can be particularly challenging for nurse executives in large health-care or educational systems. The system nurse executive, including academic deans who lead multiple programs delivered on multiple campuses, may only have a direct line of authority to chief nursing officers or program directors at individual facilities within the system and not for those who actually implement the change (Englebright & Perlin, 2008). Regardless of the organizational structure, Melnyk and Fineout-Overholt (2011) identified the importance of having a clear vision of what is to be accomplished as the initial element in leading successful organizational change, such as the creation of a new culture. Additional elements include belief, strategic planning, action, persistence, and patience.

Although various models can be used to structure environments led by nurse executives, the model of the interrelationship of leadership, environments, and outcomes for nurse executives (MILE ONE) is an evidence-based model that emphasizes continual enhancement of the professional practice/work environment (PPWE) toward empowering staff to improve outcomes (Adams, Erickson, Jones, & Paulo, 2009). The model is based on three concept areas, including (1) nurse executive influence on the PPWE, (2) PPWEs influence on patient and organizational outcomes, and (3) patient and organizational outcomes influence on nurse executives. The model is a knowledge-based framework to guide nurse executives by clarifying the role of nurse executives. Continuous measurement and evaluation, or the use of evidence, is a key component of the model. The evidence is what indicates the nurse executive's influence or leadership on organizational and patient outcomes and the work environment.

The National League for Nursing (NLN) addressed work environments for nursing faculty in academic practice. The Healthful Work Environments Tool Kit©, which was based on results from the 2003 National Study of Faculty Role Satisfaction, consists of a series of questions and resources designed to assess work environments (National League for Nursing [NLN], 2006a). DNP-prepared nurse executives in academic settings can lead the assessment process and work with faculty to interpret the results, or evidence, and design continuous improvement plans for the purpose of creating healthful work environments. Such environments facilitate a spirit of inquiry, including the use of EBP to advance practice within the realm of nursing education.

Selecting a model or framework can certainly facilitate change or transformation to a new culture. However, mentoring by a DNP-prepared nurse executive can also impact the transformation process. There is an abundance of published literature, from various disciplines, on the topic of mentoring. It is interesting that a single definition of mentoring, used across all disciplines, is not apparent. Roberts (2000) used a phenomenological approach to identify common themes among the various published definitions and yielded a comprehensive definition of the concept. According to Roberts, *mentoring* is "a formalized process whereby a more knowledgeable and experienced person actuates a supportive role of overseeing and encouraging reflection and learning within a less experienced and knowledgeable person, so as to facilitate the persons' career and personal development" (p. 162). According to Young and Wright (2001), a mentor is the experienced or skilled member of the relationship who serves as the guide. The less experienced member is referred to as the *protégé* or *mentee*. Although some mentoring relationships can consist of one mentor and mentee, others include a group approach where multiple mentors facilitate the development of a single mentee.

DNP-prepared nurse executives have the skills and competencies specific to EBP and therefore can serve as the skilled members of the mentor–mentee relationship. Effective mentoring relationships may play a key role in not only creating but also sustaining the new culture. The NLN (2006b) *Position Statement: Mentoring of Nurse Faculty* presented a mentoring framework that includes mentoring across the career continuum. Mentoring relationships consisting of practicing nurse educators being mentored by DNP-prepared executives or deans could be an effective strategy for creating a new culture of EBP within nursing education.

CONCLUSION

Leading in an environment that is filled with quality and safety concerns requires that nurse executives in clinical and educational settings create a culture in which EBP is the norm; a culture in which practice, from business practices to individualized nursing care practice and education, is based on the best available evidence and where a cycle of continuous improvement is an expectation of all care providers. Nurse executives prepared at the DNP level are well equipped to create this culture as a way of improving the quality and safety of the health-care environment and in nursing education. However, creating this culture is not an easy task. It requires an individual with the skills, knowledge, and attitudes necessary to lead complex change. DNP-prepared nurse executives are in a position to make the vision of using EBP as the basis for practice in clinical and educational settings a reality.

EXEMPLARS

The following exemplars provide rich data about the experiences of two nurse executives, including the rewards and challenges associated with their work. Pseudonyms are used in place of real names. Questions designed to facilitate analysis of the exemplars and discussion about the DNP-prepared nurse executive follow each exemplar.

Nurse Executive as a Trailblazer

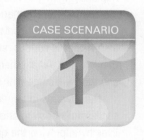

CASE SCENARIO 1

Dr. Bender is a senior-level administrator leading nursing services in privatized correctional and mental health facilities. It has been over 20 years since she held her first nurse executive position as a chief nursing officer. When asked how she felt about her work as a nurse executive, she stated, "I love it." This was evident as she described her experience, the challenges she encountered, and the rewards associated with transforming a culture and making a difference.

Dr. Bender was once described by her colleagues as a "trailblazer." She was the first psychiatric/mental health nurse practitioner in the area where she lived and wanted to practice. At that time, physicians were not familiar with the nurse practitioner (NP) role and questioned her about what she would contribute to patient care and her salary expectations, both of which they did not understand. Once she secured a position with a local physician, other physicians were able to see that an NP was a nurse who provided quality nursing care to patients, rather than a nurse trying to function as a doctor. Her actions blazed the trail for others interested in advancing their education as NPs and securing positions in this same community.

As a vice president for nursing services for a company that privatizes health services for correctional and mental health facilities in various states, Dr. Bender continues to blaze trails. Although a great deal of her work focuses on devising policies, preparing requests for proposals for new service contracts, and implementing new initiatives to ensure the provision of quality services, Dr. Bender leads the transformation of contracted state correctional and mental health facilities to a new model of care. This involves structural and cultural changes, both of which impact the provision and quality of care.

Leading such complex change is not without challenges. Transforming a facility can take 2 to 3 years and involve several hundred employees, which obviously requires patience and persistence. Dr. Bender's advice regarding leading such extensive change is to expect resistance and pushback from those involved and recognize that such behavior is part of any change, be realistic when establishing the timeline for completing the change, and have a good sense of the budget available to support the process.

However, the primary challenge Dr. Bender faces involves transforming the existing culture to one that embraces new standard of care. The quality of care is highly dependent on the skills, knowledge, and attitudes of the nursing staff. Although staff members are appropriately credentialed, they must learn and embrace a new set of cultural practices including performance standards and expectations, the use of evidence as the basis for practice and a quality improvement cycle for the ongoing enhancement of services, and the philosophy that rewards are based on performance rather than years of service. These are not minor issues. These issues, coupled with the stressors associated with working in an environment plagued with safety concerns, can impact staff recruitment and retention. Therefore, education and ongoing development of the staff is a key strategy used by Dr. Bender to facilitate the cultural transformation. She recently led a project to provide tuition support to nurses as a way to promote advanced education and lifelong learning. One of her goals is to create a staff that is curious, stimulated to learn more, and eager to improve the quality of care they provide. As another example of her trailblazing spirit, she commented, "Raise the bar and they will come with you."

The rewards of her work result from overcoming the many challenges and achieving a successful transformation. Through a successful transformation, Dr. Bender touches many lives by improving the quality of nursing care and helping people to achieve professional growth at a level they never thought they could achieve. She described the high level of pride displayed by staff at the very first facility that completed the transformation process. Their pride transcended previous beliefs that such extensive change was not possible and that they were not qualified to be part of something of such quality. This first success served as the model for future transformations and allowed involved individuals to see the trail that had been blazed under Dr. Bender's leadership. Dr. Bender stated, "To take old buildings and a staff focused on reaching retirement and transform that into a new institution run by a staff with new knowledge who are performing at a new level is wonderful."

Pursuing a DNP degree was of great importance to Dr. Bender. Prior to earning the degree, she felt underprepared in relation to her non-nursing senior-level administrative colleagues. As an NP, she wanted to advance her level of clinical practice rather than conduct research. A curriculum that represented current thinking including EBP, quality improvement, and grant writing was very important in her selection process. This was because she wanted to master the content needed to be successful in the everyday life of a nurse executive. Although she had been doing the job for many years, enrollment in the DNP curriculum was the first time she had any formal education on many of these topics. This education would round out the knowledge and expertise she had developed through her practice as an NP and nurse executive.

As a DNP-prepared nurse executive, her vision for the future is to fully integrate EBP into the nursing care delivery system that is part of the transformed culture. This is no easy task, but with her trailblazing experience, there is no doubt her vision will become a reality. She is working to secure computers and an electronic library to be used by staff to secure evidence that will eventually serve as the basis for practice. She continues to educate staff about how to integrate the evidence into all aspects of health-care delivery, including policy development. These examples are consistent with her trailblazing practice of promoting what is needed in order for one to be engaged in his or her position.

▶ **Discussion Questions**

1. Which of the nurse executive competencies identified by AONE and ANCC have been demonstrated by this nurse executive? By you?
2. In what ways is this executive creating a culture in which evidence is used as the basis for practice? Outline the steps you would need to take to create a culture of EBP at your place of employment.
3. How does this nurse executive's vision align with the five models of the Magnet Recognition Program? With your vision of excellence in nursing care?
4. How did the trails blazed by Dr. Bender impact those who entered the nursing profession after her? What trails have you blazed?
5. Would you surmise about the role that work environment plays in transforming the facilities led by Dr. Bender?

Nurse Executive as Entrepreneur

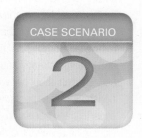

CASE SCENARIO 2

Dr. Mitchell is a DNP-prepared nurse executive who is an entrepreneur in the specialty of aesthetic medicine. She used the knowledge and skills she gained through formal education and professional nursing practice to generate a vision that included the provision of quality aesthetic care using evidence as the basis for practice. Earning a DNP degree gave her the confidence to make her vision a reality.

Becoming an entrepreneurial executive may not have been planned by Dr. Mitchell, but a look at her journey reveals how engaging in formal education programs and learning through employment led to her development as an executive. As an NP in aesthetic medicine, she learned about the standard of care within the specialty. She earned a master's degree in health services administration and held positions in a marketing department and as the chief operating officer of a health-care company that she was charged with initiating and developing. It is apparent that through these experiences she developed the competencies needed to be successful in her own business venture. However, one thing was missing. She felt she needed to earn a doctoral degree in nursing in order to ensure she could provide care and services of the highest possible quality and have the credentials necessary to be recognized as a qualified nursing leader in aesthetic medicine. Both of these reasons were essential to her future success as an entrepreneur.

As Dr. Mitchell continued to practice as an NP in aesthetics, she earned a DNP degree. She used evidence as the basis for practice while completing a practice change project specific to the nursing care in aesthetics. Aside from gaining knowledge specific to advanced nursing practice, she gained the confidence to strike out on her own. She made this career move just as she completed the DNP degree.

In anticipation of the challenges she expected to encounter from the local physicians who practice in the field of aesthetics, Dr. Mitchell was proactive. She knew that being an active member of the state NP association, including a member of the executive board, and collaborating with the state board of nursing would help her to follow all of the rules and regulations associated with being an entrepreneur and give her added support from within the discipline of nursing. Again, she learned this earlier in her career, almost in preparation for what would come in the future. Although some professional colleagues advised her to "lay low and not make yourself a target" during the early days of the business adventure, she had to initiate a marketing campaign in order to make her vision a reality. Physicians reported Dr. Mitchell to the board of medicine because they felt she was trying to function as a doctor. This caused a major stir in the community. However, Dr. Mitchell knew she was operating within the scope of nursing and realized that most of resistance resulted from physicians who did not understand the role of an NP and/or DNP-prepared nurse. The new health-care plan is playing a key role in helping all individuals, including physicians, to understand the roles that all nursing professionals can play in the provision of quality health care. However, Dr. Mitchell continues to educate individuals at the local level and through professional NP organizations.

Experiencing the challenges associated with making her vision a reality seems to have motivated Dr. Mitchell. It has been over 1 year since the doors opened to her aesthetic clinic, and she has already had to relocate to a larger space and hire additional staff. When asked how she felt about her work, she stated, "I love it." She has the opportunity to forge close relationships with patients who ultimately feel better about themselves as a result of Dr. Mitchell's expertise and her vision. EBP drives her decision making with regards to new products and services. She reviews the evidence to make safe decisions that are right rather than just looking at the bottom line. As a nurse executive entrepreneur, she continues to enhance her vision with regards to aesthetics. She continues to add to her repertoire of skills to advance her expertise and suggests that those considering a path similar to hers have a clear philosophy as the basis of practice, know and follow all regulations, be appropriately credentialed, develop support systems and rapport with key constituents, and have tough skin (no pun intended). One of her staff stated that Dr. Mitchell is her own worst enemy because she often provides free services. However, this is consistent with her business philosophy, which is, "Do the right thing regardless of cost because it will come back to you later extra, above, and beyond."

▷ **Discussion Questions**

1. Dr. Mitchell encountered many roadblocks on her journey to making her vision a reality. What roadblocks have you encountered on your journey? How have you overcome them? What could you have done more effectively after hearing about Dr. Mitchell's experience?

2. Being a member of a professional nursing organization served as a support system for this nurse executive. Identify professional nursing organizations that have a vision similar to your own. How would you use these organizations to assist you as a nurse executive?

3. Dr. Mitchell faced challenges that resulted from a lack of understanding about her credentials and/or qualifications. How should this be addressed as part of health-care reform? What contributions have you made or could you make to help others clearly understand nursing and all of the credentialing options within nursing?

REFERENCES

Adams, J. M., Erickson, J. I., Jones, D. A., & Paulo, L. (2009). An evidence-based structure for transformative nurse executive practice: The model of the interrelationship of leadership, environments, and outcomes of nurse executives (MILE ONE). *Nurse Administration Quarterly*, 33(4), 280–287. doi:10.1097/NAQ.0b013e3181b9dce3

American Association of Colleges of Nursing. (2006). *The essentials of doctoral education for advanced nursing practice*. Washington, DC: Author.

American Nurses Association. (2009). *Nursing administration: Standards and scope of practice* (3rd ed.). Silver Springs, MD: Author.

American Nurses Credentialing Center. (2013). *Magnet Recognition Program® model*. Retrieved from http://www.nursecredentialing.org/Magnet/ProgramOverview/New-Magnet-Model

American Nurses Credentialing Center. (2014). *History of the Magnet program*. Retrieved from http://www.nursecredentialing.org/magnet/programoverview/historyofthemagnetprogram

American Organization of Nurse Executives. (2013). *Certified in executive nursing practice: Candidate handbook and application*. Chicago, IL: AONE Credentialing Center.

Commission on Collegiate Nursing Education. (2013). *Standards for accreditation of baccalaureate and graduate nursing programs*. Retrieved from http://www.aacn.nche.edu/ccne-accreditation/Standards-Amended-2013.pdf

Englebright, J., & Perlin, J. (2008). The chief nurse executive role in large healthcare systems. *Nurse Administration Quarterly*, 32(2), 188–194.

Institute of Medicine. (2001). *Crossing the quality chasm*. Washington, DC: National Academies Press.

Institute of Medicine. (2003). *Health professions education: A bridge to quality*. Washington, DC: National Academies Press.

Melnyk, B. M., & Fineout-Overholt, E. (2011). *Evidence-based practice in nursing & healthcare: A guide to best practice* (2nd ed.). Philadelphia, PA: Lippincott Williams & Wilkins.

National League for Nursing. (2006a). *National League for Nursing Healthful Work Environment Tool Kit©*. New York, NY: Author.

National League for Nursing. (2006b). *Position statement: Mentoring nurse faculty*. New York, NY: Author.

National League for Nursing Accrediting Commission. (2008). *NLNAC standards and criteria. Clinical doctorate*. Retrieved from http://www.acenursing.net/manuals/sc2008_doctorate.pdf

Peters, R. M. (2002). Nurse administrators' role in health policy: Teaching the elephant to dance. *Nurse Administration Quarterly, 26*(4), 1–8.

Roberts, A. (2000). Mentoring revisiting: A phenomenological reading of the literature. *Mentoring & Tutoring, 8*, 145–170.

QSEN Institute. (n.d.). *Competencies*. Retrieved from http://qsen.org/competencies/

Young, C. Y., & Wright, J. V. (2001). Mentoring: The components for success. *Journal of Instructional Psychology, 28*(3), 202–206.

Professional Sustainability and the Nurse Executive

Sally K. Miller

Sustainability is a 21st century buzzword. There is an awareness of the lightening-speed-rate at which society is burning its resources. Whether talking about energy and external environment or human capital and internal environment, astute leaders recognize the need for conservation and optimal use of resources. For the nurse executive, professional sustainability is an important concept. It is easy to "burn out" in the professional world today. From the bedside nurse to the chief nursing officer (CNO), we hear the term *burn out* every day. Staff and management often report feeling overextended, stressed, and uninspired. Professional sustainability is a critical part of conserving human capital—both for the nurse executive personally and the human resources that he or she manages. Among the many skills required of a nurse executive is the ability to create an environment that fosters professional sustainability at all levels—from the personal to the foundational level of the organization.

What is professional sustainability? That is really the most basic question and one with not such a basic answer—and yet, before a leader is able to create an environment for sustainability, he or she needs to identify what it is. *Sustainability* by definition is "the capacity to endure" (Onions, 1964). Intuitively, most leaders would assume that "enduring" the professional role is not a goal—and yet, for some in the workforce, that is precisely the goal. Others who attempt to define professional sustainability might assume that it must include "loving" the professional role—but is that that really true? Under just a little bit of scrutiny, this concept of "professional sustainability" is a bit nebulous yet clearly an important part of strong leadership. So the question remains, "What is professional sustainability?"

The best answer is that professional sustainability is different things to different people, and a truly successful nurse executive realizes that and supports it. Sometimes it is very easy to fall into a "one-size-fits-all" approach to managing people, but that just does not work when defining and promoting professional sustainability. More important for the nurse executive is the ability to create an environment in which each employee feels free to identify his or her own definition of sustainability. The nurse executive sees sustainability from an organizational perspective, but the backbone of a strong organization is the human capital that drives it. Consequently, sustainability is at its core an individual concept and will be characterized or defined by the individual—and like all individual concepts, will vary from person to person.

If the bottom line is sustainability, then each individual must be encouraged to identify what is truly important to him or her. Is the underlying goal to keep his or her job? For some, that is the primary motivator. For others, there is a stronger desire to achieve. For those individuals, the goal might be to be good at the job; for others, sustainability might require excelling at the job. Conversely, some professionals may be more driven by emotion—he or she must like the job. It is very likely, and reasonable, that some fraction of any organizational staff will identify his or her goal as to "not hate the job." Others will say that sustainability is driven largely by liking the job, and others genuinely feel they must love their job. These are all different sustainability motivators. The person who is driven mostly by the need to excel is not sustained by the same drivers as the person who is driven by the need to love the job. A professional can dislike his or her job yet excel at it; pride is a powerful motivator, and that person will likely sustain. Conversely, there are those who love their job but do not excel at it. Everyone who has spent any time in the workforce can recall working with that person who so loved his or her job. That person may not have been all that good at it but loved it so much that he or she stayed in the position for an entire 40-year career.

The most successful organizations will be composed of a diverse collection of human capital with associated diversity of goals. Hence, the failure of any one-size-fits-all approach fosters professional sustainability.

Thankfully, not every employee or professional wants to be a "stand-out" or a star. Diversity is strength in every walk of life, from neighborhoods to stock portfolios, and the same can be said for human capital. One of the biggest barriers to professional sustainability is trying to shoehorn a person into a role that just does not fit. If excelling is important to a professional, he or she needs to be put into a role in which excelling is possible. For example, consider the professional who is positioned in an area of the organization within which he or she has a particular expertise; for example, say the director of the department of continuing education (CNE). This director, an expert in the field of CNE, has over the course of several years developed a department that, under his or her guidance and expertise, has developed a reputation for excellence in the organization and professional community. This director does an excellent job, and everyone knows it. He or she has, over the years, developed new programs, branched out into the national market, has generated lots of money for the organization, and is repeatedly recognized for his or her excellence in the role.

Then, a new chief executive officer (CEO) comes along and decides that this person has been so capable and developed this department so well that she wants to move him or her into continuing medical education (CME). CME generates a lot more money for the organization. The director is transferred from CNE to CME, and gets a new title and a big raise and lots of institutional support. However, this person is not networked in the world of CME. He or she has limited experience with CME credentialing requirements, CME needs, and the state of the competition. It is unlikely that this person will "excel" in this new role for several years—if at all. This professional was ostensibly rewarded for excellent work by being put into a position in which excelling is much less likely. If professional sustainability for this director is driven by the need to excel, he or she will likely leave the organization before very long, seeking a new position in which he or she can return to that sense of excellence—a position as director of CNE with another organization. The organization loses a valuable employee, loses a little piece of professional sustainability. So for the nurse executive hoping to foster professional sustainability (and to improve it in himself or herself), identifying the true personal definition of professional sustainability is the first critical step. Only then can strategies to maximize it be successfully identified.

If the nurse executive recognizes the diversity in his or her human capital, then recognizing and developing the diversity in each employee's sustainability requirements should not be a challenge. For some, the sustainability driver is simply to *keep* the job. Given the current economic global climate, there is an awareness that has not been apparent in decades of how difficult finding and keeping a job can be. Employees whose primary driver is to keep the job are most likely to expend the effort necessary to follow the rules. They will often always be on time, will leave when the clock strikes quitting time, and will complete assigned tasks adequately. In general, these employees will not typically be particularly enthusiastic about non-fiscal incentives. These employees will perform best when there are clearly defined expectations. Employees who are motivated by keeping their job are less likely to participate in or feel rewarded by after-hours parties or programs offered as reward; they would rather have a raise than an annual holiday party. When a person whose primary goal is to keep his or her job is hired or transferred into a position that requires an interpretation of broader guidelines, occasional after-hours activity, or participation in activities outside the direct job role, they often do not do well. Consider the following example.

A new CNO is appointed in a local health-care system. He wants very much to provide a positive environment in which good employees feel valuable. While reviewing existing vacancies, he recognizes that there is an opening for a day-shift supervisor in the housekeeping department. Wanting to reward good service, he reviews the employee records of all of members of the housekeeping department and identifies a 52-year-old employee who has been with the facility for 34 years. This employee has always had above average employee evaluations, is well regarded by peers and supervisors, and is clearly a good employee.

The CNO seeks out the appropriate mid-level manager and suggests very strongly that this employee be promoted. The mid-level manager, wanting to comply with a new CNO's wishes, strongly encourages the housekeeper to accept the promotion. The housekeeper, a veteran rule follower, does what her boss asks. Now this employee of 34 years does not have a clear set of expectations. If others do not do their jobs well, she is held accountable. As a supervisor, at times, she must stay beyond an 8-hour day. She now has to supervise other employees and discovers there are no clear-cut rules for success.

How does a situation like this end? It is unlikely that after 34 years, this employee will adapt well to the new role. As a result, in the best case scenario, the employee has the confidence to request a return to her previous position. In a more likely scenario, she becomes increasingly dissatisfied, and either her work suffers, resulting in sub-optimal performance evaluations, or she leaves her position. After 34 years, she may be able to retire, or she may go to another organization; the point, however, is that she leaves. The organization loses a valuable employee of 34 years, and the employee loses the stability of her job. This is not professional sustainability—just the opposite. Although extreme situation like this happens more than anyone realizes—and it is undoubtedly due, in part, to the fact that no one really considered the housekeeper's personal drivers in terms of her professional sustainability. Every institution needs these employees, and every nurse executive needs to recognize those conditions that will foster their sustainability.

For other employees, the sustainability driver is to be good at the job. Although these employees do tend to be rule followers, they tend to require a bit more. Their drivers include both an internal and external component. When an employee really wants to be good at the job, she needs to feel from within that she is good; however, this employee also usually needs to feel as though that good performance is recognized externally as well. This person is not satisfied unless employee evaluations are truly above the average. If most people get "above average," this employee needs "excellent." If most people get "excellent," this employee needs "outstanding." An occasional employee of the month recognition or personal accolade from peers and superiors is important. To sustain in the organization, this employee, unlike the last example, needs to be in a position in which she is good and needs to have that occasionally recognized by those around her. An employee who is driven to be good at the job will always maintain a continuous, if relaxed, effort toward improvement. This type of employee sustains by staying just a bit ahead of the crowd.

Different from the employee who wants to be good at the job is the employee who must excel. Excelling is not the same as liking or even loving the role. The professional who needs to be identified as truly excelling is best used in position that fosters the ability to achieve excellence. This person will not be a rule follower, although he or she may offer rationale when the rules are broken. The person who needs to excel is not a "9-to-5" employee and will not do well when presented with what he or she perceives as arbitrary or general rules that have no true foundation in achieving the organizational mission. Often, the work product of these employees is so strong that the leadership tolerates some degree of "lone ranger" approach. Again, from the perspective of a CNO trying to achieve organizational sustainability, it is important to recognize that some fraction of the human capital must include this type of employee; the successful CNO will make reasonable allowances to support this employee's achievement while maintaining organizational harmony.

Another subset of the employee population is driven by a more emotional level of satisfaction; the goal is to either "not hate the job," "like the job," or even "love the job." For this type of employee, an important factor is the job environment; the people, support services, and physical environment. Unlike those who are driven by achievement, where the work itself is the primary issue, those who are driven more by emotion must enjoy those ancillary or peripheral factors. People who need to like their job will need to like the majority of people with whom they interact on a daily basis and must like the boss.

This type of employee will often personalize his or her work space with pictures, possessions, pillows on chairs, space heaters, or music. Whether the personal space is a desk, cubicle, locker, or office, personal touches are likely to be apparent. Relationships in the workplace are important. This employee will often know just who to call in another department to get a thing done. An employee whose primary driver is to like the job will not do well in high-stress environments. Consider a front office receptionist. One who is driven by liking the job will do best in an environment in which the phone rings occasionally and she gets to talk with several people daily. Most are fairly pleasant, but occasionally, someone is not. Appointments come in, the receptionist has equipment that works properly, and she is doing well managing the day's events. Her desk will have personal touches such as flowers, pictures, a nameplate, and often a sweater on the back of the chair. This person becomes easily stressed when presented with tasks that are labeled important; as long as they are intermittent and manageable, all will be well.

Conversely, someone who is driven by excelling at the job will become bored in the previously described environment. A receptionist who wants to excel will do best with a fast-paced and diverse environment. She has phones ringing all day, frequently has calls on hold, is trying to field messages, and ensures responses by difficult-to-reach executives. This employee will thrive on being trusted with important tasks such as ensuring that a critical document be prepared and shipped high priority. Unlike the person who needs to like the job, this employee does not necessarily need to like everyone with whom she interacts but does need to know that they are reliable. At the end of the day, this employee needs to feel that her performance has been excellent.

Finally, consider the employee that really must love the job. To this person, the job itself is the primary driver—not the environment. This person loves what he or she does. An employee who must love the job does not necessarily need to like the people around him or her; the passion is for the work. Consider the in-service nurse educator who just loves to work with new graduate nurses (GNs). She has a passion for helping new GNs transition in to the nursing role. This educator may have carved a niche over the years into her role in which most programs she develops and delivers target GNs. As long as this employee is able to stay in a role that focuses on GNs, she will remain happy and productive. New administrators may come and go; there may be challenges at times in scheduling rooms, supplies, or with other employees in the department, but these are all secondary as long as she can continue to work with GNs. This employee may have designed and developed highly successful programs for training and transitioning GNs; transfer her to work with another population, and she will not sustain.

In a parallel example, another employee may not love GNs per se but loves developing and implementing programs. This employee may have been hired to design and implement the first nurse extern program in the facility. Two or 3 years later, the program is running flawlessly with a clear record of success. The employee, however, needs another program to develop. If she is required to stay with this nurse extern program to provide ongoing administrative support, the aspect that she loved is gone, and the employee will not sustain. If she is not used for program development elsewhere in the organization, she will probably leave—another loss to sustainability.

Professional sustainability has two implications for nurse executives: from a personal perspective, the CNO needs to identify his or her own sustainability driver, and from a professional or role perspective, the CNO needs to recognize the diversity of sustainability drivers that exist within the human capital of an organization. Supporting that diversity of drivers is a separate challenge, but just recognizing that they exist is the first step. In recognizing that a diverse staff inherently means a diverse set of sustainability drivers, the most successful CNOs thus recognize that one blanket approach to people management cannot be successful. Of course, it is not practical to expect an individual approach to the management of each individual employee—the challenge for the successful CNO is to find the balance.

REFERENCE

Onions, C. T. (1964). *The Shorter Oxford English Dictionary*. Oxford: Clarendon Press.

Health-Care Informatics: Essential and Necessary in the 21st Century

Carol Patton

INTRODUCTION AND OVERVIEW OF COMPUTERS AND HEALTH CARE

There is no doubt that there is a major impetus to integrate health-care technology into health-care delivery in the 21st century. Having health-care technology provides opportunity to foster and facilitate information and to inform health-care providers with critical, timely, and relevant information to inform care and make data-driven decisions.

One way to envision the relevance and criticality of health-care information systems in today's health-care delivery systems is to think of it in the paradigm of information-rich environments in which sharing has to occur moment to moment and in some cases second to second. For example, in a critical care unit, patient status is monitored and regulated with smart technology with recordable data that can be stored and examined in the aggregate for quality improvement purposes. Information-rich health-care systems must be supported with state-of-the-art technology and informatics to be responsive and support data-driven decisions. The purpose of this chapter is to provide an overview of use of health-care informatics and technology in contemporary health-care delivery settings, examine essential components of health-care systems and information technology to guide and shape quality improvement in patient safety and quality, and describe the criticality of nursing leadership in shaping and advocating for health-care information technology supports to inform data-driven decisions.

Every health-care provider must be knowledgeable and on-board with information systems and health-care technology. It is not an option to not engage in health-care informatics and technology. For example, one of the major areas that is exploding with interest in the health-care section related to health-care technology is the use of electronic health records (EHR). With the explosion of interest in electronic medical records (EMRs), there are claims and assertions about how the use of EMRs will improve patient safety and outcomes. For example, there are contemporary sources that purport that the adoption of EMRs will improve quality of care, reduce medical errors, and reduce costs in addition to providing an electronic database of an individual's health information (Ennis, Rose, Callard, Denis, & Wykes, 2011, p. 117).

One glimpse at the magnitude of the coming of EMRs is that in the United States, there is incredible federal support for health-care informatics. For example, President Obama has pledged $50 billion over 5 years to achieve the goal of having an EMR for every American by 2014. With this enormity of federal support, there is no doubt that health-care informatics systems is a major federal initiative and here to stay in all health-care systems, large and small, but as often is the case, "the devil is in the details."

There are many issues and challenges to be addressed regarding the health-care informatics, and certainly, it is an exciting time to think about how the many issues and challenges related to health-care informatics will be addressed in diverse health-care systems.

Government and Regulatory Influences on Health-Care Informatics and Technology

It is quite interesting to know that the first EMR was developed on 1950s and early 1960s. The first EHRs were developed as clinical information systems (Atherton, 2011, p. 187). The federal government began using EHRs in the U.S. Department of Veterans Affairs (VA) in the 1970s. Today, the VA hospital has one of the most sophisticated EHR systems, and it largely grew out of concerns for patient safety and quality. The present VA EHR system allows any health-care provider to access patient health data regardless of location and provides exemplary integration of EHR data (Atherton, 2011, p. 187).

SYSTEM DECISIONS

The key components for a success health-care informatics system consist of three major components. The three major components are people, hardware, and software.

People

Perhaps one of the greatest challenges in planning, designing, implementing, and evaluating a comprehensive health-care informatics system is knowing how to successfully engage key people (stakeholders) in the change process. Change leading to successful planning, designing, implementation, and evaluation of health-care informatics systems must embrace interprofessional collaboration (Lorenzi & Riley, 2010). For example, the information technology support (ITS) person must fully understand the complexity of the processes happening simultaneously between the health-care provider and the patients they care for. It is not an easy task to try to upgrade a health information system when the health-care provider is trying to save a life in the emergency department. This means all change involving health-care informatics systems and upgrades must include and embrace the people (stakeholders) who are using the system and without whom the system will never be successful or fully operational.

Hardware

Hardware consists of the physical components of a health-care informatics system. For example, system hardware is composed of computers, servers, and all necessary components for a fully functional and operational system (Kaminski, 2009). Software allows users to conduct specific functions, and there are four main categories typically seen in health-care informatics systems. Without software, the computer cannot purposively function in any applications in a relevant or meaningful manner.

Table 13.1 indicates the four main categories of software essential to health-care informatics systems and accompanying characteristics.

TABLE 13.1. The Four Main Categories of Software Essential for Health-Care Informatics Systems and Characteristics

Category of Software	Characteristics
Operating system (OS) software	• The most fundamental and important software of the computer • Is fundamental for the operation of the computer and for capacity to add all additional software and hardware (e.g., printer, fax capability)
Productivity software	• Typically referred to as *office suites* • The most common software used on any computers (e.g., word processing, spreadsheets, databases) • Programs are usually bundled together
Creativity software	• This software allows the user to draw, record sounds and voice, integrate video and other multimedia
Communication software	• Software that allows communication via different mechanisms (e.g., instant messaging, e-mail, connecting to Internet browsers, conferencing)

One of the issues with operating system software is that it must be updated frequently and can be costly not only in the purchase of new software; however, there are indirect costs associated with downtime to integrate new software and teach users and support integration of the new system. For example, not all computers have the newest software and will need updates at different times. For example, maybe all employees working in the system need a computer upgrade with software updates every 3 years. This can be quite a challenge working with the key stakeholders to determine how best to integrate the updates and software upgrades and also provide support for the users.

Software

Open-source system are software systems developed to be shared between and among users of a system, and typically, there is little or no charge for using or downloading an open-source system.

Commercial software is software that requires a site license and payment and may be restricted to certain numbers of users of the software. For example, a health-care organization might have to subscribe to commercial software for the specific EHR system they want to subscribe to. Commercial software may be available in the form of "add-on" to a system that is used for the health-care organization information technology infrastructure. For example, a commercial software may be able to be purchased at the time of the initial purchase of the technology system, and later, the organization can add an upgrade or a new feature to the software for additional monies. An example would be adding a software that allows patient call back within 24 hours after same-day outpatient surgery to see how the patient is doing.

LINKAGES BETWEEN HEALTH-CARE INFORMATION SYSTEMS AND PATIENT QUALITY AND SAFETY

There are many claims and assertions that using health-care informatics systems will improve patient care through enhanced quality and safety, although there is scant research data to date supporting this claim. What is clear and readily apparent is that health-care informatics does provide opportunity through systems design to identify patterns of adverse events through aggregate data.

Through examination and analysis of patient outcomes, health-care organizations can analyze trends in patient safety and issues as well as identify strategies to minimize safety risks and hazards (Agency for Healthcare Research and Quality, 2008). The Patient Safety and Quality Improvement Act of 2005 (Public Law 109-41) was signed into law on July 29, 2005. This initiative was the result of the findings of the 1999 Institute of Medicine report, *To Err is Human: Building a Safer Health System.* It is hypothesized that integration of health-care informatics into the U.S. health-care system will improve patient quality and safety.

TABLE 13.2. Essential Criterion for Decision Making When Selecting a Health-Care Information System

- Plan and thoughtfully design the health-care informatics system focusing on the strategic plan for the organization.
- Focus on mission and philosophy of the organization to determine the scope of the health-care information allowing for needed scope and potential expansion.
- Determine system access and ability to interface with other inter– and intra–health-care informatics systems.
- Consider interface with patients and health-care consumers.
- Facilitate systems that allow aggregation of data for quality assessment and improved quality and safety outcomes.
- Consider integration of all systems into the health-care informatics system infrastructure.

Computerized physician order entry (CPOE) is providing a strategy to enhance patient quality and safety by improving legibility of physician and other health-care provider orders. Historically, there have been many untoward patient outcomes including sentinel events for patients across the life span due to illegible handwriting in paper-based medical records.

The costs of health-care informatics systems are not a small ticket item and selection of the system cannot be underestimated. The decision to purchase or upgrade the health-care information system must be careful, thoughtful, and include input from health-care information technology personnel, health-care providers, nursing leadership, and the finance department. These decisions cannot be made in isolation because it will be several years most often before the system can be upgraded or changed. The last thing any nurse leader or senior health-care system executive wants is to spend time and money choosing and implementing a system that does not meet organizational needs.

Table 13.2 includes essential criterion for decision making when selecting a health-care information system to support an information-rich health-care environment to inform data-driven clinical decisions that enhance patient quality and safety.

QUALITY ASSURANCE AND DEVELOPING HIGH-RELIABILITY ORGANIZATIONS

Regardless of the model of quality assurance a health-care organization subscribes to, it is clear that health-care information systems and technology play a crucial role in allowing the organization or quality improvement team to examine aggregate data to update systems and inform data-driven system changes at the micro-, macro-, and mesosystems levels (Nelson, Batalden, & Godfrey, 2007).

Quality does not just happen in health-care organizations, and it must be a purposeful, thoughtful, and well-designed plan with sustained commitment to become high-reliability organizations with high-reliability teams with each patient encounter. The health-care organizations that embrace quality by design at the micro-, macro-, and mesosystems levels will be the preferred organizations of the future. For example, it is the interprofessional health-care teams that drive quality and change on the sharp end of care in health-care organizations and that have the capacity to lead change based on the use of technology to examine aggregate data to inform change (Sollecito & Johnson, 2013).

EVIDENCE-BASED PRACTICE

Evidence-based practice requires the nurse leader to be able to critique and interpret research findings and determine if the findings can be integrated into nursing practice. There is still a gap between research and getting research from bench to bedside in every health-care setting (Patton, 2011). Health-care informatics and computers provide access to critical research data and contemporary databases that provide contemporary and current research to change and shape nursing and specifically focusing on patient quality and safety. In addition, staff and health-care providers need to feel comfortable looking for evidence-based practice to shape and inform clinical policies so contemporary care meets the standards of care. Nurses must have input in systems and processes that shape and inform IT systems and upgrades in the 21st century.

SECURITY AND CONFIDENTIALITY WITH ELECTRONIC MEDICAL RECORDS AND INFORMATION SYSTEMS

Although there are numerous benefits to having EMRs, health-care information systems and easy access to confidential and secure patient data presents challenges in contemporary health-care settings like never before (Patton, 2011). For example, staff and health-care providers have a user identification and passcode that signifies their ability to enter secure health-care information systems such as the EMR. Some of the greatest challenges faces in contemporary health-care information systems are protection of patient's privacy and confidentiality of all health information. Information security ensures that protection of information is guaranteed at all times. Information security also is intended to foster and protect the highest level of security as a defense and avoid attacks on health-care information systems that have potential for entire network and system collapse (Ciampa & Revels, 2013, p. 209).

BARRIERS AND CHALLENGES OF HEALTH-CARE INFORMATICS FOR HEALTH-CARE PROVIDERS

There is no doubt that with the amount of money the federal government is expending on health-care information technology that EMRs are here to stay, and it is intuitively clear that EMRs will eventually be adopted in every health-care organization providing patient care in the United States. An EHR is also referred to as an EMR.

EMRs are part of the larger health-care system information technology infrastructure and system. By 2013, the federal government has indicated this federal budget request represents the current federal administration's priorities for guiding the U.S. Department of Health and Human Services (HHS) to enhance the health and well-being of all Americans, and this includes investment in federal dollars to enhance and upgrade IT and EHRs in every health-care delivery setting. The current federal initiatives foster and promote resources needed to guide nationwide implementation of interoperable health information technology, including secure EHRs. The request also increases funding for the Office of the National Coordinator for Health Information Technology to help create a nationwide health information technology infrastructure (U.S. Department of Health and Human Services [HHS], 2013).

There are many claims and assertions that using EHRs will increase transparency in health-care delivery and also that it will enhance patient safety and outcomes (Etzioni, 2010). Table 13.3 indicates some of the key contributions of EMRs to enhance patient safety and outcomes.

TABLE 13.3. Key Contributions of Electronic Medical Records to Enhance Patient Safety and Outcomes

Key Contributions of Electronic Medical Records to Enhance Patient Safety and Outcomes	Results and Impact on Patient Safety and Quality
Multiple health-care providers can access the EMR simultaneously	Enhanced access to critical patient information by multiple providers simultaneously
Ability for early identification of critical laboratory values	Enhanced capacity to communicate critical or life-threatening laboratory values to the health-care provider for immediate action or changes in the plan of care
Clarity of orders with CPOE system	Orders are placed in a legible and complete manner and leave no room for interpretation of illegible handwritten orders
Early identification of possible drug-to-drug interactions or potential side effects	There are alerts within EMRs that provide alerts particularly with certain drug-to-drug interactions or potential side effects (e.g., Coumadin and Bactrim) Alarms inherent within the EMR system will not allow the order to be submitted until the issue is corrected, and this usually cannot be done with a silence of the alarm or a "work around"

CPOE, computerized physician order entry; EMR, electronic medical record.

ELECTRONIC MEDICAL RECORDS AND ACCESS TO CARE

Although there are many claims and assertions regarding how EMRs will improve transparency in health-care delivery and that EMRs will enhance patient safety and outcomes, there is still no clear or compelling data-driven research to support these assertions. One major concern with integration of EMRs and technology into health-care delivery is that it may not be embraced or adopted by all health-care providers specifically at a time when many primary care providers are in short supply (Crilly, Keefe, & Volpe, 2011). For example, there are still many challenges and issues in the United States getting primary care providers into some areas due to social isolation, and one of the fears with integration of EMRs into rural health-care areas is that rural primary care providers already in short supply may further negatively impact health-care providers who are unsure or in doubt regarding EHR systems.

CHALLENGES AND BARRIERS TO INTEGRATION OF ELECTRONIC MEDICAL RECORDS FOR HEALTH-CARE PROVIDERS

One of the greatest challenges for health-care providers with integration of EMRs is the need to support and infrastructure (Crilly et al., 2011). For example, there is data that indicates some health-care providers are leaving practice and retiring early either because they do not embrace the use of EMRs or because they feel it is not worth the effort to change at this point in their career.

Lack of Standards for Electronic Medical Records

One of the major issues and challenges with EMRs particularly confronting rural Appalachian primary care providers is the lack of support and education for advancing to integration of EMRs in primary care. Although physicians may support the concept of EMRs, these providers are often so engaged in patient interactions and care delivery that they must have support from various sources to really advance their skills and competencies in integration and use of EMRs (Grossman, Zayas-Caban, & Kemper, 2009). Not only do health-care providers need support and infrastructure when working with EMRs but they must also educate and explain these concepts and how EMRs are used to their patient populations who may or may not embrace technology and related concepts.

Usability and Flexibility

There is no doubt that the EMRs and those using the technology must embrace adopted software supporting EMRs. Specifically, there is a need for flexibility and suitability of the software selected in a health-care delivery setting (Ward, Stevens,

Brentnall, & Briddon, 2008). For example, any health-care organization wishing to have health-care providers embrace software to be used for an EMR suggests that health-care providers are major stakeholders in this change process and they need to be at the tables for discussion and hear the critical conversations that occur. Health-care providers, including, but not limited to, physicians and nurses, must have support for time away from direct patient care to engage in these discussions and know their voices and concerns are heard prior to decision making at the health-care systems organizational level. For example, having an IT decision made at the organizational level without considering the needs and views of the health-care providers typically does not result in a favorable outcome most of the time. It would be foolish to adopt a new computer system or software program without discussing the needs of health-care providers who will be using the technology.

Trends in Adoption of Electronic Medical Records by Family Physicians

It would seem reasonable that there are many variables influencing health-care providers to adopt EMRs. EMRs are currently being integrated into all health-care delivery systems as a result of major U.S. government initiatives to integrate health-care technology and informatics to improve access to patient care data through EMRs (Stream, 2009). There is a growing body of literature examining EMR adoption, and one specific study conducted in Washington state with a robust research design and methodology indicates EMR adoption in Washington state by family physicians is strongly associated with the practice size (Stream, 2009). For example, barriers to implementation of the EHR in Washington state by primary care physicians are largely linked to financial and that adoption of EMRs is expected to be at approximately 68% in the next 4 years. It does not matter how large or small a health-care system is; technology is never easy to integrate, and one cannot assume it will be positively embraced.

Meaningful Use

Currently, many health-care organizations are still using paper-based charting and documentation. It is clear that EHRs can enhance patient care and benefit health-care providers and more importantly the patients and populations they serve. Table 13.4 highlights days in which EHRs provide provider and patient benefits and rationale.

The Health Information Technology for Economic and Clinical Health (HITECH) Act provides HHS authority to establish programs to improve health-care quality, safety, and efficiency through the promotion of health information technology (HIT), including EHR and private and secure electronic health information exchange. As a result of the HITECH Act, eligible health-care professionals and hospitals can qualify for Medicare and Medicaid incentive payments when they adopt certified EHR technology and use it to achieve specified objectives.

TABLE 13.4. Benefits of Electronic Health Records and Rationale

Benefits for Health-Care Providers and Patients Having Electronic Health Records	Rationale
Complete and accurate information for providers to provide the most accurate and timely care	EHRs allow health-care providers to learn about, analyze, and synthesize patient information in the medical record prior to entering the patient room, prior to a patient encounter.
Increased access to patient data and health-care information	Information in the medical record is accessed and shared between and among the interprofessional health-care team. With paper-based medical records, there is much copying of information or multiple members of the interprofessional health-care team may need to access the medical record or components of it at the same time, delaying patient information or accurate updates in the plan of care.
Patients are empowered by assuming a more active and integrated role as a health-care consumer in holistic and comprehensive care and in their past and current medical treatment plan.	There is potential in some electronic medical record systems allowing patients to share all or components of their EHR with family members, health-care providers, or specialist providers over the Internet. Some IT systems also provide opportunity for health-care providers to e-mail and schedule appointment times with patients and provide appointment reminders for patients.

EHR, electronic health record; IT, information technology.

Two recent regulations released by Medicare and Medicaid focus on one regulation that defines "meaningful use" objectives and what health-care organizations and health-care providers must do to meet qualifications for bonus payments, and the other regulation identifies the technical capabilities required for health-care organizations to meet requirements for certified EHR technology. The impact of the HITECH Act is that health-care informatics is here to stay, and it is not an option for health-care organizations and health-care providers to say whether or not they embrace the technology.

PERSONAL HEALTH RECORD

In addition to EMRs, personal health records are another area of impetus for health-care technology. A *personal health record* (PHR) is defined as a strategy to "increase patients engagement in their health treatment and health options" (Ennis et al., 2011, p. 117). "A PHR is an individual's electronic record of health-related information that conforms to national standards and interoperability standards that is managed, shared, and controlled by the individual patient" (Kahn, Aulakh, & Bosworth, 2009, p. 369). PHRs allow individuals to assume accountability for adding information from multiple sources into one document. The individual owns the health-care data and determines how it will be used and also determines who has access to it.

TABLE 13.5. Commonly Used Commercial and Open-Source Personal Health Records

Revolution Health	http://www.revolutionhealth.com/
iHealth Record	http://www.ihealthrecord.org/
KP Online	https://www.kaiserpermanente.org/
MS HealthVault	http://healthvault.com/
My Health*e*Vet	http://www.myhealth.va.gov/
My Family Health Portrait	http://www.hhs.gov/familyhistory/
WebMD Personal Health Record	http://www.webmd.com/phr

The PHR is typically designed to be patient-driven and managed by the patient for the patient. It is challenging to imagine that many patients cannot even record and track their medications so it seems there will be a clear and compelling need to offer extensive support for patients with regard to updating and managing a PHR. For example, when a medication is changed, the patient would need to access and update his or her PHR with the new information.

PHRs may be available to patients through their insurance providers and may be accessed on the insurance provider website through a server. The downside would be that if a person changed insurance carriers, he or she would lose access to the PHR he or she had developed. Other PHRs are available through open access through web-based Internet sites. These web-based Internet sites include commercial and open-source/public domain sites for PHRs. Table 13.5 highlights sights of commonly used commercial and open-source PHRs.

ISSUES AND CHALLENGES WITH ELECTRONIC PERSONAL HEALTH RECORDS

As one might imagine, there are challenges and issues with respect to patient's privacy and confidentiality as well as issues with keeping electronic PHR (ePHRs) up-to-date and current. It is interesting to note that one open-source ePHR sites were quickly used by health-care consumers, so it appears that the concept of ePHRs is attractive as a means of keeping one's personal health information from multiple sources in one location that is easily accessible through the Internet. It appears that computer savvy health-care consumers are able to embrace and use ePHRs; however, it is equally intuitive to assume that health-care consumers who are not computer savvy need support, encouragement, and assistance to become computer literate to be able to add their personal health information and update changes in health status and plans of medical care including medications. There is clearly a compelling need for all health-care providers to assess use of ePHRs and provide support and encouragement for health-care consumers using ePHRs to improve quality and safety through quick and easy access to critical health-care information and patient data.

THE FUTURE

There is no doubt that health-care technology is an integral part of health-care systems now and will become even more so in the future. Realistically, staff and health-care providers will experience even more technology and that technology will come at the speed of light no doubt. For example, it is realistic to expect increased integration of social media as communication systems in health care given that many health-care organizations are already using Facebook, Twitter, and other social media to communicate with patient populations and market health-care goods and services.

Health-care workers will not only be care providers but they will also be knowledge workers who need support and assistance with technical skills to navigate the many phases and nuances of health-care information technology. There will always be newer and more improved computer systems and technology updates, and the half-life of information will be perhaps months and not years. Technology support and enhancement skills will be needed for staff and health-care provider support, and these skills and competencies will be more and more in demand for new hires.

CONCLUSION

Health-care technology and informatics is complex but a necessary and integral component of staff and health-care provider roles. Health-care leadership must plan, design, implement, and evaluate health-care technology and provide input from frontline interprofessional health team members to interface in relevant and purposive ways to create the most efficacious, cost-effective, health-care technology systems. There are many components of health-care technology that beg for input from interprofessional health-care teams and those who are working with the technology at the bedside. Health-care providers also must be prepared to advocate for support and resources necessary to implement a successful health-care technology infrastructure and partner with health-care technology specialists and health-care informatics practitioners. To delegate or relegate these important and essential roles to health-care technology specialists and health informatics practitioners is not honoring professional accountability.

REFERENCES

Agency for Healthcare Research and Quality. (2008). *Patient Safety and Quality Improvement Act of 2005*. Retrieved from http://www.ahrq.gov

Atherton, J. (2011). Development of the electronic health record. *Virtual Mentor, 13*(3), 186–189.

Ciampa, M., & Revels, M. (2013). *Introduction to healthcare information technology*. Boston, MA: Cengage.

Crilly, J. F., Keefe, R. H., & Volpe, F. (2011). Use of electronic technologies to promote community and personal health for individuals unconnected to health care systems. *American Journal of Public Health, 101,* 1163–1167.

Ennis, L., Rose, D., Callard, F., Denis, M., & Wykes, T. (2011). Rapid progress or lengthy process? Electronic personal health records in mental health. *BMC Psychiatry, 11,* 117.

Etzioni, A. (2010). Personal health records: Why good ideas sometimes languish. *Issues in Science and Technology, 26*(4), 59–66.

Grossman, J. M., Zayas-Caban, T., & Kemper, N. (2009). Information gap: Can health insurer personal health records meet patients' and physicians' needs. *Health Affairs, 28*(2), 377–389.

Kahn, J. S., Aulakh, V., & Bosworth, A. (2009). What it takes: Characteristics of the ideal personal health record. *Health Affairs, 28*(2), 369–376.

Kaminski, J. (2009). Computer science and the foundation of knowledge model. In D. McGonigle & K. Mastrian (Eds.), *Nursing informatics and the foundation of knowledge* (pp. 29–52). Sudbury, MA: Jones and Bartlett.

Lorenzi, N. M., & Riley, R. T. (Eds.). (2010). Reviewing the problem. In *Managing technological change: Organizational aspects of health informatics* (2nd ed., pp. 3–18). New York, NY: Springer.

Nelson, E. C., Batalden, P. B., & Godfrey, M. M. (2007). *Quality by design: A clinical microsystems approach.* San Francisco, CA: Jossey Bass.

Patton, C. M. (2011). Evidence-based practice and research. In T. Hebda & P. Czar (Eds.), *Handbook of informatics for nurses & healthcare professionals* (5th ed., pp. 545–577). Philadelphia, PA: Prentice Hall.

Sollecito, W. A., & Johnson, J. K. (2013). *McLaughlon and Kaluzny's continuous quality improvement in healthcare* (4th ed.). Sudbury, MA: Jones & Bartlett.

Stream, G. R. (2009). Trends in adoption of electronic medical records by family taxonomy of critical factors for adopting electronic health record systems by physicians: A systematic literature review. *BMC Medical Informatics & Decision Making, 10,* 60–77.

U.S. Department of Health and Human Services. (2013). *Fiscal year 2013. Justification of estimates for appropriations committee.* Washington, DC: Author.

Ward, R., Stevens, C., Brentnall, P., & Briddon, J. (2008). The attitudes of health care professionals: An interview study. *Health Services Research, 11,* 256–266.

Leadership Succession Planning and Development

Virginia Wilson

Health care in the 21st century is a tapestry of providers, insurers, suppliers, and payers. In this complex environment, health care is big business with total spending in 2007 at $2.7 trillion (Ferman, 2009; Sisko et al., 2009). Nurse executives in independent roles in practices or in health-care organizations struggle with issues related to cost containment, quality care, and excellence on a day-to-day basis. The focus on day-to-day operations is a tactical approach to delivering care, but there just as great a need to plan for the future to avoid endangering effectiveness and cost containment strategies for success of the organization. Nurse executives in the health-care industry, especially in patient care delivery systems, are in a position to recognize and prepare for transition of care providers by identifying others with leadership potential within their organizations, improving bench strength internally, increasing diversity of candidate pools, sharing talent internally and more efficiently, and increasing organizational flexibility and employee job satisfaction (Bondas, 2006). This leadership competency of succession planning and development goes beyond just individual practice and reaches out into the organization to prepare for the undeniable fact of upcoming leadership transition.

Succession planning is more than just an organizational chart that shows who is holding what job and the next person on the dotted line trail. Overall, the best-practice organizations in business and industry use succession planning and management to develop and maintain strong leadership. In doing so, skills and competencies are identified and developed to be ready for the foreseeable and inevitable future with workforce retirement rends. Succession planning and development is also an organizational tool to motivate and retain leadership within the organization. The intellectual capital that the organization contains is an asset that takes years to develop and can be lost in a short time period when opportunities present in other locations or planned for or unplanned talent exodus occurs.

Succession planning and development is an ongoing and dynamic process that aligns human capital needs with end goals and objectives of the practice or organization. Challenges such as restructuring, mergers, acquisitions, and/or bankruptcy are possible for every practice or health-care organization today. The plan and response of a good leader is to continually work at selecting, developing, and retaining the members of an organization who have the skills needed to sustain and move the practice or organization forward.

Census data indicates a graying of the United States. Practices and organizations without succession planning are at risk of not being prepared when the retirement wave begins. In addition to foreseen leadership vacancies, there is always the possibility that unforeseen events such as disease, automobile crashes, natural disasters, or terrorist acts may occur. A practice or organization with a plan that maps out a chain of command and the transition of leadership will be better prepared to continue operations in a normal manner than one that does not.

Turnover and recruiting is expensive for any organization. Recognizing succession planning and development as a key talent initiative displays a vision for the future. Leaders in organizations have an opportunity to discover employee career aspirations and abilities that can be developed into ready individuals to attend to upcoming vacancies. Being prepared for inevitable change in leadership is a sign of action and not reaction. Organizations are better prepared to respond quickly and effectively to major changes when there is a talent management system in place that matches development and training with the purpose and business of the practice or the organization. Without a succession plan in place, few organizations are fully prepared to continue operations with as little disruption as possible when leadership turns over.

Leadership succession for nurse executives is more than a replacement strategy and is one that needs continual attention for the ongoing success of practices and organizations (Beyers, 2006; Bonczek & Woodard, 2006; Sherman, 2005). Turnover for nurse executives may result from the aging of the population, illness, catastrophic events, job satisfaction issues related to the work environment, or retirement. To provide for a smooth transition in practice environments, leadership succession planning includes the ability to attract, retain, and develop the leadership talent within the practice or organization.

To develop the talent pool is to build a practice or organization's bench strength. Looking to the sports world, a perfect analogy is to have a backup for key positions so that a sports team is prepared to replace a key player when an unforeseen event occurs (Aroian, Meservey, & Crockett, 1996). There is always a cost involved in building and developing the skills of employees, but the benefits outweigh the costs in both human capital and dollars. A practice or organization will be short-sighted if it does not create internal bench-building programs based purely on dollars and cents. There is ample evidence in business and industry that organizations that invest in developing their internal bench over time outperform the organizations that have not. Organizations that have been identified as clock-building such as General Electric, Procter & Gamble, Walmart, 3M, and Sony develop and grow their bench strength from within. As a result, these companies are seen as role models for keeping their organizations at the forefront of change resulting in sustainability and profitability (Collins, 2001; Collins & Porras, 2002).

Keeping the focus on delivering quality patient care, managing costs, and reducing waste presents nurse executives with challenges that can be viewed as opportunities to create a strategic plan for continuity and success into the future. This trinity of challenges presents opportunities for nurse executives to contribute to the decision making and continuous success in health-care organizations today. Although the time has come for health-care practices and organizations to be lean and mean in their operations to ensure fiscal continuity of the quality of patient care, a core objective of practices and organizations alike cannot be overlooked. Nurse executives will need to address the development of their successors to respond to the changing environment of evidence-based practice and complex reimbursement strategies. Mayfield (as cited in Birk, 2010) states that "revenue is being peeled away by external forces. It is imperative that we manage the internal costs, much of which can be attributed to inefficiency and rework. As a result, health-care leaders are having to quickly absorb the tools and techniques that contribute to the effectiveness in this realm" (p. 15). In the newly defined practice realm, there needs to be a plan for transition and succession to maintain a stable care environment.

Changing the culture of health-care delivery in practices and organizations requires new ways of thinking. Identifying talent that not only knows the health-care landscape but also displays a knack for sensing opportunity and seizing the moment should be potential leaders that an organization makes an effort not to lose. The time now is not to cut leadership development programs and succession plans but to embrace the concepts, fashion the plan, and set a practice or organization on a path that can withstand the economic challenges and leadership turnover that will come.

There is a need to challenge the established practices and develop new systems of care delivery in an environment where reimbursements are being cut and quality outcomes cannot be sidestepped. Bisognano (2010) defined six changes that would help improve health-care quality and safety through nursing's practices:

- Focus on transformational leadership at all levels.
- Redesign care to optimize nurses' professional expertise and knowledge.
- Collaborate with all personnel to work together to ensure safe and reliable care for patients in acute settings.
- Build systems and a culture that encourage, support, and spread vitality and teamwork in all areas of nursing.

- Put in place structures and processes that ensure patient-centered care.
- Develop a national learning system to make all models and prototypes accessible to nurses at all levels throughout the United States.

Nurse executives in organizations require preparation for upcoming changes in health-care financing that will challenge even the most experienced practitioners. The redesign and refinancing of health care under the Obama administration will ultimately have a great impact on the reimbursement to the health-care providers, especially private practices and health-care organizations. The truth is that few organizations are prepared to weather the storm with experienced leaders in place, let alone in a time of uncertainty in leadership change.

The current changes in the health-care plan target practices and organizations in the form of spending reductions and reduced payments in Medicare and Medicaid tied to readmission rates. Forget about the past, the challenge today is to prepare leaders with competencies that address current and future changes in health-care delivery and reimbursement. Bundling, for example, which has always been a cost containment strategy in managed care will continue as a method to consolidate payments into one lump sum. The danger in increased demands for bundling of services in delivering care is that it does not reflect the true line item cost to deliver safe, quality, and efficient health-care services. Working with such cost containment strategies require competencies that go beyond basic accounting principles but a full understanding of what the shrinking reimbursement dollar means to continue to provide quality and efficient care.

Nurse executives in leadership roles are essential and effective to the long-range sustainability if not profitability of a practice or a health-care organization underscoring the emphasis on the need to begin succession planning as soon as possible. Considering the current climate and culture where quality and cost-effectiveness are closely intertwined, the nurse executive responsibilities include setting priorities, focusing on the business of care delivery inclusive of quality outcomes and cost-effectiveness, and measuring and benchmarking outcomes and planning for succession to ensure the sustainability and continuity of care delivery (American Organization of Nurse Executives Education Committee, 2005). Directly linked to the sustainability of the outcomes is the need to develop and implement a succession plan to continue quality patient care and fiscal returns.

According to Gandossy and Verma (2006), a 2005 study by the Corporate Leadership Council found that "72 percent of companies predict that they will encounter an increasing number of leadership vacancies over the next 3 to 5 years" (p. 38). The challenge for nurse executives in health-care organizations or practices is in recognizing that leadership is increasingly more stressful due to the demands to meet corporate objectives and turn a profit for shareholders or just to have a positive profit margin. The leadership demands are the same as for other member of the health-care leadership team, but those demands also include balancing the responsibilities of clinical or patient care ethics along with the business objectives.

Vacancies for identified nurse executives may be on the rise, and without a succession plan in place, there will be a challenge to excellence and continuity for a practice or any health-care organizations.

The first challenge to consider is the imperative need to continually deliver quality excellent health care when the workforce is aging. Since Census 2000, the population has continued to grow older, with many states reaching a median age over 40 years old (U.S. Census Bureau, 2011). According to Rothwell et al. (2005), workforce statistics alone should be a major force in motivating health-care leaders, including nurse executives to promote long-term stability for their practice or their health-care organizations. The evidence from industry and other businesses is clear that all organizations should be preparing for both their aging workforce as well as their aging leadership teams because leadership positions are as susceptible to vacancies for the same reasons as the workforce when considering retirement, illness, disabilities, terroristic acts, or death.

The average age of a nurse in the United States is a major factor in the consideration of who will replace current leaders if a succession plan is not in place. According to the U.S. Bureau of Labor Statistics' *Occupational Outlook Handbook, 2010–2011 Edition,* "employment of RNs is expected to grow much faster than the average and, because the occupation is very large, 581,500 new jobs will result, among the largest number of new jobs for any occupation. Additionally, hundreds of thousands of job openings will result from the need to replace experienced nurses who leave the occupation" (U.S. Bureau of Labor Statistics, 2010). Nursing practice will be affected in the near future because greater than 55% of nurses in leadership roles report planning for retirement beginning in 2011. The need for succession planning and development of nursing's potential leaders should be on the radar of every nurse charged with leadership responsibilities.

Maintaining the high levels of quality care delivery will depend on succession that is planned for in light of the decreased numbers of practicing nurses, the age of the practitioners, and the continued drive in health care to provide cost-effective and quality health care in today's health-care model of managed care. The problem of leadership succession in most clinical practices and organizations is that it depends on planning. In addition to the informal mechanisms in place, there needs to be leadership development programs with an identified process in place to identify, educate, and provide for the next generation of leaders. Responsible and appropriate leadership is mandatory and essential if health care in its current incarnation is to survive at the levels practitioners have come to expect and patients have come to rely on.

Nurse executives know they will not be in providing care or directing clinical operations forever, and like the public at large, they will be preparing for retirement over the next few years. Considering the need for continuity in the organization is a large reason for nurse executives to look beyond the interpersonal or operational needs currently in the practice environment and attend to the future. Research studies in both the United States and Canada address the magnitude of the problem related to executive retention and turnover, and without an identified plan in place, a practice or an organization will be exerting a good deal of time, effort, and dollars for the search and hiring of replacement.

Leadership development is best achieved on the job with real-time learning experiences as opposed to job training experiences. A good maxim is to avoid the trap of developing leadership competencies that fit past needs. Leadership development is dynamic, and the competencies needed will change as the practice or organizations change. Leadership skill and competency development is based on adult learning principles that require active participation and experiences in the day-to-day operations. The bench strength of the practice or organization will be improved by developing as many people as possible who are willing and able to undertake the challenges. Practices and organizations with succession plans will be better positioned to compete in the future without disruption of normal operations in the face of an unknown reimbursement economy.

Succession planning and management is not limited to a single individual or action. Within a practice or organization, there needs to be a combined effort to integrate succession planning throughout. Successful succession plans involve senior partners and chief executives, human resource involvement, and leaders and managers from all corners of the organization. Nurse executives can lead the succession planning process by the following:

- Devoting more time and attention on the job development
- Devoting more time and attention to planned leadership training
- Developing various experiences to build competencies related to each individual organization

Successful succession planning results from an integration of work effort throughout the practice or organization. This includes the board or the senior partners, human resources, and every member of the management/leadership team. Human resources has a crucial role in developing the tools for leadership development, facilitating the overall process, identifying and tracking the assessment of the high performers and those with high potential, structuring the learning experiences, and leading the discussion of the work learned. The management/leadership team is responsible and held accountable for helping their employees develop to their fullest potential by mentoring, coaching, and challenging them to integrate concepts and theories into real life applications.

In the changing landscape of health care today, succession planning and development is a strategic priority for practices and health-care organizations. As a core strategy for any organization, delivering health-care services succession planning will provide the direction and prepare for the future success for a practice or a health-care organization. Succession planning provides an opportunity to proactively address and plan for continued effective performance of the organization by attention to developing, replacing, and using new leaders over time. Without a succession plan, a practice or organization will find itself faced with disruptions that change the current and the future strategic direction. The need is now to support a change in culture, to recognize the value of succession planning, and to meet the strategic challenge and plan for the future of the practice or organization.

A BRIEF HISTORY OF SUCCESSION PLANNING

Succession planning is not new. Secular and religious historical literature presents the concept of succession planning as noted leaders continued their work and power. Children often succeeded parents in the Chinese, Egyptian, and Roman dynasties and empires; successors to power through bloodlines. Religious leaders planned for succession by teaching disciples or devotees to carry on the message and practices beyond the death of the religious leader. For example, Christian teachings were continued with succession planning by Jesus who sought out 12 men to become apostles, learners in the tenants of a new religion who developed into the new leaders of the religion upon the death of Christianity's leader. This strategic plan for succession planning permitted the continued growth and development of this new, and at the time, controversial religion. Preparing the next generation of leaders kept a message alive, continued a power dynasty, and provided for continuity.

However, not all power transition in history was planned or ran smoothly when succession ran through historical family bloodlines. History provides multiple examples where the leadership succession occurred as result of turmoil and often bloody strategies to the throne among siblings, no planning involved (Edwards & Mazzatenta, 2004).

Carlyle (1888) provided some of the first theoretical support for the process of family succession in one of the oldest leadership theories, that of the "great man" theory. A leader is great based on his or her family background, DNA, or upbringing not on learned skills or behaviors. Strategic planning, leadership development, and leadership grooming was not a part of the up and coming next generation leader. About the turn of the 20th century, the transition to a position of power occurred as a result of familial power and a source of resources within the family history. Sustainability and continuity, as well as profitability, were left to chance and history documents that not every family beyond the patriarch maintained its growth and presence.

During the 20th century, the right of bloodline succession in dynasties began to fade as industry began to rival throne dynasties for power, and the continuity of organizations began to take a place on the world stage. At its simplest definition, *succession planning* can be seen as "a means of identifying critical management positions . . . extending up to the highest position in the organization" (Carter, 1986, p. 3). This is a simple beginning but one that the needs to be expanded; a practice or an organization needs to go beyond identifying key positions, and their human capital needs to realistically fill the leadership pipeline.

There are early and successful examples that blended family succession and industry succession in families such as Ford, Rockefeller, Morgan, and Carnegie that saw to their passage of leadership and power through succession that assured continuity and continued dominance in industry. Communicating goals and objectives for succession planning as a method to sustain an organization began about the turn of the 20th century.

Fayol in 1916 was one of the first authors to describe objective needs of any organization in planning for succession and leadership turnover (Fayol, 1916/1949). Fayol's work was further examined by Rothwell et al. (2005), who wrote that Fayol identified generic needs to protect an organization's core and continuity including the development of talent, having talent in place that was prepared and ready to assume the mantle of leadership when the need arose.

In a more contemporary vein, Rothwell et al. (2005) define *succession planning* and *management* as

> the process that helps ensure the stability of the tenure of personnel. It is best understood as any effort designed to ensure the continued effective performance of an organization, division, department or work group by making provision for development, replacement and strategic application of key people over time. (p. 10)

In the culture of evidence-based practice, assumptions about practice are assessed and evaluated in the research. Early research on the subject of succession planning evaluated sports teams, school superintendents, manufacturing organizations, and Forbes 500 companies. Early research questions about succession planning was an attempt to identify the impact on organizations when an executive or key leaders leave because common practice "knows" that change disrupts an organization, especially at the top. Four themes emerged that are still valid today when considering leader succession and evaluating an organization's sustainability and profitability:

- Successor origin
- Organizational size and rate of succession
- Succession and post-succession performance
- Succession contingencies or antecedents such as leadership style and organizational characteristics

The concept of succession planning and the outcomes on organizations began with an assessment of professional baseball teams. This early research provided data that lead to a position that succession was not planned so much but occurred as a result of a vicious cycle. Vicious cycle theory described succession as a natural and disruptive force in organizations that changed the norm or caused a shakeup in organizations and their practices (Grusky, 1960). Succession as a common approach to resolving performance issues resulted in the cause and effect line of thinking that evolved into the common sense theory for replacing leadership. Poor performance was seen as the motivational factor that leads to a need to replace a poor manager, and external pressures outside of the teams forced a team to do something about poor management (Grusky, 1963).

Last, a baseball team will result to scapegoating as a mechanism to force leadership succession when performance is poor. Scapegoating theory is at the root of sports team leadership changes when a team is losing, and someone has to go to make things better, generally the coach (Gamson & Scotch, 1964). Interestingly enough, baseball teams were not the only organizations that ousted a leader (coach) if performance was poor. Business organizations found support for the scapegoating theory if there was a chief executive officer (CEO) with a low-power base and a poor performing organization (Boeker, 1997). The leader is the one to take the fall when an organization is not doing well, yet, what made the study of succession and performance interesting was and still is that a change at the top does not always lend itself to a fresh beginning in the post-change era.

Post-succession performance research in the major sports of baseball, football, basketball, and hockey found that although succession would change performance in the remaining season immediately after succession, there was no sustained impact that extended into the following sports season (McTeer, White, & Persad, 1995). However, as is the case with descriptive and exploratory research, the early succession theories of common sense, vicious cycle theories, and scapegoating can be viewed as foundational work to set the stage for the later economic indicator studies that expand into research using multiple variables and controls. Even in the 21st century, scapegoating is common in organizations and continues to be the basis of additional sports and business studies seeking to evaluate succession and organizational performance.

The importance of reviewing the early and continued research into succession planning is that the results provide an opportunity to see the importance of planning for leadership transition whether planned or unplanned and its impact on an organization. No single succession theory or single model can be applied across all industries and settings, but the research in succession planning seems to come together around clusters that include the following:

- Successor origin
- Organizational size and rate of succession
- Succession and post-succession performance
- Succession contingencies or antecedents

To date, there seems to be no succession theory or plan that can be applied across all industries and settings. However, the message is clear that the health-care landscape is changing, the population as a whole is getting older, and that the future endeavors of an organization lie in its ability to be prepared for leadership transition in as smooth as possible process to support continuity of its goals and mission and promote profitability for survival.

Like a crisis management plan that allows the continuity of delivering health-care services in a time of a disaster or an unforeseen event, succession planning is not only a process but also a survival plan for practice organizations into the 21st century.

Nurse executives are as much at risk for a leadership crisis in the ranks as all other leaders. Among nursing's authors, Hader, Saver, and Steltzer (2006) and Johnson and D'Argenio (1991) address the facts that to consider replacing nursing's leaders for continuity and sustainability, organizations need to include the following:

- Preparation
- Education
- Development

Nurse executives share the responsibility for clinical and professional leadership described in their core competencies, a part of which includes preparing for the future with the knowledge that health care as an industry has not prepared well for the impending retirement of its leaders lacking behind business and industry when it comes to succession. The next generation of nursing leaders must be ready to fill the void in the near future to assure continuity of quality patient outcomes and cost containment.

A 2008 study by the Aberdeen Group in Talent Acquisition Strategies defines *succession management* as "a combination of process, tools and disciplines that enable an organization to plan for anticipated leadership needs as well as identify, develop and retain and allocate key talent" (p. 1). If indeed as the topic is argued by Butler and Roche-Tarry (2002) that "succession planning is an ongoing, dynamic process that helps an organization to align its business goals and its human capital needs" (p. 201), then where is the research to support that advanced practice nurse (APN) leadership succession plans are in place and support the strategic plans that integrate succession planning and management to continue health-care delivery practices and organizations as best in class?

Succession planning as a strategic initiative has added benefits for the practice or the organization. Succession planning is known to the following:

- Increase organizational flexibility
- Increase employee job satisfaction
- Result in a more efficient sharing of internal talent

Success for succession planning and development as a strategic initiative results from support shared across any organization by the governing body or board, chief executive officers, and human resources. An organization's human resources is actively involved in the efforts to identify internal stakeholders with leadership potential, improve bench strength internally, and increase diversity of candidate pools. Even in the 21st century, any organization needs to pay special attention to gender-leveraging diversity in its efforts to leverage human capital. Disparities exist in both training and development as well as compensation scales throughout industry and business.

There is a growing body of literature to support the importance of leadership succession planning in nursing. Nurse leaders in general recognize and verbalize the importance of succession planning and development, but there is little evidence to support the fact that plans are active and in place. Redman (2006) and Drenkard (2010) both described succession planning as a key business strategic initiative in health-care organizations to continue the mission of quality health-care delivery and protecting the organization for its future leadership replacement needs. The time is now to begin to talk the talk and walk the walk when planning for the future through succession planning and development.

It is essential that nurse executives take a strategic approach to position their practice environments for success in the 21st century by taking stock of their practice environments and begin by identifying key leadership positions within the organizations, identifying potential successors to those in current leadership roles, and creating actionable leadership development plans for nurse executives as appropriate. Working collaboratively with other disciplines in the care delivery system is a role in which the nurse executives will provide leadership, which is as important for health-care organizations as in other forms of industry in the changing environment of patient care delivery.

One thing is for certain, health care is an ever-changing environment, and bench strength in succession planning and development can help offset the disruption in centers of excellence for patient care. Therefore, with the impending retirement of nurse leaders, a change in potential candidate pools of prepared nurse leader replacements and the question of continuity of excellence, the presence and breadth of leadership succession planning and development needs to be determined and shared with the nursing leadership population at large. This must begin with recognizing that health care is a consumer product and a big business that requires continuity for essential health and well-being of patients, their families, the community, and the nation at large. Nursing leaders in practice are charged with the exploration of succession planning and development in organizations not only as a practice competency but also in preparing for the future health of the nation.

BARRIERS TO SUCESSION PLANNING AND DEVELOPMENT

The journey to succession planning and development is not without challenges. General barriers to succession planning in organizations come from multiple sources, such as the governing body or board, the CEO, partners with controlling shares in a practice, or the organization itself. In addition, barriers can arise from not only one source but also any combination of the three when it comes to the question of a leadership vacancy and whether to promote an internal candidate or hire an external candidate.

A barrier specific to a nursing-led development of a leadership succession plan might be in the organization's culture. The role of a nurse executive as well as the overall perception of nursing may generate resistance in promoting, developing, and executing a succession plan and development lead by nursing that begins with the composition or the age of the board or senior members of the practice or organization. Nursing as a discipline and profession continues to suffer from the residual public perspective that nursing is women's work and therefore places a lesser value and recognition of nursing's work (Mason, Leavitt, & Chaffee, 2007). In some cases, this perception and lack of recognition for the profession and practice of nursing has led to the invisibility of nurses as well as nursing's leadership contribution to the performance of the organization. This cultural barrier manifests itself in a lack of an executive team and board strong commitment to the cost and resources necessary to develop and execute a succession plan for nursing leaders in the organization.

Overcoming the perception and lack of recognition barrier takes an ongoing effort to educate senior leadership or senior partners and to assertively advocate for nursing and succession planning. Nursing leaders must launch an active campaign to inform and educate those members of the executive leadership who control the flow of internal resources in order to facilitate a change in beliefs about nursing's role in the 21st century health-care practice or organization and the importance of nursing to the to the organization's bottom line (Brady-Schwartz, 2005). It is the role of nursing leadership to "strategically align the priorities of the organization with the framework for nursing excellence" (Drenkard, 2010, p. 264) to continue nursing's proven impact on the organization's cost, services, quality and safety, and human resource initiatives. Leadership succession planning for health-care delivery organizations is essential to the mission and continued accomplishment of the organization's goals.

There may also be the simple issue that a practice or organization does not have the necessary bench strength internally to fill a leadership position when one arises. An additional barrier or challenge may be the laissez-faire approach to filling vacancies when they occur. This challenge of attending to the vacancy when it occurs can be a recipe for disaster and disruption in the forward motion of an organization. The first mention of this impact on organizations was described as a vicious cycle theory in that leadership succession by Grusky (1960) as a natural and disruptive force in organizations that changes the norm or shakes up organizations and their practices.

The CEO of the organization or partners with controlling shares in a practice can become a barrier to succession planning by simply taking one day at a time and operating from a philosophy where the prevailing focus is on the here and now. This forces an organization to operate and run the day-to-day business from a tactical instead of a strategic approach. Hutton (2003) states, "Because the vast majority of health-care organizations do not have formal succession plans in place, it is possible that most CEO's are poorly informed about how a succession plan can benefit them and their organization" (p. 21). Finally, although in a position of power, a chief officer is human, and openly supporting and planning for replacement is an acknowledgment that the chief officer is not immortal or irreplaceable. A wise leader would do well to keep in mind the laws of leadership that state the 21st Law of Legacy is that a leader's lasting value is measured by succession (Maxwell, 1998).

Although the nurse executives in an organization is generally not considered the organization's chief officer, the responsibility of operations relating patient care delivery, a core component of the health-care business, rests with nursing's leaders. As such, the nurse executive in an organization may also be a barrier to the support, creation, or execution of a succession plan for the same reason as the CEO. The same resistance or failure to plan for succession reported in CEO's may affect nurse leaders in general.

A second impediment to the creation and execution of a succession plan for nursing may be the board of directors or senior practicing partners. Because most nurse leaders in an organization are not sitting members of the board, a nurse leader will need to increase the political endeavors to have an official voice to the board or senior practicing partners. The inertia and avoidance of the importance of planning for leadership transition through succession planning by a board are key impediments that can stand in the way of succession planning.

Interpersonal dynamics in and among the executive members of the leadership team may lead to an unspoken desire to support the status quo and not disturb the current operations. Overall, there may be a general lack of knowledge about the role that a nurse leader plays in the organization or what talent pipeline exists that can be developed and tapped when the time is necessary. Last, the board or the senior practicing partners may simply not consider succession planning and development an open item to transparently discuss. Whatever the reason, ensuring that there is a succession plan in place to replace leadership with as little disruption as possible and to address all of the organization's leadership needs including key job replacements is the board's or practicing partner's responsibility to ensure the continuity of the organization.

Additional barriers to succession planning and development from the organization come in one of two ways. A one-size-fits-all is not a productive approach for development and training because this is simply not true. If an organization believes that a one-size-fits-all can be the standard approach to development and training, the approach will fail. Organizations and practices must be aware of and prepared to remove the mitigating factors that contribute to the one-size-fits-all approach including the failure to assign accountability and monitoring of the program beyond that of human resources (HR). HR is an integral component of any training and development program for succession planning but is not the sole owner of all things succession.

Training program issues and challenges need to be recognized early on to avoid adding another barrier to the succession process. Issues that are not addressed early will lead to time lapses in building internal bench strength. The end result of failing to constantly assess and monitor the leadership development and training programs can result in failing to adjust the programs in time to prevent an organization's loss of forward motion or possibly even a loss of a competitive edge.

Finding the right person for the right job is an essential part of succession planning, but finding the right job fit cannot be limited to only hiring internal candidates if the requirements of the job are not met. Even the best training programs are not always able to supply the leadership talent needed or there may be internal mitigating circumstances that the internal candidates do not meet the needs of the practice or organization at that moment in time.

Building internal bench strength and preparing internal talent through leadership development and training programs are examples of best practices that health care in general has not yet fully embraced. Recent work in industry and business for succession planning has been about removing as many barriers as possible in recognition of the need to sustain and have a ready to fill pipeline of talent to fill leadership positions. An example beyond industry and business of a bureaucratic organization that is ready to fill openings in leadership positions for planned or unplanned reasons is that of the U.S. military.

The military have long known and provided for development of personnel ready for transition into key leadership roles. From the lowest new recruit to the top generals, the military prepares for leadership change through a succession plan that could be best summed up as a readiness model (Grusky, 1964). The model assesses the needs of its members and provides the opportunities to fill the gaps and weaknesses through education and experience.

One final barrier to succession planning and development for a practice or organization would be to acknowledge that many variables in the plan or process can lead to ineffective or failed initiatives. Things can and do happen that are not according to plan; no plan is perfect, but having an assessment/evaluation loop will keep development and training plans on track.

Failures in succession planning may arise from the human factor of current leadership avoiding planning for their replacements, or it may be that a board that fails to address the issue of succession for leadership because of cost and resources, or last, that the culture of the organization does not inherently value communication, talent sharing, and development. Whatever the cause, the signs of resistance or failure to embark on the journey toward a succession and development plan should raise a red flag in a practice or organization to prevent an overall organizational failure in future leadership turnover.

A failure to identify potential leadership candidates within the organization, to support or encourage ongoing internal leadership development, and to plan for the possibility of unplanned vacancies will have a long-range impact of ensuring the continuity of health-care delivery in the future. All of the reasons cited for failure and unresolved barriers are an antithesis to the leadership competencies, the business benefits preparing for leadership transition, and the need to prepare for the continuity of the care delivery system as a whole (Bolton & Roy, 2004). Recognizing the nurse executive responsibilities of setting priorities, focusing on the business of delivering care in a quality outcomes and cost-effective manner, measuring and benchmarking outcomes, and planning for succession to ensure the sustainability and continuity of care delivery are all a part of the single leadership competency.

The argument can be made that having a succession plan as part of an organization's genetic makeup will strengthen an organization's ability to continue to function and that succession planning should be a part of the organization's DNA. Yet as late as 2009, "approximately 50 percent of major companies lack a realistic strategic plan for replacing their CEO" (Cheloha, 2009, p. 12). The need continues throughout health care as well as industry to begin to prepare for that leadership transition and to make the succession plan and development a core component of an organizations makeup.

The DNA approach is a logical way to embed the plan and process in the organization's makeup. That way, the characteristics of effective succession planning and management will no longer be a special project or an added burden to the goals and objectives of a practice or organization. Succession planning and development to build bench strength will be a natural function of the organization that engages and ensures leadership participation and commitment. There would be no question in expanding the view of talent, leveraging human capital, and creating opportunities for education and application. All of these assumptions and beliefs would be integrated into the practice or organization's DNA and would be the chromosomes for continuity. The DNA approach removes barriers, prepares for the future, and provides for a smooth transition during changes in leadership.

INTERNAL AND EXTERNAL SUCCESSION

There are risks and benefits associated with both internal and external leadership successors. Organizations struggle with the dilemma of making a choice from an internal pool of talent or choosing someone from the outside. Several meta-analysis research studies of the literature have examined internal versus external leadership succession and the impact on the organization and have not come up with a conclusive body of evidence to direct an organization's choice (Bommer & Ellstrand, 1996; Giambatista, Rowe, & Riaz, 2005; Kesner & Sebora, 1994).

An organization might first consider an internal successor if there is one available. Looking through the lens of the employees in an organization internal succession would be viewed as leadership's vision for continued success and a cost–benefit return on the development of internal talent.

An internal successor brings value to the new position in the practice or organization that an external successor cannot. The value is seen as intellectual capital that includes a working knowledge of the organization, the culture, and the climate. The internal successor has already developed a network of interpersonal relationships that provide inside information and provide channels for informal communication. However, as previously noted, the meta-analysis researches of succession by Kesner and Sebora (1994) and Giambatista et al. (2005) are not conclusive that that is indeed the case.

Filling a leadership position from within the organization also displays to internal and external stakeholders that the current leadership team supports and is developing talent from within. When an internal candidate fills a leadership position, the effect goes beyond that one singular appointment. A ripple effect is created throughout the ranks of the practice or organizations when the position just vacated opens up and new opportunities are created for more than one individual.

Choosing an external successor for the organization or practice may be the only choice if there are mitigating factors such as a history of legal, ethical, or fiscal violations. If this is the case, then choosing an external successor could be seen as an opportunity to clean house and start the organization on a fresh path of ethical and legal behaviors. However, choosing an external successor can be risky business and requires careful consideration. As opposed to an internal candidate, the external successor candidate's overall history should be carefully evaluated, checking references beyond a simple review of a resume or curriculum vitae. The practice or organization needs to consider the candidate's leadership track record, the availability of the external candidate, and the cost of hiring the external candidate. In addition, all stakeholders should feel comfortable that external candidate is a better choice than an internal candidate or the hiring may result in stakeholder backlash from failure, the possibility of negative press, or the possibility of turnover in incumbent leaders (Goldsmith, 2009). Ultimately, the hiring responsibility will fall to the board or the senior practicing partners, but before the final contract is signed, a talent cost–benefit analysis is necessary so that all objective information for the external successor candidate can be examined closely before the appointment is made.

A single leadership successor hire can have implications far beyond just the one hire of an external individual. Looking inward for the leadership successor should be the first choice, unless the practice or organization finds that the talent pipeline is insufficient or that the environment is forcing an outside search. If that is the case, then choosing the external successor should be done with caution and only after the talent cost–benefit analysis to ensure that the right successor is chosen for the job. A wrong choice would contribute to the disruption of the organization's workflow and have far-reaching complications beyond that of just the wrong hire.

Choosing a successor is a challenge and an opportunity to provide for an organization's desire for sustainability, but it cannot be undertaken without commitment and participation from all corners of the organization. Leaders in business and industry recognize that the succession plan and process is a living document that changes as the needs of the organization and its environment change. Succession planning and development can support leadership transition in an organization if the plan and execution of the plan makes use of the normal life cycle in managing the talent within. A talent management life cycle includes the facets of identifying, developing, and managing talent to build an organization's bench strength for leadership replacement. A talent management life cycle must be a part of leadership in nursing that uses succession planning and development as part of the strategic plan to promote continuity, sustainability, and profitability, yet the challenge may not be the succession plan itself but the absence of an adequate pipeline within the organization where nurses are available and interested in transitioning into true nurse leadership roles.

Succession planning as a strategic plan and not a replacement strategy helps to ensure that the organization will receive a return on their investment in their employees and provide a pipeline of talent to fill upcoming vacancies in leadership roles. According to Kristick (2009),

> By understanding the skills and talents of employees and mapping them to the needs and requirements of the business, organizations can identify critical roles within the organization, determine staffing needs, and then target specific learning and development activities to groom specific employees for managerial and leadership positions. (p. 51)

SUCCESSION PLANNING PREVENTS PROMOTION WITHOUT PREPARATION

Promoting an internal successor without preparation will lead to its own set of challenges. The organization may be faced with more high performers than high-potential employees forcing an outside selection of a successor. However, until there is a clear assessment of internal talent, an organization is working at a disadvantage when subjective discussion and criteria are used to categorize the organization's bench strength.

The differentiation between high-potential employees and high performers is important in the early development of a succession plan because the description objectively describes those who display leadership talent not just talent in the work environment. Nursing's history has not always been selective in dividing potential leaders into two groups, but a realistic plan for succession targets those who are able to be groomed for the next level of responsibility in leadership, remembering that clinical excellence does not automatically transfer into leadership excellence.

High-potential individuals display leadership traits and have a desire to undergo the necessary education and training to develop leadership competencies. Leadership skills can be taught, but the basic leadership traits of the ability to communicate well, to problem solve, to reason, and to be social and display honesty and integrity are visible naturally in high-potential individuals.

In contrast, high performers are those who consistently meet the job responsibilities and competencies. High performers are visible not only in their completion of job tasks and responsibilities but also can be tracked through performance appraisals that evaluate their performance over time. High performers may even fulfill a position that would be more difficult to replace than a leadership position in an age when technical specialization is a part of the health-care delivery landscape. In addition, not every nurse or high performer aspires to be groomed or move up into an executive position, so an honest assessment of interest or desire to undertake the training and change of job category is a necessary part of the criteria for training and development.

The practice or organization needs a developed leadership strategy in place to set the stage for developing education and training programs. The leadership strategy for succession planning and development should contain a realistic picture and analysis of the current status of the organization as well as a vision of what the future should look like. This strategy should contain recommendations to bridge the gap between the current environment and the future environment. The recommendations will need to suggest not only the number of prepared leaders that are needed but also the competencies they will need. This is the time to state the desired leadership characteristics that will move the organization forward and what behaviors and skills will be necessary to facilitate that forward motion. Without a defined and developed leadership strategy in place for the practice or organization, there is a peril in promoting internal successors into an undefined future.

Another peril of promotion without preparation can be found in the unrealistic and subjective expectations that occur when a high performer is placed into a new a leadership position. A disconnect will result if a high performer is promoted into a leadership position without the necessary training and development. The right tool belt is required for any job and providing objective information about job requirements and realistic performance goals will translate into better performance.

Succession planning and development plans also require measurement metrics. A measurement plan should include the number of positions that have bench-ready candidates as well as the overall number of high-potential employees who have completed development cycles. Without measurement metrics, the organization will suffer from guesstimates and not have an accurate accounting of the status of what otherwise may be an excellent succession plan.

BEST PRACTICES FOR SUCCESSION

Recent general industry studies, peer-reviewed journal articles, and trade publication articles have identified best practices for succession planning, although there is clearly not one size fits all. Succession planning can be viewed as the means to close the gap between the current organization and the desired future, a continuity of excellence. As a key talent management initiative, succession planning and development does not happen by chance, and procrastination will only contribute to chaos in the transition of power if the organization's potential leaders are not prepared to take on the responsibilities and the challenges. Successful organizations using succession planning and development for leadership transition strategically track critical roles within the organization and proactively develop their internal talent pools of high performers for bench strength in filling leadership positions as the need arises.

Best practices in succession planning begins with the commitment of the top leadership team, a board or senior practicing partners, and the commitment extends throughout the organization as a known strategic initiative.

Effective and successful succession planning and development characteristics include the following:

- Engaging and ensuring executive participation and commitment
- Expanding the view of talent available
- Promoting transparency
- Leveraging human capital
- Creating a culture of talent sharing
- Creating opportunities for education and application
- Creating and maintaining measurement metrics

Once succession planning and development is embraced by the organization or the practice, the best practices include developing objective steps to the process that will ensure the success. With an end goal in mind, the development of an action plan sets the stage for all other steps. The action plan will personalize the succession activities to the individual organization—an important step to avoid falling into the one-size-fits-all trap. The action plan becomes the visual commitment of the organization to identify and develop talent because building bench strength for smooth leadership transition is a critical priority.

Top leadership and executive commitment and participation in the process goes beyond lip service and involves a display of real buy-in. Senior practicing partners or top leadership teams play an active role in driving succession planning and development as a critical strategic initiative. This process requires leading by example so that the words of commitment at the top of the organization can be viewed in their actions. Succession planning and development is not without a cost, and one way to display commitment through action is make sure that adequate financial and people resources are allocated to the effort.

Commitment and participation extends to all levels of leadership in an organization planning for succession. Managers at the day-to-day operations levels are held accountable to identify and develop talent in their work areas. Objective measuring metrics lend themselves to driving this participation and accountability as managers are assessed in these areas in their performance appraisals that form the basis of salary increases or promotion.

Creating the environment for the succession plan and development process requires a change in the culture that must take place to facilitate successful and nondisruptive leadership transition. A change in the practice or organization's culture will change the way an organization operates. This new culture is more transparent and approaches the end goals and operating objectives from a proactive stance. For some practices or organizations, this may be a change from the tactical day-to-day approach to a today and tomorrow approach, but in the end, the organization and its members will benefit.

Transparency is practiced not just talked about. It is this transparency in succession planning and development that keeps things visible, open to all, and in the end leads to a building of trust. Trust within the organizational culture requires access to information, consistency in what will constitute success in training and development, and openness in the promotion and upward mobility processes. Transparency in a succession planning and development culture lends itself to an organization's ability to keep its intellectual capital of high-potential talent and reduce or eliminate costly hiring cycles.

Best practice organizations are always looking inward. They analyze the work needing to be accomplished and the people available to get the job done. Identifying key positions or critical positions that are needed for achieving the organization's goals and objectives is an ongoing process. Talent is assessed beyond those already in leadership positions to expand the pool. Recognizing that leadership transition is a disruptive force, best practice organizations avoid allowing key positions to remain vacant for long periods of time. On the same note, interim leadership is not forever but viewed as a short-term stop gap to maintain normal operations until the prepared internal successor or external successor can step in.

Talent reviews go beyond the current leadership level throughout the organization. Cultivating existing talent is analogous to farming rather than hunting. Best practice organizations use objective assessment criteria, focus in on the high performers with specialized skills, avoid favoring individuals who are like their current managers, promote respect for differences in personalities and working styles, and avoid subjectivity. There is still greater effort needed in expanding the view of talent relating to gender issues as the literature reports that more men than women continue to receive specialist development in organizations.

A best practice to address the gender disparity in leadership development includes increasing the opportunities for growth for women to teach and develop them into higher level leaders. The responsibility for leadership development for women goes beyond just the organization. As long as a gender balance disparity exists in leadership development, women who are high performers must make their intentions known and not wait for opportunities to be handed to them. If the lack of training and development opportunities stem from a misconception that women are not interested in leadership positions due to other life and social obligations, it is up to the woman to step up and voice interest. As identified in barriers to succession planning, nurses are at risk for gender development disparity due to the residual public perspective that nursing is women's work and therefore places a lesser value and recognition of nursing's work resulting in lack of recognition for the profession and the invisibility of nurses in an organization. If there are no standards for development opportunities and training programs, assumptions and unconscious biases may result in an unequal development and playing field.

From an organizational perspective, providing equal opportunities for leadership development creates a robust and diverse talent pipeline. Succession planning is objective and well defined including the process of recognizing performance equally among the identified high performers and making HR policies more family-friendly. In addition to best practice organizations, the process and opportunities for leadership development are transparent and lead to opportunities for additional mentorships and provide more transitional support into a leadership role.

Best practice organizations develop leadership skills in a range of experiences. The targeted goal of training and development is to enhance the capabilities of the high performers toward the end or destination job. Once again, the training and development programs are organization-specific and may provide opportunities for external training as well as internal training. High performers are challenged and stretched in their competencies to accelerate development and provide the opportunities to exhibit skills beyond their current responsibilities. The high-potential individual is not developed in a vacuum, and current leadership participation includes mentoring and coaching to provide support to the learning environment.

Look to the future for redefining the needs of the practice or the organization. Build in an assessment and reevaluation loop so that the current needs do not overshadow the future needs of the organization. The fact is that change is constant, and what is needed for today's success and sustainability may not be the same as for the near future. Human resource needs as well as volume and product delivery may change based on the health-care services needs in the population. Health-care delivery systems like other industry must keep a watchful eye on conditions that may lead to restructuring, mergers, acquisitions, reimbursement changes, or bankruptcy. Like a sound fiscal philosophy, when the forecast has been based on comprehensive data collection, the actual outcomes equal or come closest to predicted outcomes.

The culture of talent sharing across an organization builds high-performance teams. The organization's goals and objectives are better served in the best practice organizations that link processes across the organization. This involves effort in integrated leadership as well as employee development programs. A culture of talent sharing promotes a learning environment for development that matches employee skill and training to the organization's goals and objectives and strengthens this culture by aligning performance with financial reward and returns. Organizations that have a culture of talent sharing find that they are able to respond quickly to disruptions to operations and are better positioned to adapt to the changes in the marketplace and business environment.

Technology plays a strong partner in supporting the training and development of high performers. In the 21st century, mentoring is not only face-to-face but can take place through podcasts, social networking, blogs, or e-mails to support the mentor–mentee relationship. Using social networking provides a window of real-time mentoring to share knowledge, offer guidance, share informal learning moments, and guide the development experiences. In addition to supporting the high performers in their training and development, technology supports the organization's efforts in the overall succession planning process by maintaining updated records in a data storage area and tracking the progress of those in the leadership pipeline with their accomplishments to date.

Every best practice organization makes use of evaluation and feedback loop that uses measurement metrics for objectivity to modify the plan and process as needed and to have a mechanism in place to monitor, record, and report individual progress. The mantra for this is to measure, measure, and measure. Measurements provide an assessment of the development and training programs as well as track the individual progress of the high performer.

The individual characteristics of each organization should determine the evaluation criteria and benchmarks. Using measurement metrics in the plan and development supports the objectivity of the process. The measures that are used to assess the end results will vary, but the measurement metrics help to make sure that the desired outcomes of the process are achieved. Common measurements include the average number of qualified candidates that are available for each defined leadership position, the ethnic and gender diversity in the talent pool, the ethnic and gender diversity in promotions, and the extent to which leadership positions can be filled with internal talent when the need arises. Tracking attrition rates from the training and development programs provides an opportunity to determine, assess, and evaluate the programs as well as the nature of the attrition. Measurement is not static in nature but is designed so that the data supports decisions which will ensure continuous improvement of the process.

Measurement is not just about those in the pipeline and ready to fill leadership positions but also about success of those promoted to leadership positions. High performers should be reassessed regularly to gather data on their transition to the role and their job performance. This cycle of reassessment and evaluation is an objective process to determine continued high performance at the appointed leadership level.

SUCCESSION PLANNING AND EMPLOYEE DEVELOPMENT AS A CORE STRATEGY

Succession planning and development is a sound approach to strategic management of any practice or organization as it is a reflection of the leaders in climate, culture, and outcomes. The strategic process takes place over time, just as the development of leadership talent does. Leadership development plans and programs ensure an organization's continuity and growth. In addition, succession planning and development supports individual growth and development, which leads to enhanced retention, job satisfaction, and a commitment to the organization.

The strategic process can be summed up in the five phases of strategic vision: objective setting, strategy crafting, implementation and execution, performance monitoring and evaluation, and a feedback loop to revise strategy as a result of changing conditions or new information (Thompson, Strickland, & Gamble, 2005, p. 20). This mirrors the process of succession planning that begins with an idea to improve the talent pool of an organization and ends with a feedback and revision loop. The strategic process is a necessary shared partnership between the board or senior practicing partners, the chief executive, nursing leadership, and the organization.

Employees remain the number one input into the open system of any health-care organization. Retaining those employees with specialized skills and talents is a crucial component of success for an organization in planning for its future. In the succession planning and development process, the identification and recognition of employees is directly related to an employee's job satisfaction and commitment to the organization. Succession planning and development as a strategic initiative is the practice or organization's process to see an end return on its investment or sustainability and profitability. Focusing on both high performers and high potentials provides an opportunity for the organization to recognize its workforce and help maintain high levels of retention. Learning opportunities have been identified as important to employees in that learning opportunities translate as a return on investment for the employee in the form of worth and marketability.

As a result of succession planning and development as a strategic initiative, employees are valued, and the culture of the organization shifts for the employee from just being a job to becoming a valued stakeholder in the organization's achievement of its end goals and objectives. High performers and high potentials alike engage in the organization's operations at higher levels. They become more involved, communicate through all channels, interact across the organization beyond the work group, and participate actively. Successful clockwork organizations link training and development to action-oriented results in meaningful projects and initiatives (Collins, 2001).

The role of the leader in an organization that develops and uses succession planning as a strategic initiative operates from a platform of facilitating change and growth within both the organization and the employees. This transformational approach to leadership inspires, motivates, and encourages collaborative effort to move the organization and individuals forward and in doing so strengthens the organization.

This leadership approach and style is good for the organization as a business. If the practice or organization's current overall performance is strong, there is less likelihood for a need to make radical changes in strategy, but without a succession plan, there will be a gap that in the future will affect its performance and sustainability.

Succession planning as a core strategy for nurse leaders also needs a competitive analysis of the marketplace to better prepare the practice or organization to determine its own overall business performance. Nursing leaders are an economic force for any practice or organization, and the failure to plan for the strategically plan for the future may result in a change of leadership, a loss of knowledge capital, and failure of the organization.

Succession planning and employee development as a core strategy provides the setting for the ability to measure improved business performance in the industry and marketplace. In health-care delivery systems, this can be measured not only in quality outcomes but also in fiscal ones. Over the long term, succession planning has been proven to save money and provide a continual level of operations. Replacing those in leadership positions is an expensive process with search fees and search firms charging large dollar amounts to fill the vacancies. Practices and organizations spend less while daily operations continue at nondisruptive levels, and best in class organizations that have achieved national recognition through credentialing and accrediting bodies that embrace succession planning continue their excellence in delivering health-care services.

A PRIMER FOR SUCCESSION PLANNING AND DEVELOPMENT

Beginning to build a practice or organization's succession and development plan is not an as daunting a task as it may seem. Following the direction of best practice organizations gives a template that can be customized for each individual organization. Begin by structuring the plan to be flexible enough to accommodate the changing needs of the organization and industry. Focus the plan on leadership development programs that anticipate the planned for and natural turnover of leadership positions. If one does not exist, create and include in the practice or organization a board- or senior partner–approved policy that addresses succession planning for the organization and is detailed enough to clearly spell out the roles and responsibilities of everyone who is involved in the process.

Include the assessment step for all employees including high performers, high potential, and also for current leaders. Work and job responsibilities should be clearly stated in position descriptions with competencies that flow from the objective statements therein. Competencies necessary for nurse executives include being a skilled communicator and a change agent, which should be addressed in training and development programs.

Development plans are unique to each practice or organization's needs, but in the early stages of succession and development planning, there is an opportunity to consider adding leadership training that is geared to the interests of potential leaders in the form of classes, coaches, mentors, or new work assignments. Translating the class or learning workshop materials in to the real world brings learners back to reality. Providing real-life experience with the concepts from the classroom makes the learning more effective. Action learning brings the high-potential individuals and current leadership together and provides an opportunity to plan, develop, execute, and evaluate projects that can benefit both the learner and the organization, which makes the learning experience more relevant.

Development plans are most successful when they contain a list of realistic goals, a description of the learning process, a description of support mechanisms, and how the learning can be used in the current work environment. Development is the first step, but there needs to be opportunities to manage the expectations of the high-potential individuals as real-time internal candidates for leadership vacancies. Transparency needs to extend to actual position appointment opportunities including how they will be advertised, what if any limitations are placed on the opportunities and in all reality, a mechanism to openly discuss with the candidates in private their readiness for the position, or the need to continue in targeted areas of development.

Once the development and design are in place, it is time to deliver or execute the plan. Although this will present challenges at the start, a succession and development plan will position a practice or health-care organization in a stronger survival position. Industry and business provide many examples of organizations that have thrived in poor economic conditions in part due to their internal talent initiatives and maintaining a commitment to leadership development programs. Long-term viability for health-care delivery organizations is as important to the health of the nation as the organizations that have set the standard for succession planning and development such as IBM, DuPont, Intel, ExxonMobil, and others. Successful, sustainable, and profitable organizations provide the proof that imbedding leadership talent and improving internal bench strength into the culture and the strategic plan works.

Last, evaluating the process and outcomes of a leadership and training plan is essential. An organization needs to determine what works and what does not in order to adjust and change the plan and programs. Like performance improvement in clinical practice, the questions asked will provide the data to revise what will make succession planning and development most effective and efficient. Some general areas to assess might include how have the internal candidates fit into their new roles, what is their success rate, or have the programs expectations met the realities of the organization.

Moving from a replacement strategy to a succession planning and development plan will be a new way of thinking and requires a learning curve throughout the organization. Making this an actionable strategic plan will result in changes for the organization and employees where the effect is:

- Knowledge acquisition
- Appreciation of knowledge
- Learning appraisals
- Application possibilities (current and future)
- Process evaluation for effectiveness
- Process evaluation for efficiency
- A reward process for achievements

Keeping the process and plan simple and transparent will provide the opportunity to measure the outcomes of building internal bench strength and preparing for the future leadership needs. High performers can be evaluated on areas such as emotional intelligence, relationship building, communication skills, and/or analytical thinking. Nurses today are knowledge workers in the clinical environment, and making that transition to being an effective leader using new and specialized knowledge will require training and development in the core competencies to lead health-care practices and organizations in the near future. Succession planning and talent development is an extension of who nurses are. Nurse executives make use of planning, development, delivery, and evaluation of care, leading organizations through the transition of leaders is no different in succession planning and talent development.

SUMMARY

Succession planning and development prepares a practice or an organization to keep pace with changes in the industry and business in light of leadership changes. Developing and maintaining a prepared strong talent pool helps ensure that organizations are informed and competitive in their marketplace (Crosby & Shields, 2010; Marshall & Heffes, 2004). Engaging, empowering, and encouraging employees to go beyond their current reality creates a win-win situation for both the employee and the organization helping to ensure sustainability along with profitability.

Growing great leaders as a part of succession planning and talent development begins with a policy that encourages everyone to develop expertise and vision outside of their work unit. The organization expands its view of talent and seeks candidates for training, development, and ultimately promotion from diverse units or departments in filling leadership positions. Recognizing that organizations are political animals at heart provides an opportunity to set the stage for integration by creating formal mechanisms to openly discuss the natural conflicts and tensions that develop within organizations.

As a part of growing new leaders from within to build bench strength, the culture needs to encourage integration to meet the organization's goals and objectives. Managers and leaders need to be formally rewarded in a manner that works for the organization as they send valued employees to other work units to gain more experience and/or as they welcome other employees in the training and development programs into their work units for the experience. The organization is responsible to provide peripheral support to not only the learning high performers but also to the leaders and manager who risk changes in their work units through participating in an open exchange and talent sharing culture.

Not everyone will make it to the final senior positions of leadership, so the organization will need to have a process and system in place to make the promotion process possible. Objective criteria and measurement throughout the training and development cycle will provide information to strengthen the final decision regarding who is ready and capable to attend to the leadership needs of the organization and who is not. A transparent succession and development plan reflects the ethical principle of humanitarianism or fairness with the full knowledge that fairness may not be the same as equality in being promoted to leadership positions.

A succession and development plan can be a holistic approach to the organization's talent and management life cycle. Developing talent, managing the program, and optimizing and rewarding talent all work toward sustaining an organization when leadership needs arise. The end result of building bench strength as opposed to replacement strategies is that the organization can maximize its internal talent, increase employee satisfaction, loyalty, and retention, all of which have an impact on an organization's bottom line and sustainability.

Succession planning and talent development is not just one strategy that fits all practices and organizations but a combination of the following:

- Cultivating internal talent
- Improving employee satisfaction
- Planning for future leadership needs
- Actionable strategic planning

This combination is a prescription that delivers long-term results in the prepared organization. Organizations that look to the future and are prepared will be better positioned to minimize the loss of internal talent, to save dollars in costly search efforts, and to react and adapt to the changing health-care delivery landscape.

Organizations that hold the key for continued success will be those that recognize the strength of their internal talent, that see their employees not only as the most valuable input and asset to the organization, and that are willing to commit and invest in employee development to prepare for upcoming leadership vacancies. Succession planning and talent development organizations know that their employees are the key to long-term success, sustainability, and profitability by tailoring their program to their needs, defining the necessary qualifications to fill the leadership vacancies, and providing objective criteria and transparency in all aspects of the process.

Now more than ever, there is a need for nurse executives to recognize and prepare for transition of leadership in care providers to ensure continuity in health-care organizations in the form of succession and development planning (Fig. 14.1).

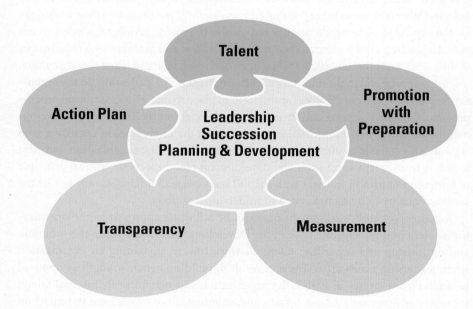

FIGURE 14.1. Leadership succession planning and development.

Nurse executives as leaders are the key to addressing the development of their successors who must be well prepared to respond to the changing environment of evidence-based practice and complex reimbursement strategies.

REFERENCES

Aberdeen Group. (2008). *Talent acquisition strategies*. Retrieved from http://www.aberdeen.com

American Organization of Nurse Executives Education Committee. (2005). AONE nurse executive competencies. *Nurse Leader, 3*, 15–21. doi:10.1016/j.mnl.2005.01.001

Aroian, J., Meservey, P. M., & Crockett, J. G. (1996). Developing nurse leaders for today and tomorrow: Part 1. Foundations of leadership in practice. *Journal of Nursing Administration, 26*(9), 18–26. Retrieved from CINAHL with full text database.

Beyers, M. (2006). Nurse executives' perspectives on succession planning. *Journal of Nursing Administration, 36*(6), 304–312. Retrieved from CINAHL with full text database.

Birk, S. (2010). Quality cost efficiency: The new quality-cost imperative. *Healthcare Executive, 25*(2), 14–24. Retrieved from Business Source Premier.

Bisognano, M. (2010). Nursing's role in transforming healthcare. *Healthcare Executive, 25*(2), 84–87. Retrieved from CINAHL with full text database.

Boeker, W. (1997). Strategic change: The influence of managerial characteristics and organizational growth. *Academy of Management Journal, 40*(1), 152–170. Retrieved from Business Source Complete database.

Bolton, J., & Roy, W. (2004). Succession planning: Securing the future. *Journal of Nursing Administration, 34*(12), 589–593. Retrieved from CINAHL with full text database.

Bommer, W. H., & Ellstrand, A. E. (1996). CEO successor choice, its antecedents and influence on subsequent firm performance: An empirical analysis. *Group and Organization Management, 21*(1), 105–123. Retrieved from Business Source Complete database.

Bonczek, M., & Woodard, E. (2006). Who'll replace you when you're gone? *Nursing Management, 37*(8), 30–34. Retrieved from Academic Search Premier database.

Bondas, T. (2006). Paths to nursing leadership. *Journal of Nursing Management, 14*(5), 332–339. Retrieved from CINAHL with full text database.

Brady-Schwartz, D. C. (2005). Further evidence on the magnet recognition program. Implications for nursing leaders. *Journal of Nursing Administration, 35*(9), 397–403. Retrieved from CINAHL with full text database.

Butler, K., & Roche-Tarry, D. E. (2002). Succession planning: Putting an organization's knowledge to work. *Nature Biotechnology, 20*, 201–202. Retrieved from Business Source Complete database.

Carlyle, T. (1888). *On heroes, hero-worship, and the heroic in history*. New York, NY: Frederick A. Stokes & Brother. Retrieved from http://www.questia.com/read/1444983#

Carter, N. (1986). Guaranteeing management's future through succession planning. *Journal of Information Systems Management, 3*(3), 13–14. Retrieved from Business Source Complete database.

Cheloha, R. S. (2009). Barriers to CEO succession. *The Corporate Board, 30*(177), 12–16. Retrieved from Business Source Corporate database.

Collins, J. (2001). *Good to great*. New York, NY: Harper Business.

Collins, J., & Porras, J. (2002) *Built to last*. New York, NY: HarperCollins.

Crosby, F. E., & Shields, C. J. (2010). Preparing the next generation of nurse leaders: An educational needs assessment. *Journal of Continuing Education in Nursing, 41*(8), 363–368. Retrieved from ProQuest database.

Drenkard, K. (2010) The business case for Magnet. *Journal of Nursing Administration, 40*(6), 263–271. Retrieved from CINAHL with full text database.

Edwards, M., & Mazzatenta, L. O. (2004). Han Dynasty. *National Geographic,* 2–29. Retrieved from Academic Search Premier.

Fayol, H. (1949). *General and industrial management.* London, United Kingdom: Pitman Publishing. (Original work published 1916)

Ferman, J. (2009). Paying for health care reform. *Healthcare Executive,* 49–51. Retrieved from http://findarticles.com/p/articles/mi_hb5693/is_200907/ai_n32334065/?tag=mantle_skin

Gamson, W., & Scotch, N. (1964). Scapegoating in baseball. *American Journal of Sociology, 70,* 69–72. Retrieved from JSTOR database.

Gandossy, R., & Verma, N. (2006). Passing the torch of leadership. *Leader to Leader, 2006*(40), 37–44. Retrieved from Business Source Complete database.

Giambatista, R. C., Rowe, W. G., & Riaz, S. (2005). Nothing succeeds like succession: A critical review of leader succession literature since 1994. *The Leadership Quarterly, 16*(6), 963–991. doi:10.1016/j.leaqua.2005.09.005

Goldsmith, M. (2009). Who's next: Choose your successor. *Leadership Excellence, 26*(4), 9. Retrieved from Business Source Complete database.

Grusky, O. (1960). Administrative succession in formal organizations. *Social Forces, 39,* 105–115. Retrieved from JSTOR database.

Grusky, O. (1963). Managerial succession and organizational effectiveness. *American Journal of Sociology, 69,* 21–31. Retrieved from JSTOR database.

Grusky, O. (1964). The effects of succession: A comparative study of military and business organizations. In M. Janowitz (Ed.), *The new military* (pp. 83–111). New York, NY: Russel Sage Foundation.

Hader, R., Saver, C., & Steltzer, T. (2006). No time to lose. *Nursing Management, 37*(7), 23–48. Retrieved from Academic Search Premier database.

Hutton, D. H. (2003). Succession planning: Dress rehearsal for the understudies. *Trustee, 56*(10), 14–22. Retrieved from Business Source Complete database.

Johnson, K. R., & D'Argenio, C. (1991). Management training effects on nurse manager leadership behavior. *Nursing Economics, 9*(4), 249–254. Retrieved from CINAHL with full text database.

Kesner, I. F., & Sebora, T. C. (1994). Executive succession: Past, present and future. *Journal of Management, 20,* 327–372.

Kristick, J. (2009). Filling the leadership pipeline. *Training and Development, 63*(6), 48–52. Retrieved from Business Source Complete database.

Marshall, J., & Heffes, E. M. (2004). Tips for judging quality of training. *Financial Executive, 20*(6). Retrieved from Business Source Complete database.

Mason, D. L., Leavitt, J. K., & Chaffee, M. W. (2007). *Policy and politics in nursing and health care.* St. Louis, MO: Saunders.

Maxwell, J. (1998). *The 21 irrefutable laws of leadership.* Retrieved from http://www.u-leadership.com/the_21_irrefutable_laws_of_leadership-w.pdf

McTeer, W., White, P. G., & Persad, S. (1995). Manager/coach mid-season replacement and team performance in professional team sport. *Journal of Sport Behavior, 18*(1), 58–68. Retrieved from Business Source Database.

Redman, R. (2006). Leadership succession planning: An evidence-based approach for managing the future. *Journal on Nursing Medication, 36*(6), 292–297. Retrieved from CINAHL with full text database.

Rothwell, W. J., Wang, W. A., Jackson, R. D., Payne, T. D., Knight, S., & Lindholm, J. E. (2005). *Career planning and succession management: Developing your organizations talent for today and tomorrow.* Westport, CT: Praeger.

Sherman, R. (2005). Growing our future nursing leaders. *Nursing Administration Quarterly,* *29*(2), 125–132. Retrieved from CINAHL with full text database.

Sisko, A., Truffer, C., Smith, S., Keehan, S., Cylus, J., Poisal, J. A., . . . Lizonitz, J. (2009). Health spending projections through 2018: Recession effects add uncertainty to the outlook. *Health Affairs, 28*(2), 346–357. doi:10.1377/hlthaff.28.2.w346

Thompson, A., Strickland, A., & Gamble, J. (2005). *Crafting and executing strategy: Text and readings* (15th ed.). New York, NY: McGraw-Hill.

U.S. Bureau of Labor Statistics. (2010). Registered nurses. In *Occupational outlook handbook, 2010–2011 edition.* Retrieved from http://www.bls.gov/oco/ocos083.htm

U.S. Census Bureau. (2011). *Age and sex composition 2010: 2010 census brief.* Retrieved from http://www.census.gov/prod/cen2010/briefs/c2010br-03.pdf

15

Teambuilding: Insights, Strategies, and Tools

Faye A. Meloy

"Teamwork is the ability to work together toward a common vision. The ability to direct individual accomplishments toward organizational objectives. It is the fuel that allows common people to attain uncommon results."

—Andrew Carnegie

The rapidly changing face of the health-care environment and realities of limited human and capital resources have resulted in the need for nurse executives to have a breadth of skills, insights, and knowledge like never before. To compete effectively, health-care organizations must have a strong sense of community, highly functional teams and networks of individuals that support each other in achievement of organizational goals, and the delivery of seamless, high-quality, cost-effective health-care services. Contemporary nurse leaders must not only understand the theoretical and clinical foundations of nursing practice but must also be able to bridge the chasm between the business and human elements of health-care delivery. Social and economic forces such as the aging of the population, ongoing advances in technology managed care, dramatic changes in reimbursement, and a changing workforce necessitate the use of highly integrated strategies from multiple disciplines in the actualization of effective nursing leadership. The Doctor of Nursing Practice (DNP) provides a unique blend of advanced knowledge and clinical research skills that transcend traditional levels of educational preparation. This chapter's focus on teambuilding that provides an overview of insights, strategies, and tools that will assist the advanced practice nurse executive in capitalizing on the collective wisdom of teams in promoting collaborative practice while proactively shaping quality, cost-effective delivery systems now and in the future.

TEAMBUILDING

High-performing organizations achieve results through the knowledge, skills, and unique perspectives from individuals at all levels. In a survey of job satisfaction/ retention in a cross-section of staff nurses and nursing leaders employed in a multi-hospital system teamwork and coworker support ranked highest among all groups (Kuhar, Miller, Spear, Ulreich, & Mion, 2004). Lack of teamwork in an intensive care unit (ICU) setting has also been shown to have a direct impact on patient mortality (Aiken, Clarke, Sloane, Sochalski, & Silber, 2002). Teambuilding among multiple disciplines poses additional challenges due to the lack of a common vocabulary, long-standing organizational/professional hierarchies, role confusion, and fear of change. New mandates linking health-care reimbursement to quality outcomes and coordination of care have heightened the awareness of teamwork as a critical element in health-care delivery; however, the important foundational elements and inherent challenges associated with teambuilding are often overlooked (Jansen, 2008).

Characteristics of Teams

Trust, respect, and mutual accountability are essential components of highly effective team in which members share a common vision and demonstrate strong collaboration and interdependence. Team members are able to engage in open, unfiltered dialogue and focus on achievement of collective results rather than individual agendas or need for recognition. There is shared accountability for both group process and outcomes (Huber, 2010). All too often, due to various predisposing factors, functioning is hampered by a lack of commitment, competing agendas, conflict, mistrust, inattention to results, and the absence of shared accountability for team process and outcomes by one or more team members. It is important for the nurse executive to differentiate between genuine team collaboration and dysfunctional pseudo teams in which individuals refer to themselves as a *team* but infuse personal agendas, toxic communication patterns, and dysfunctional interpersonal personal interactions into group activities (Katzenbach & Smith, 2003). The lack of accountability for team achievement combined with an inability to recognize the need for change in behavior often results in proliferation of a viscous cycle of dysfunction over time. Resistance to change and lack of accountability can often be traced to situations where individuals are uninformed, jaded by prior negative experiences, over-rewarded and under-coached, stagnant in their career path, protected due to specialized knowledge or technical skills, and predominantly focused on self-interests. In these instances, it is imperative that the source(s) be readily identified and remedied through education, support, and/or reconfiguration of team membership.

Conflict Management

Conflict is defined as an expressed struggle between at least two independent parties who perceive that incompatible goals, scarce resources, external variables, and interference from others are preventing from achieving their goals (Wilmot & Hocker, 2001, p. 41). Conflict is inevitable in any work environment due to inherent differences in goals, needs, desires, responsibilities, perceptions, and ideas and can be manifested as intrapersonal, interpersonal, or intergroup (Almost, 2005). Katzenbach and Smith (2003) assert that conflict, such as trust and interdependence, is a foundational element of evolution in high-performing teams as individuals blend their unique experiences, perspectives, values, and expectations into a common purpose and plan of action. Historically viewed in negative contexts, there is a tendency among individuals to avoid conflict whenever possible. However, contemporary views recognize the multidimensional aspects of conflict with both constructive and destructive effects depending on the source of conflict, the task at hand, and how the conflict is managed. New paradigms for constructive conflict resolution include (1) replacement of old attitudes of competition with new approaches that foster collaborative problem-solving, shared accountability, humility, honesty, and respect; (2) open and honest communication; (3) willingness to let go of the past and emphasis on creating new possibilities; and (4) developing a mutually agreed on plan of action (Katzenbach & Smith, 2003).

Figure 15.1 depicts the personal preferences in the use of conflict resolution strategies as categorized by Thomas and Kilmann (1978), which include avoidance, accommodation, competition compromise, and collaboration. Avoidance is typically manifested by ignoring the issue, postponing action until a beret time, or withdrawing from the source of conflict and is evidence of a passive, unassertive communication

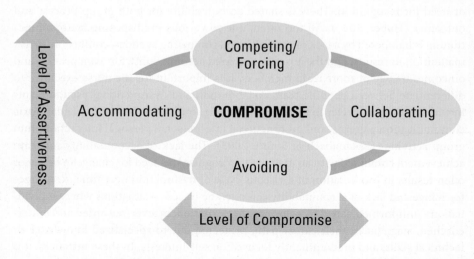

FIGURE 15.1. Conflict management styles. (From Thomas, K. W., & Kilmann, R. [1978]. Comparison of four instruments measuring conflict behavior. *Psychological Report, 42,* 1139–1145.)

strategy. Accommodation, a cooperative but unassertive strategy, involves neglecting personal concerns to satisfy the needs of others and may be useful in situations where preserving harmony and avoiding disruption are paramount or when one party has a vested interest that is unimportant to the other. Use of accommodation may take the form of selfless generosity or charity, obeying an order despite reluctance to do so, or yielding to another's point of view. Competition typically focuses on winning and losing as a primary concern where one party's needs are satisfied at the other's expense. Although a competitive strategy may be useful in situations when quick, decisive action is needed, this highly assertive but uncooperative approach is typically used when an individual feels that defending a particular position, standing up for one's rights, or when "winning" is the primary motivating factor. Compromise, is often described as a "splitting the difference" approach to conflict resolution wherein both parties exchange concessions in favor of a timely resolution. Compromise is characterized as an intermediate-level assertive, cooperative strategy and is most often used to identify a middle ground position that can be effective in situations where opponents have equal power and are strongly committed to mutually exclusive goals. Collaboration encompasses a high degree of assertiveness and cooperation and is characterized by an attempt by all parties to find a mutually satisfying outcome. Collaboration is viewed as a win-win strategy in which individuals focus disagreements on issues and problems rather than personalities. Collaboration entails trust, respect for all parties, and cultivates a sense of empowerment among team members. The collaborative approach to problem-solving and conflict resolution works best in an environment that supports transparency and equality (Huber, 2010; Sportsman & Hamilton, 2007; Thomas & Kilmann, 1978).

Conflict management techniques stress the importance of open and honest dialogue characterized by and sensitivity to others. Unfortunately, all too often, conflict among team members emerges in the case of strong opposing positions, heightened emotions and in situations that are perceived to be "high stakes" for the parties involved. In these crucial situations, individuals typically demonstrate their worst behaviors. Coaching and mentoring in individuals and teams in "crucial conversations" will provide insights and skills that will proactively assist in the mitigation and resolution of conflict in a collaborative manner and facilitate ongoing team performance. The essential elements of crucial conversations include (1) identifying the most important outcome to be achieved while seeking mutual purpose; (2) taking time to analyze what is really going on in the situation; (3) creating a respectful environment that makes it safe to discuss without risk; (4) learning how to take charge of your emotions and exert influence over your own feelings; (5) refining personal stories; (6) speaking persuasively not abrasively; (7) listening for genuine understanding; and (8) moving forward with a clearly articulated, mutual plan of action (Patterson, Grenny, McMillan, & Switzler, 2012).

In a study of conflict management styles of undergraduate and graduate nursing and health-professions students, Sportsman and Hamilton (2007) identified that the prevalent style for both groups was compromise followed by avoidance, with only 9.8% of participants choosing collaboration at that level. Although further study is needed, these preliminary results underscore the need for ongoing development and refinement of conflict resolution skills with an emphasis on collaboration in both nursing education and practice.

Setting the Stage

Teambuilding is a process of raising awareness and fostering a sense of shared accountability that helps individuals to move from a focus on "self" by enabling them to recognize the power of cooperation and collaboration while fostering a genuine appreciation of others. There are often concomitant tasks of overcoming prior conditioning related to ego development and a willingness to allow interdependence and vulnerability. No small task at best. Consequently, it is important to ensure that the organizational culture, alignment of corporate objectives with team-related activities, and educational/technical supports are available to assist individuals in achieving that goal.

It is impossible to promote high-performing teams without true organizational commitment to the elimination of organizational hierarchies at all levels. Shared vision, open dialogue, trust, and a sense of belonging are critical elements for cohesiveness in overcoming organizational challenges and ongoing strategic development. Unfortunately, all too often, organizations implement teams but confine important information and critical dialogue to a few key individuals. Long-standing paradigms of organizational hierarchies must be replaced by an organizational climate that fosters equalization of power, shared governance, participative management, and individual contributions to organizational goals. Team members must understand how their contributions align with corporate objectives and receive positive reinforcement that their work is valued. However, in the face of uncertainty, there is often a perceived dichotomy between trust and conflicting goals (restructuring, downsizing, cost containment, and quality care). Drawing on extensive empirical research, an irrefutable case can be made that the culture and capabilities of an organization—derived from the ways it manages its people—are the real and enduring sources of competitive advantage. Transparency, free flow of information, and a strong track record of high-performance management strategies include a commitment to job security, selective hiring practices, extensive training/support systems, elimination of status differences between stakeholder groups, and decentralization of authority and self-managed teams as basic elements of organizational design (Pfeffer & Veiga, 1999).

A critical element of effective teambuilding is cohesiveness and alignment between team-related activities and organizational objectives. Important elements for consideration in the early stages of team development relate to clarity of team "purpose" and goals, rules of engagement, and interpersonal relationships. Synergy of vision and desired outcome is essential. Team members must understand how their efforts fit in the scheme of organizational priorities and agree that their efforts can contribute to a preferred future state. Strategies such as gap analysis may be beneficial in establishing these critical linkages (Persily, 2013). Important question for consideration may include the following:

1. What problem or gap is the team addressing?
2. What is the impact of the gap on the organization and its "stakeholders"?
3. What are the compelling reasons for addressing the gap?
4. What are the confounding variables contributing to the gap?
5. What are the outcome metrics that will be used to monitor progress?
6. How will success be measured?

Team norms and expectations related to communication, interpersonal relationships, decision making, and resolution of conflict must also be clearly articulated. Trust, mutual respect, collaboration, and interdependence are integral components of highly effective teams. Team members must engage in unfiltered dialogue around ideas, focus on achievement of collective results, and hold one another accountable for team process and outcomes. As a means to this end, it is becoming increasingly more common for teams to operationalize rules of engagement in a formal written agreement. Components of such agreements include behavioral objectives, which stipulate the following:

- All communication must be open, honest, and direct.
- There will be disclosure regarding specific team member interests and bias.
- Individuals will defer personal needs and priorities for the common interest of the team.
- Feedback is expected when individual behaviors create difficult or uncomfortable situations for others.
- There is agreement to work through difficult issues until a mutually agreeable resolution is identified.
- Team members will support each other and offer assistance as needed.
- Confidentiality will be maintained at all times, and sensitive information will not be shared without permission.
- Commitment will be demonstrated by honoring meeting commitments, loyalty to absent team members, and presenting others in the best light possible (Huber, 2010).

Valuing the Individual

The inherent strength of an effective team is correlated with balanced contribution and participation from its members. Although a well-known adage associated with teambuilding (T-together E-everyone A-accomplishes M-more) aptly describes the synergistic effects of collaboration and cohesiveness among team members, it oversimplifies the unique talents, skills, and personalities that individuals contribute to overall team function and outcomes. Valuing individual differences, capitalizing on associated strengths, and compensating for areas of weaknesses are often overlooked, yet integral, components of team function and performance. The power of synergy evident in team activities is in direct proportion to the skills members possess and the initiative demonstrated by team members. Individuals who feel valued as team members are more likely to be actively engaged in group activities. Work teams need people with strong technical and personal skills, who have the courage and conviction to look beyond the status quo. Teams also need self-identified leaders who take responsibility for getting things done. However, an imbalance in involvement, in which a few team members dominate group activities, predisposes the team to member burnout and disenfranchisement. Tools such as the Myers-Briggs Type Indicator (MBTI), the Belbin Self-Perception Inventory (SPI), the Profiles of Organizational Influence Strategies (POIS), and the Bartol/McSweeney Conflict Management Attitude Scale provide valuable insights into personality traits, team member characteristics, role preferences, and conflict resolution strategies that facilitate inclusiveness, self-confidence, engagement, and empowerment among group members.

Teambuilding, as conducted with the help of the MBTI tool, is the process by which a group of individuals are encouraged to learn about themselves, each other, and their leader(s) and to gain an awareness of how these components fit together to enhance team success (Hirsh, Hirsh, & Krebs-Hirsh, 2003). As a complement to the MBTI, the Belbin SPI focuses on individual personal role preferences and within team settings and assists in identifying both gaps and imbalances in critical team functions. The POIS evaluates an individual's preferred influence strategies used in personal and professional interactions. The Bartol/McSweeney Conflict Management Attitude Scale, specifically developed for nurses, offers insights to preferred conflict resolution strategies and provides a starting point for educational strategies that increase the repertoire of conflict resolution skills among team members, thereby enhancing the opportunity for meaningful dialogue and collaboration.

Myers-Briggs Type Indicator

The MBTI is a personality trait assessment based on Carl Jung's theories of personality type. The MBTI has been widely used to explain the ways in which various combinations of personality traits influence both an understanding of self and interactions with others, so it can provide valuable insights related to team development and effectiveness. The MBTI uses four contrasting dichotomies (depicted by letters) which categorize individuals into one of 16 personality types. The four opposing poles are extroversion (E) versus introversion (I), sensing (S) versus intuition (N), thinking (T) versus feeling (F), and judging (J) versus perceiving (P). The E/I scale identifies how individuals direct and receive energy. The S/N scale indicates personal preference for taking in and processing information. The T/F scale describes attributes related to decision making. The J/P scale focuses on how individuals organize their work. Characteristics commonly associated with each of the 16 personality types (Myers, 1998) are outlined in Figure 15.2.

	Sensing Types		Intuitive Types	
Introverts	**ISTJ** Quiet, serious, earn success by thoroughness and dependability. Practical, matter-of-fact, realistic, and responsible. Decide logically what should be done and work toward it steadily, regardless of distractions. Take pleasure in making everything orderly and organized—their work, their home, their life. Value traditions and loyalty.	**ISFJ** Quiet, friendly, responsible, and conscientious. Committed and steady in meeting their obligations. Thorough, painstaking, and accurate. Loyal, considerate, notice and remember specifics about people who are important to them, concerned with how others feel. Strive to create an orderly and harmonious environment at work and at home.	**INFJ** Seek meaning and connections in ideas, relationships, and material possessions. Want to understand what motivates people and are insightful about others. Conscientious and committed to their firm values. Develop a clear vision common good. Organized and decisive in implementing their vision.	**INTJ** Have original minds and great drive for implementing their ideas and achieving their goals. Quickly see patterns in external events and develop long-range explanatory perspectives. When committed, organize a job and carry it through. Skeptical and independent, have high standards of competence and performance—for themselves and others.
	ISTP Tolerant and flexible, quiet observers until a problem appears, then act quickly to find workable solutions. Analyze what makes things work and readily get through large amounts of data to isolate the core of practical problems. Interested in cause and effect, organize facts using logical principles, value efficiency.	**ISFP** Quiet, friendly, sensitive, and kind. Enjoy the present moment, what's going on around them. Like to have their own space and to work within their own time frame. Loyal and committed to their values and to people who are important to them. Dislike disagreements and conflicts, do not force their opinions or values on others.	**INFP** Idealistic, loyal to their values and to people who are important to them. Want an external life that is congruent with their values. Curious, quick to see possibilities, can be catalysts for implementing ideas. Seek to understand people and to help them fulfill their potential. Adaptable, flexible, and accepting unless a value is threatened.	**INTP** Seek to develop logical explanations for everything that interests them. Theoretical and abstract, interested more in ideas than in social interaction. Quiet, contained, flexible, and adaptable. Have unusual ability to focus in depth to solve problems in their area of interest. Skeptical, sometimes critical, always analytical.
Extraverts	**ESTP** Flexible and tolerant, they take a pragmatic approach focused on immediate results. Theories and conceptual explanations bore them—they want to act energetically to solve the problem. Focus on the here-and-how, spontaneous, enjoy each moment that they can be active with others. Enjoy material comforts and style. Learn best through doing.	**ESFP** Outgoing, friendly, and accepting. Exuberant lovers of life, people, and material comforts. Enjoy working with others to make things happen. Bring common sense and a realistic approach to their work, and make work fun. Flexible and spontaneous, adapt readily to new people and environments. Learn best by trying a new skill with other people.	**ENFP** Warmly enthusiastic and imaginative. See life as full of possibilities. Make connections between events and information very quickly, and confidently proceed based on the patterns they see. Want a lot of affirmation from others, and readily give appreciation and support. Spontaneous and flexible, often rely on their verbal fluency.	**ENTP** Quick, ingenious, stimulating, alert, and outspoken. Resourceful in solving new and challenging problems. Adept at generating conceptual possibilities and then analyzing them strategically. Good at reading other people. Bored by routine, will seldom do the same thing the same way, apt to turn to one new interest after another.
	ESTJ Practical, realistic, matter-of-fact. Decisive, quickly move to implement decisions. Organize projects and people to get things done, focus on getting results in the most efficient way possible. Take care of routine details. Have a clear set of logical standards, systematically follow them and want others to also. Forceful in implementing their plans.	**ESFJ** Warmhearted, conscientious, and cooperative. Want harmony in their environment, work with determination to establish it. Like to work with others to complete tasks accurately and on time. Loyal follow through even in small matters. Notice what others need in their day-by-day lives and try to provide it. Want to be appreciated for who they are and for what they contribute.	**ENFJ** Warm, empathetic, responsive, and responsible. Highly attuned to the emotions, needs, and motivations of others. Find potential in everyone, want to help others fulfill their potential. May act as catalysts for individual and group growth. Loyal, responsive to praise and criticism. Sociable, facilitate others in a group, and provide inspiring leadership.	**ENTJ** Frank, decisive, assume leadership readily. Quickly see illogical and inefficient procedures and polices, develop and implement comprehensive systems to solve organizational problems. Enjoy long-term planning and goal setting. Usually well informed, well read, enjoy expanding their knowledge and passing it on to others. Forceful in presenting their ideas.

FIGURE 15.2. Characteristics frequently associated with MBTI personality type. (Modified and reproduced by special permission of the publisher, CPP, Inc., Mountain View, CA 94043 from *Introduction to Type*, Sixth Edition, by Isabel Briggs Myers. Copyright 1998 by Peter B. Myers and Katharine D. Myers. All right reserved. Further reproduction is prohibited without the publisher's written consent.)

Insights gained about self and others can be useful in the developmental stages of team formation or as a resource to enhance cohesiveness and productivity of existing team activities. Hirsh et al. (2003) suggest that the MBTI tool specifically assists teambuilding by the following:

- Fostering openness and trust
- Providing a neutral affirmative language with which to discuss differences
- Underscoring the value of diversity
- Teaching team members to value and work with the strengths of others
- Helping increase productivity by aligning individual MBTI preferences to particular team functions
- Identifying team assets and blind spots
- Providing a framework to enhance group effectiveness

Davies and Kanaki (2006) examined predictions about team effectiveness based on the diversity of personality types inherent among team members. Their results suggest that organizations might improve the functioning of teams by analyzing the mixture of roles existing in their teams and by focusing training and development strategies accordingly. Although personality inventories have not traditionally been used in educational or practice settings of health professionals, the enhanced awareness and enriched insights of interpersonal interactions has the potential to enhance teambuilding, communication, and collaboration at all levels.

Belbin Self-Perception Team Role Inventory

In order for effective team collaboration, there must be clearly delineated roles and responsibilities (Carson & Issac, 2005). As a result of extensive research on team effectiveness, Belbin (2010) suggests that a mix of different team skills, rather than individual talent/expertise, is a primary determined team performance. The specific team roles that individual exhibit to varying degrees are integral to team success. The nine essential roles as defined by Belbin are shaper, company worker (implementer), completer/finisher, coordinator, team worker, resource investigator, plant, monitor/evaluator, and specialist. The SPI consists of a self-report questionnaire that asks how an individual deals with various work situations. The self-report is correlated with responses from external observers who evaluate what behaviors they see the person displaying in the workplace. The correlation of these results is used to determine relative strengths, preferences, and weaknesses related to the nine identified team roles (Fig. 15.3) and can be used to gain insight on behaviors and maximize the effectiveness of team function (Belbin, 2012).

Davies and Kanaki (2006) also examined interpersonal traits associated with specific team roles and concluded that organizations can improve team effectiveness through identification of specific strengths, weaknesses, and role preferences inherent in individual team members. Insights gained can be useful in team formation, identification of gaps in essential skills in existing teams, and in coaching/mentoring activities in support of team achievement.

Team Role		Contribution	Allowable Weaknesses
Plant		Creative, imaginative, free-thinking. Generates ideas and solves difficult problems.	Ignores incidentals. Too preoccupied to communicate effectively.
Resource Investigator		Outgoing, enthusiastic, communicative. Explores opportunities and develops contacts.	Over-optimistic. Loses interest once initial enthusiasm has passed.
Co-ordinator		Mature, confident, identifies talent. Clarifies goals. Delegates effectively.	Can be seen as manipulative. Offloads own share of the work.
Shaper		Challenging, dynamic, thrives on pressure. Has the drive and courage to overcome obstacles.	Prone to provocation. Offends people's feelings.
Monitor Evaluator		Sober, strategic and discerning. Sees all options and judges accurately.	Lacks drive and ability to inspire others. Can be overly critical.
Teamworker		Cooperative, perceptive and diplomatic. Listens and averts friction.	Indecisive in crunch situations. Avoids confrontation.
Implementer		Practical, reliable, efficient. Turns ideas into actions and organises work that needs to be done.	Somewhat inflexible. Slow to respond to new possibilities.
Completer Finisher		Painstaking, conscientious, anxious. Searches out errors. Polishes and perfects.	Inclined to worry unduly. Reluctant to delegate.
Specialist		Single-minded, self-starting, dedicated. Provides knowledge and skills in rare supply.	Contributes only a narrow front. Dwells on technicalities.

FIGURE 15.3. Belbin team role summary descriptions. (Copyright Belbin 2012 used with permission from http://www.belbin.com)

Profiles of Organizational Influence Strategies

The strategic and influential use of power and knowledge is critical if the nursing profession move forward to support teambuilding and effect change to more collaborative and interdisciplinary service delivery models (Jansen, 2008). The POIS tool, developed by Kipinis and Schmidt (1999), is an evidence-based, reliable, and valid instrument that evaluates personal preferences related to the use of influence strategies among individuals in organizational contexts. There are three forms of the POIS, including (1) form M, which is developed for use by managers that focuses on exploring barriers to effective upward communication and influence; (2) form S, which is designed to facilitate improved patterns of influence used by managers with subordinates; and (3) form C, which is designed to reflect influence strategies used by individuals with coworkers and is especially useful in teambuilding activities. The POIS instruments were developed through a series of research projects designed to evaluate commonly used methods of influence and which ones work best in specific situations. These studies identified seven basic influence strategies: reason, friendliness, bargaining, assertiveness, coalitions, appeal to a higher authority, and sanctions. The POIS helps individuals understand not only their preferred influence styles but also provides valuable insight into both past and future choices of influence strategies. It should be noted that all influence strategies have the potential to be used effectively depending on specific circumstances. However, overreliance or avoidance of any given strategy may lead to inflexibility or ineffectiveness in team-related dialogue and debate (Table 15.1).

Bartol/McSweeney Conflict Management Scale

Although individuals are inherently capable of using multiple conflict resolution methods, there is a tendency to rely on some strategies more heavily than others as a result of personal preference or past experiences. Effective conflict management is a vital skill that can be learned; however, when under duress, frustrated individuals often resort to ineffective automatic responses that inhibit opportunities for constructive resolution and growth. Identifying one's usual response to conflict is an important first step in developing a repertoire of conflict management skills essential as a foundation for teambuilding and collaboration (Bartol, Parrish, & McSweeney, 2001; Boggs, 1999). There are multiple assessment inventories available to assist individuals in identifying personal response and preferred conflict resolution strategies. One such example, specifically developed for nurses, is the Bartol/McSweeney Conflict Management Attitude Scale. This inventory consists of 80 statements that reflect attitudes toward conflict management strategies that may be deeply engrained form early life, which may and may not unconsciously influence habits of responding to conflict under duress. It is generally accepted that individuals have a preferred style for managing conflict but will revert to other strategies when the preferred style is unsuccessful. Although the Bartol/McSweeney Conflict Management Scale does not

TABLE 15.1. Influence Strategies, Behaviors, and Common Uses

Influence Strategy	Behavior Used to Achieve Results	Common Uses
Reason	Relies on data, discussion, and logic	Selling ideas
Friendliness	Demonstrated interest, goodwill, and esteem to create a favorable impression	To acquire desired personal favors or assistance, or to compensate for a weak power base
Coalition	Use of peer pressure as means of persuasion	Applicable for personal and organizational uses; can be used for both personal benefit and selling ideas
Bargaining	Relies on negotiation and exchange of benefits/favors	Used when seeking personal benefits
Assertiveness	Uses a forceful and persistent manner to communicate demands	Used to overcome resistance
Higher authority	Invokes influence of those in higher organization levels to support requests	Used when resistance is expected
Sanctions	Use of reward/punishment derived from organizational position	Used to influence subordinates

Adapted from Kipinis, D., & Schmidt, S. M. (1999). *Profiles of organizational influence strategies*. Retrieved from http://www.mindgarden.com/products/pois.htm. Used with permission from http://www.mindgarden.com

identify how quickly an individual moves from one conflict style to another, it does identify the pattern of choices (Bartol et al., 2001). Insights gained provide a starting point for ongoing development and refinement of conflict management strategies that will maximize both individual group potential inherent in teambuilding and other collaborative personal/professional endeavors.

Inventories such as MBTI, SPI, POIS, and the Bartol/McSweeney Conflict Management Attitude Scale have not traditionally been used in the education of health professionals; the enhanced self-awareness and enriched insights into interpersonal interactions has the potential to enhance communication, collaboration, conflict resolution, development of overall team effectiveness at all levels. They also provide a foundation for ongoing activities related to mentoring, coaching, and leadership development.

Emphasis on Team

Successful teams need the right mix of technical, problem-solving, decision-making, and interpersonal skills to maximize effectiveness (Katzenbach & Smith, 2003). In addition, it is imperative that all team members have a common understanding of why the team exists as well as the alignment with organizational priorities. Old paradigms of winning and losing must be replaced with an attitude of collaborative problem solving which focuses on shared accountability, humility, honesty, and respect. Team members must be willing to let go of past realities, focus on creating a preferred future, develop strategies to achieve desired objectives, and feel empowered throughout the process. The use of appreciative inquiry strategies may facilitate a much needed shift in team focus from "what is not working" to uncovering the positive core of team strengths as a basis to move forward. Roles and responsibilities of individual team members in support of overall group function must be clearly articulated, and there must be shared accountability for team function and outcomes. There should also be a shared understanding and agreement regarding how decisions will be made, how conflict will be managed, and resources available to the team for guidance and support. Evaluation of both individual and overall team performance should be conducted on an ongoing basis and create a rich repertoire of "lessons learned" as a foundation for personal development and enhancement of future team initiatives (Huber, 2010; Katzenbach & Smith, 2003).

Putting It All Together

Recognizing the inherent complexities associated with effective teambuilding, the nurse executive is in a unique position to develop and support team initiatives by helping individuals to align personal goals with organizational priorities in a cooperative and collaborative manner. The marketplace imperatives care for quality, innovation, cost-effectiveness, and customer satisfaction needed for sustainable competitive advantage in the rapidly changing health-care environment highlight the need for enhanced collaboration and cooperation among key stakeholders and a heightened dependence on the wisdom of teams in addressing organizational challenges. Long-standing habits of individualism, rampant confusion about teams and teamwork, and negative prior experience with teams undercut the possibilities that teams offer at the very moment that the need has become so critical (Katzenbach & Smith, 2003). Consequently, it is important that nurse executives can readily identify nonfunctional pseudo teams and ensure that valuable resources and support are redirected to committed individuals and meaningful work products.

It is impossible to direct individuals to become a "team," rather the focus should be on creating a natural evolution of team commitment by providing a sense of purpose and a set of performance goals to which they will hold themselves accountable. The Drexler-Sibbet Model of Team Development (Fig. 15.4) illustrates the phases of team development and highlights the dynamic nature of team interactions where regression is as possible as moving toward greater maturity and self-actualization (Grove Consultants International, 2014). Because changing circumstances and opportunities may profoundly impact team function and outcomes, alignment of these foundational elements should be assessed on an ongoing basis (McKnight, Kaney, & Breuer, 2010).

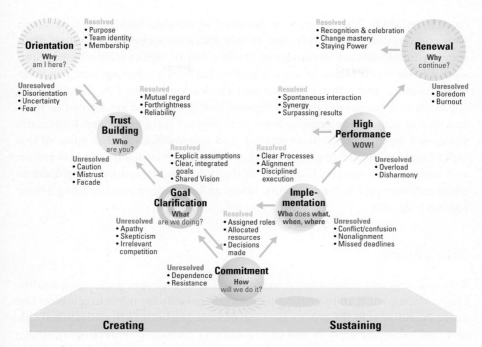

FIGURE 15.4. Dynamic nature of team interactions. (Used with permission from The Grove Consultants International, http://www.grove.com. For more information on the Model and TP System, please visit http://www.grove.com)

Even under the best of circumstances, desired outcomes will not always be realized. However, it is important to celebrate "failures" as well as "successes" because both instances provide a wealth of experiences on which to build future teambuilding and collaborative endeavors. It is also important to identify when teams hit seemingly insurmountable barriers to performance and need management intervention. In these instances, the power of planned abandonment or modifications to team membership can be weighed against strategies that will assist teams in overcoming obstacles and moving forward. Strategies for getting "unstuck" include (1) revisiting the basics (review purpose, strategy, and performance goals), (2) identifying opportunity for small wins that have the potential to overturn the cycle of frustration and stagnation, (3) injecting new information and approaches, (4) using facilitators and mentors as needed, and (5) considering changing the teams' leadership or membership in an effort to remove obstacles to team achievement (Katzenbach & Smith, 2003).

In recognition of the importance of a team approach to health-care delivery, a national teamwork improvement initiative exists in the TeamSTEPPS program developed and available through the Agency for Healthcare Research and

Quality (AHRQ). The program is designed to develop highly effective teams who communicate effectively and reduce the consequences of human error (Agency for Healthcare Research and Quality, 2014). This evidence-based teamwork system trains teams to work together; back each other up; and promotes quality, safety, and efficacy for the best clinical outcomes. The TeamSTEPPS approach to team development recognizes that good teams are trained to work together to achieve the competencies that support team behaviors: leadership, situational monitoring, mutual support, and communication. The value of this type of national initiative program is that it is publicly available, comprehensive, and customizable to meet the needs of the individual health-care organization while maintaining a focus on quality, safety, and efficacy in practice using a team approach to care.

SUMMARY

Teambuilding and collaborative-based practice in the rapidly changing health-care environment is an increasingly important priority for nurse executives. The nurse executive is in the unique position of fostering both an organizational culture that values the wisdom and contribution of teams and in developing strategies that support meaningful team development and achievement. Teambuilding is in many ways a mechanism to actualize collaboration, and team-based models of care and decision making have been identified as an essential mechanism for evolving models of health-care delivery. Although teambuilding and interdisciplinary practice are viewed as generally agreed to be a worthy goal, Jansen (2008) asserts that there are a myriad of historical, economic, political, and professional socialization challenges to achieving that aim. This chapter's focus on teambuilding provides an overview of the myriad of insights, strategies, and resources available to facilitate teambuilding and foster collaboration. However, due to the complexity of personal, organizational, and environmental influences, there is no clear course for success. Ongoing dialogue, practice-based research, and widespread dissemination of findings among disciplines will enhance understanding of how best to facilitate the collective wisdom of teams in proactively shaping quality, cost-effective health-care delivery systems that are operationalized through collaboration among stakeholders at all levels. An understanding that the essence of teambuilding is grounded in personal relationships complemented by the broad-based knowledge and perspectives gained through education for advanced practice roles in positions nurse executives to be catalysts in breaking down traditional barriers to collaboration and facilitate meaningful teambuilding efforts that will develop the best of "what is," envision "what might be possible," share perspectives of "what should be," and facilitate innovation and creating the "preferred future."

Important "Takeaways"

Putting it all together ...
Value and nurture both the "I" and "We" in teams
Focus on oppurtunities not problems
Make it real-align values; create a sense of urgency
Take away the blame
Manage conflict
Walk the talk
Provide the tools
Step up to the plate
Celebrate both success and failures
Know when to get out of the way

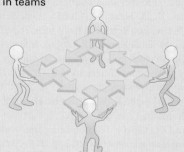

Thoughts to Ponder ...
Does the culture of the organization value teams?
Does the "walk" match the "talk"
Are there adequate resources to support team development and function?

Think about experiences with teambuilding ...
What worked and why?
What didn't work and why?
What could have been done differently to enhance team effectiveness?

Reflect on your role (both as a team member and nursing executive)
What are your strengths and areas for improvement in teambuilding efforts?
- How can you contribute to creating a "preferred future" of collaboration among all stakeholders?
- What are the resources and supports needed to accomplish that goal?
- Where will you begin?... when?... and how?

REFERENCES

Agency for Healthcare Research and Quality. (2014). *TeamSTEPPS*. Retrieved from http://teamstepps.ahrq.gov/

Aiken, L. H., Clarke, S. P., Sloane, D. M., Sochalski, J., & Silber, J. H. (2002). Hospital nurse staffing and patient mortality, nurse burnout, and job dissatisfaction. *Journal of the American Medical Association, 288*(16), 1987–1993.

Almost, J. (2005). Conflict within nursing environments: Concept analysis. *Journal of Advanced Nursing, 53*(4), 444–453.

Bartol, G. M., Parrish, R. S., & McSweeney, M. (2001). Effective conflict management begins with knowing your style. *Journal of Nursing Staff Development, 17*(1), 34–40.

Belbin. (2012). Team role summary descriptions. In *Team role report* (p. 2). Retrieved from http://www.belbin.com

Belbin, R. (2010). *Management teams: Why they succeed or fail* (3rd ed.). Burlington, MA: Elsevier.

Boggs, K. U. (1999). Resolving conflict between nurse and client. In E. Arnold & K. U. Boggs (Eds.), *Interpersonal relationships* (pp. 323–345). Philadelphia, PA: W.B. Saunders.

Carson, K., & Isaac, M. (2005). *A guide to team roles: How to increase personal and team effectiveness*. Retrieved from http://belbinimprovingteams.com

Davies, M. F., & Kanaki, E. (2006). Interpersonal characteristics associated with different team roles in work groups. *Journal of Managerial Psychology, 21*(7), 638.

Grove Consultants International. (2014). *The Drexler/Sibbet team performance level*. Retrieved from http://www.grove.com

Hirsh, E., Hirsh, K. W., & Krebs-Hirsh, S. (2003). *Introduction to type and teams* (2nd ed.). Mountain View, CA: CCP.

Huber, D. L. (2010). Teambuilding and working with effective groups. In *Leadership and nursing care management* (4th ed., pp. 215–234). Maryland Heights, MO: Saunders.

Jansen, L. (2008). Collaborative and interdisciplinary health care teams: Ready or not? *Journal of Professional Nursing, 24*(4), 218–227.

Katzenbach, J. R., & Smith, D. K. (2003). *The wisdom of teams: Creating the high performance organization*. New York, NY: Harper Collins.

Kipinis, D., & Schmidt, S. M. (1999). *Profiles of organizational influence strategies*. Retrieved from http://www.mindgarden.com/products/pois.htm

Kuhar, P. A., Miller, D., Spear, B. T., Ulreich, S. M., & Mion, L. C. (2004). The meaningful retention strategy inventory: A targeted approach to implementing retention strategies. *Journal of Nursing Administration, 34*(1), 10–18.

McKnight, R., Kaney, T., & Breuer, S. (2010). *Leading strategy execution: How to align the senior team, design a strategy-capable organization, and get all employees on-board*. Philadelphia, PA: True North Press.

Myers, I. B. (1998). *Introduction to type: A guide to understanding your results on the Myers-Briggs Type Indicator*. Palo Alto, CA: CPP.

Patterson, K., Grenny, J., McMillan, R., & Switzler, A. (2012). *Crucial conversations: Tools for talking when the stakes are high* (2nd ed.). New York, NY: McGraw Hill.

Persily, C. A. (2013). *Team leadership and partnering in nursing and healthcare*. New York, NY: Springer.

Pfeffer, J., & Veiga, J. F. (1999). Putting people first for organizational success. *Academy of Management Executive, 13*(2), 37–48.

Sportsman, S., & Hamilton, P. (2007). Conflict management styles in the health professions. *Journal of Professional Nursing, 23*(3), 157–166.

Thomas, K. W., & Kilmann, R. (1978). Comparison of four instruments measuring conflict behavior. *Psychological Report, 42*, 1139–1145.

Wilmot, W., & Hocker, J. (2001). *Interpersonal conflict* (6th ed.). Boston, MA: McGraw-Hill.

Evidence-Based Approach to Novice Nurse Orientation in Perianesthesia Units

Seun O. Ross

INTRODUCTION AND OVERVIEW OF THE PROBLEM OF INTEREST

At the forefront of effective treatment for ailing patients, specialized nurses continue to gain importance and momentum. On a daily basis, specialized nurses care for terminally ill patients and are required to give accurate, timely, and individually tailored responses to each patient. This specialty care requires a standardized training approach for nurses entering this detail-oriented work setting. A standard blueprint for specialized didactic nurse orientation should be implemented with a minimum 8-week timeline, according to Benner's (1984) stages of competency: novice, advanced beginner, competent, proficient, and finally expert.

Novice nurses are frequently plagued by occupational stress from lack of nursing experience and individual factors (Kelly & Mynatt, 2000). Advanced nurses tend to perform in a more fluid, focused, and informed approach based on patient knowledge and skilled involvement, whereas novice nurses are too absorbed with organization, priority setting, and task completion (Elbright, Urden, Patterson, & Chalko, 2004). Nurses learn and refine their clinical knowledge from socially determined aspects of

193

their work environment, initially through orientation. However, inadequate orientations can unfortunately inhibit novice development of expertise (Elbright et al., 2004).

Background

Sixteen years ago, recently graduated nurses who desired to work in specialized units were first required to work on a medical-surgical (med-surg) floor. However, due to the current and growing nursing shortage, the practice of serving on med-surg prior to entry into critical care nursing has been supplanted by a new phenomenon of novice nurses in the critical care units. Hospitals attempted to curtail their lack of experience by developing nursing internship programs to transition graduate nurses into specialized nursing (Reddish & Kaplan, 2007). When novice nurses are first hired, the primary need is to orient them to nursing as a profession as well as to the specifics of the unit. These orientations include instructive classes to update or introduce the nurse to the prevailing health problems and nursing issues seen on the unit. Included in this is an introduction on technology used in the units, including ventilators, central lines, monitors, and so forth (Ihelenfeld, 2005). Over the course of 15 weeks, these orientations are often criticized as insufficient because they do not provide new nurses with the requisite education to work effectively and independently in their selected units.

At the conclusion of the customary didactic orientation program (typically ranging from 2 to 4 weeks), new nurses are still not comfortable with initiating physician orders, implementing new procedures, or in demonstrating confidence (Olson et al., 2001). Given the proper education, training and skills, stress levels, burnout, and undesirable coping mechanisms can be mitigated by having a mentorship or intensive didactic orientation program for the new nurse (McCall, 2002).

Significance of the Problem

Safe nursing practice in specialized areas requires a body of knowledge and skills distinct from that required of other nursing specialties (Pooler, Slater-MacLean, Simpson, & Giblin, 2005). A strong knowledge base enhances the standard of care and reduces undesirable coping mechanisms and portentous patient outcomes (i.e., falls, medication errors) for nurses on specialized units. The results of a recent study by Laschinger and Leiter (2006) showed that patient safety outcomes are associated with the quality of nursing practice and that the stress/burnout process plays an important mediating role.

Stress is a major component of burnout and must be managed in a healthful manner. Coping mechanisms are those behaviors that determine how well we adapt and move on when confronted with stressful events. Those who cope in a rather passive, defensive way are more prone to burnout than those who actively confront the events (Davies, 2008). Being adequately prepared is vital in giving the novice nurse the necessary tools to identify problems/issues in the care of a patient.

This subgroup of critical care nurses is particularly vulnerable, owing to the presence of certain stress-related risk factors such as inadequate preparation due to the nursing shortage, inadequate orientation, lack of education, inadequate staffing, and burnout (Kelly & Mynatt, 2000). The nature of critical care practice places those nurses at the front line, which can be aggressive, demanding, challenging, and unrelenting. Eventually, the burden of cumulative stress is compounded by meager coping skills on the job, which contribute to unproductive coping mechanisms and compromised patient safety. These outcomes complicate patient's progress, have a negative effect on their well-being, and can lead to an untimely death (Blegen, Goode, & Reed, 1998).

Nurses who are extremely stressed leave their jobs, abuse substances, and become financial and legal liabilities to their employers because of increased use of health benefits, absenteeism, workplace accidents, associated workman compensation, disability claims, theft, security problems, decreased productivity, and high turnover rates. In addition, low morale and poor communication within the department and diverted supervisory and managerial time increase liabilities to employers (Dunn, 2005). It has been estimated that the cost of replacing a specialized nurse was 25% of his or her base salary, plus 30% of his or her benefit compensation. Each year, this cost increases because of rising hourly wages and cost benefits for employers (Peterson & Van Buren, 2006).

PICO Question

Without current best evidence, practice is rapidly outdated, often to the detriment of patients. Evidence-based practice (EBP) is an approach that enables clinicians to provide the highest quality of care in meeting the multifaceted needs of their patients and families (Melynk & Fineout-Overholt, 2005). In addition, there is evidence to indicate that health-care providers who use an evidence-based approach to delivering patient care experience higher levels of satisfaction than those who deliver care based in tradition. Foreground questions are essential to finding the right evidence to answer them. The four components are PICO: P—population of interest, I—intervention of interest, C—comparison of interest, and O—outcome of interest (Melynk & Fineout-Overholt, 2005).

The purpose of the study is to analyze whether specialized nurses who undergo 10 weeks of didactic orientation are at decreased risk for stress, burnout, turnover intention, and ominous patient outcomes compared with nurses who undergo shorter orientations. The population includes new nurses participating in the perianesthesia orientation program at a hospital in suburban Maryland. The facility is one of the largest health-care facilities in the nation and treats approximately 10,000 patients in its critical care units yearly. The objective of the intervention is to increase the (preceptor-led) clinical aspect of didactic critical care unit orientation to a minimum of 10 weeks compared to the standard time of 4 weeks. The outcome is to increase the level of knowledge of these nurses, which will decrease the levels of stress, burnout, and undesirable coping mechanisms among specialized nurses, and translates into increased patient safety by reducing adverse and near-miss events (i.e., medications errors, falls, and cardiopulmonary resuscitation [CPR] occurrences) and turnover by the novice nurse.

Summary

Part and parcel of clinical care excellence is superior care providers, most notably identified as implementing a critical care team to streamline care and optimize outcomes; the critical care nurse is central to these efforts (Mirski, Chang, & Cowan, 2001). Contextually, the transition to expert nurse must be placed and evaluated. It is essential to embrace an objective that can be reproduced for successive professional development and optimize outcomes from training programs (Reddish & Kaplan, 2007). Given the core mission of the nursing profession and the daily interactions with patients experiencing a myriad of serious and complicated health problems, an inadequately prepared nurse is a significant risk to patients.

Interest in the impact of nursing working conditions on patient safety outcomes has grown since the Institute of Medicine report in 1999 (Institute of Medicine, 1999). There have been numerous studies linking work life characteristics particularly new nurse orientation to patient outcomes such as adverse events and patient mortality (Whitman, Kim, Davidson, Wolf, & Wang, 2002). Understanding the best approach to support novice nurses in their transition will be essential on providing a treatment and wellness environment that is safe for the patient while maturing the specialized nurse.

REVIEW OF LITERATURE EVIDENCE

New nurses are often conflicted with their reality. They must immediately navigate through performance standards learned in the university setting contrasted with their ability to provide on-site quality care, as they adjust to higher work volumes. The time to learn and practice basic nursing skills in a student role has long passed, and new nurses must now focus their attention on gaining competency in clinical skills (Boswell & Wilhoit, 2004). In a recent national survey, the American Association of Critical Care Nurses (AACN) found that 80% of responding critical care units had an educator-developed orientation program (Kirchhoff & Dahl, 2006). Unfortunately, critical care orientation practices vary widely. Insufficient information exists on national practices related to current methods of orientation instruction, orientation outcome measures, and post-orientation support programs (Boswell & Wilhoit, 2004).

Research studies show that EBP leads to higher quality care, improved patient outcomes, reduced costs, and greater nurse satisfaction than traditional approaches to patient care (Melynk, Fineout-Overholt, Stillwell, & Williamson, 2010). EBP is defined as the process of making decisions about patient care and care delivery integration using the best evidence, clinical expertise, and patient values (Sackett, Straus, Richardson, Rosenberg, & Haynes, 2000). After almost 20 years of EBP, it is apparent that reducing variations in practice and following evidence-based guidelines improves quality of care and patient outcomes (Hampton, Griffith, & Howard, 2005). With this focus, EBP has gained importance for delivering clinical patient care (Stevens & Staley, 2006). The key strategies to improve patient care quality and safety are selecting interventions based on scientific evidence and developing protocols to reduce variations in practice (Wells, Free, & Adams, 2007).

Methodology of the Literature of Evidence

For the purposes of this review of evidence, the articles and studies used were limited to the time frame of 1999 to 2010. The Jennie King Mellon Library online databases (CINAHL, Ovid, EBSCOhost) were used to select articles for the capstone, using the key words: *nursing orientation*, *specialized care*, *EBP*, *drug abuse*, *stress*, *medication errors*, *falls*, and *turnover*. The studies used in this paper are quantitative and qualitative with interpretive, retrospective, descriptive, phenomenological, and correlational designs. The studies used multiple variables and descriptive statistics to summarize these variables.

Findings

Specialized nursing care requires a standardized training approach for nurses entering the work setting. Vast health-care money is being invested in strategies aimed at recruiting and retaining an energized, well-educated, critically thinking workforce (McGirr & Bakker, 2000). However, there are minimal studies to inform what constitutes an optimal work environment for the acute care, hospital-based novice nurse. Even less evidence exists to detail the factors that exhaust, alienate, and discourage those nurses and its effect on the patient population.

The studies conducted on novice nurses demonstrated that new nurses are susceptible to feelings of inadequacy in rendering quality patient care (Boswell & Wilhoit, 2004). According to Foley, Kee, Minick, Harvey, and Jennings (2002), qualitative research has demonstrated that nurses' ability to recognize subtle changes and initiate appropriate action is enhanced by their experience and expertise. Those nurses who are able to independently recognize subtle changes in the patient, unit, or system prevent ominous events and take corrective action and increase positive outcome. Blegen et al. (1998) examined the impact of nursing education and experience on quality of care by measuring indicators of adverse occurrences, including the patient care unit rates of medication administration errors, patient falls, nosocomial infections, patient complaints, pressure ulcers, cardiopulmonary arrests, and death.

Results from the two studies provide consistent support for the prevailing belief that more experienced nurses provide higher quality care. Units with more experienced nurses had lower medication error rates in both studies and lower patient fall rates. It can be concluded that the results of these studies support critical concern for better orientations, which will in turn install more experienced nurses in hospitals.

The inadequacy experienced by novice nurses have negative implications, including decreased levels of self-confidence and increased levels of stress during the transition period from novice to professional nurse. If unresolved, the outcome of this negative work experience has the potential to lead to increased levels of stress/burnout, unwanted coping mechanisms, and ultimately adverse effects on patient treatment (Boswell & Wilhoit, 2004).

This section will review the current literature and research studies on the effects of inadequate nursing orientation on patients in critical care areas. The areas to be discussed are inadequate nursing orientation in relation to nurse stress/burnout, inadequate nursing orientation in relation to undesirable coping mechanisms, and inadequate nursing orientation in relation to nurse turnover. In each of these topics, their relationship to patient outcomes will be identified.

Inadequate Nursing Orientation and Nurse Burnout/Stress

Stress, by its most common definition, is a condition or feeling experienced when a person perceives that demands exceed the personal and social resources the individual is able to mobilize (Lazarus & Folkman, 1984). Professional burnout is a syndrome manifested by emotional exhaustion, depersonalization, and reduced personal accomplishments; it commonly occurs in professions such as nursing (Maslach, Jackson, & Leiter, 1996). The stress experienced in the beginning of professional nursing practice is well documented in literature (Hamel, 1990; Jasper, 1996; Kelly, 1996; Oermann & Moffitt-Wolf, 1997; Speedling, Ahmade, & Kuhn-Weissman, 1981).

Symes et al. (2005) conducted a study of stress in new graduates. The study used a nonexperimental, descriptive research design. A convenience sample of 99 participants was recruited and seven instruments (Demographic Data Collection Tool, Social Readjustment Rating Scale, Stressful Life Events Screening Questionnaire, Impact of Event Scale, Help Experiences, Symptom Checklist-6, and the SF-12v2 Health Survey) were used to collect data. The results of the study revealed that over 58% of respondents were highly stressed when dealing with the pressures of being an inexperienced nurse.

Interest in the impact of nursing working conditions on patient safety outcomes has grown since the Institute of Medicine report in 1999 (Institute of Medicine, 1999). There have been numerous studies linking work life characteristics (i.e., stress/burnout) to patient outcomes such as adverse events and patient mortality (Blegen et al., 1998; Kovner & Gergen, 1998; McGillis-Hall et al., 2003; Needleman, Buerhaus, Mattke, Stewart, & Zelevinsky, 2002; Tourangeau, Giovanetti, Tu, & Wood, 2002).

According to Oermann and Moffitt-Wolf (1997), the more predominant stresses in inexperienced nurses arose from a lack of organizational skills and the newness of clinical situations and nursing procedures. Work stress and burnout are associated with negative work attitudes and performance. In health-care settings, these conditions threaten the quality of patient care and patient safety.

A study conducted by Laschinger and Leiter (2006) consisted of a subset from a larger study, the International Survey of Hospital Staffing and Organization of Patient Outcomes. The study was designed to explore relationships between hospital work environment characteristics, nurse staffing, and nurse and patient outcomes. A stratified random sample of 17,965 nurses were surveyed and returned useable questionnaires. The instruments used were the Practice Environment Scale of the Nursing Work Index and the Maslach Burnout Inventory. They found that patient safety outcomes were associated with the quality of the nursing practice work environment, and nurses' burnout played a mediating role. These results suggested that a nurse's perception of his or her work environment correlated to the professional practice. Positive perceptions translated into more engaged attitudes of their work and increased safety in patient care.

Studies by Kim et al. (2005) and Greco, Laschinger, and Wong (2006) showed more than half, 58% and 64%, respectively, of nurses who worked in acute care settings reported severe levels of burnout according to the Maslach Burnout Inventory. As a result of these high percentages, the nurses studied demonstrated increases in falls, nosocomial infections, and medication errors in their patient population.

Inadequate Nursing Orientation and Undesirable Coping Mechanisms

Despite the best efforts to prepare nurse interns for immersion into the critical care arena, significant clinical challenges await, and it is unknown how individual nurse interns will react under stressful situations (Badger, 2008). The prevalence of alcohol and drug abuse in the nursing population has not been fully documented, but it is believed to parallel the general population (Dunn, 2005). It is suspected that 10% of the nursing population has substance abuse problems, and 6% of nurses have problems that are serious enough to interfere with their ability to practice (Dunn, 2005).

The American Nurses Association (ANA) has estimated that 6% to 8% of nurses use either alcohol or drugs to an extent sufficient to impair their professional judgment. Among nurses, prescription-type medication use has been noted to be higher, and illicit drug use has been noted to be lower than in the general population (Dunn, 2005). Although several studies have shown that substance abuse in nursing may mirror the general population, there are subgroups within nursing that are more prone or vulnerable to substance abuse (Dunn, 2005). Nurses who work in critical care settings report more prescription-type substance abuse and easier access to substances in the workplace than noncritical care nurses. One study demonstrated that critical care nurses were more likely than their peers to report using marijuana, cocaine, and binge drinking (Dunn, 2005).

Inadequate Nursing Orientation and Nurse Turnover

The American Association of Critical Care Nurses specifically warns that the impact of nurse turnover has serious implications for the field of critical care because the sickest patients in the hospital require the highest nurse-to-patient ratio. These critically ill patients are likely to need the attention of the most highly trained nursing personnel (National League for Nursing, 2001). Because of their influence on patient safety and health outcomes, nurse turnover has received considerable attention worldwide (Stone et al., 2003). Providing comprehensive orientation programs that prepare the new specialized nurse for his or her role is essential. An effective orientation can provide dividends in staff retention and satisfaction (Thomason, 2006).

Beecroft, Dorey, and Wenten (2007) conducted a study finding that inadequate nurse staffing doubles the risk of unfavorable clinical outcomes. The prospective survey design, in the study, used multiple instruments (over 13) and was conducted from 1999 to 2006 with 889 new nurses. The aim of the study was to determine the relationship of new nurse turnover intent with individual characteristics, work environment variables, and organizational factors. The study also compared new nurse turnover with actual turnover in the 18 months of employment following completion of residency.

The effects of nurse staffing patterns on patient care have stimulated a number of studies that reports links between staffing levels on critical care units and adverse patient outcomes (Archibald, Manning, Bell, Banerjee, & Jarvis, 1997; Blegen et al., 1998; Blegen & Vaughn, 1998; Fridkin, Pear, Williamson, Galgiani, & Jarvis, 1996; Sovie & Jawad, 2001). Recent research has shown that improved nurse staffing ratios can be linked to sizable and significant effects on preventable hospital deaths (Aiken, Clarke, Sloane, Sochalski, & Silber, 2002; Blegen et al., 1998). Aiken et al. (2002) found, in a study of 10,184 staff nurses, that a higher patient–nurse ratio was linked to increased risk of patient mortality. A systematic review of studies conducted by Lang, Hodge, Olson, Romano, and Kravitz (2004) found substantial evidence to support the relationship between adequate staffing levels and lower hospital mortality levels, failure to rescue ratios, and shorter length of stay. A report by McGillis-Hall, Doran, and Pink (2004) found that the use of less experienced nurses resulted in higher numbers of medications errors. The Agency for Healthcare Research and Quality (AHRQ), in its study, revealed the financial burden of adverse events can raise the cost of total treatment by 84%, increase length of stay by 5.1 to 5.4 days, and probability of death by 4.67% to 5.5%.

Replacing a newly oriented nurse is very expensive and affects hospital efficiency. The cost of replacement encompasses recruiting and orienting the new nurses, hiring temporary agency nurses, and supervising new nurses. Turnover rates for new nurses have been reported to be between 35% and 60% (Mathews & Nunley, 1992). The price of such high turnover rates range from 1.2 to 1.3 times the average nurse salary (Jones, 2005). Furthermore, changes in nurse staffing decrease the effectiveness of team-based care on patient units, resulting in less effective working relationships between nurses and physician, and thus ultimately affect patient care (Cangelosi, Markham, & Bounds, 1998; Hassmiller & Cozine, 2006).

Limitations

The lack of scholarly work and research discussing nursing orientation was the biggest limitation to the study. Narrowing the results to correlate with burnout/stress, turnover, and undesirable coping mechanisms increased the difficulty of locating articles.

Summary

The focus on safety by The Joint Commission on Accreditation of Healthcare Organizations and on quality by two reports—*Crossing the Quality Chasm* and *To Err is Human: Building a Safer Health System*—has created public awareness that errors in health care have a large and unacceptable impact on the patient, cost, ethics, and public confidence (Batcheller, Burkham, Armstrong, Chappell, & Carelock, 2004; Hart & Davis, 2011). Critical care nurse interns will be challenged with various stressful clinical situations and dilemmas. Maintaining psychological equilibrium, health, and well-being is an essential part of being a critical care nurse. Nurse interns need to be given the tools and the opportunity to reflect on their work, process their experiences with mentors or trusted peers, and have access to more formal support resources.

The appropriate quality and length of orientation has the potential to increase the novice nurses sense of belonging in the organization and work satisfaction (Winter-Collins & McDaniel, 2000). Studies have shown that new graduate nurses benefit from a structured, customizable, and standard orientation program that focuses on development of critical thinking skills, patient care management, and the enhancement of self-esteem (Thomason, 2006). As the novice nurses develop and gain confidence, they are better able to provide quality care, and everyone wins: nurse, patient, and agency.

CONCEPTUAL MODEL AND ORGANIZATIONAL FRAMEWORK OF THEORY

Patricia Benner began what she described as an articulation project of the knowledge embedded in nursing practice almost 30 years ago. Profound exemplars of nursing practices were uncovered from observations and interviews with clinical nurses during this project that demonstrated that clinical nursing practice was more complex than theories of nursing predict. This constituted a paradigm shift in nursing by claiming that knowledge can be developed in practice, not just applied, and signifying that practice is a way of knowing in its own right. Her work indicated a growing concern with the development of explanatory frameworks for understanding the nature of nursing practice and the development of nursing expertise (Altmann, 2007).

Patricia Benner's participation in the AMICAE research project had two direct outcomes: Her interpretation of the Dreyfus model of skill acquisition led to the theory from novice to expert and to the description of the concepts and competencies of nursing practice. The concepts of novice, advanced beginner, competent, proficient, and expert nurse are relational; and each interrelated step is marked by a progressive increase in clinical knowledge and critical thinking (Benner, Tanner, & Chesla, 1992). Although she continued to explain each step in her theory, she never changed the description for each stage, which is outlined in the following text.

Novice to Expert: Stages of Clinical Competence

Stage 1: Novice

Beginners have had no experience of the situations in which they are expected to perform. Novices are taught rules that help them perform. The rules are context-free and independent of specific cases; hence, the rules tend to be applied universally. The rule-governed behavior typical of the novice is extremely limited and inflexible. As such, novices have no "life experience" in the application of rules.

Stage 2: Advance Beginner

Advanced beginners are those who can demonstrate marginally acceptable performance, those who have coped with enough real situations to note, or to have them pointed out by a mentor, the recurring meaningful situational components. These components require prior experience in actual situations for recognition. Principles to guide actions begin to be formulated. The principles are based on experience.

Stage 3: Competent

Competence, typified by the nurse who has been on the job in the same or similar situations 2 or 3 years, develops when the nurse begins to see his or her actions in terms of long-range goals or plans of which he or she is consciously aware. For the competent nurse, a plan establishes a perspective, and the plan is based on considerable conscious, abstract, analytic contemplation of the problem. The conscious, deliberate planning that is characteristic of this skill level helps achieve efficiency and organization. The competent nurse lacks the speed and flexibility of the proficient nurse but does have a feeling of mastery and the ability to cope with and manage the many contingencies of clinical nursing. The competent person does not yet have enough experience to recognize a situation in terms of an overall picture or in terms of which aspects are more important.

Stage 4: Proficient

The proficient performer perceives situations as a whole rather than in terms of chopped up parts or aspects, and performance is guided by maxims. Proficient nurses understand a situation as a whole because they perceive its meaning in terms of long-term goals. The proficient nurse learns from experience what typical events to expect in a given situation and how plans need to be modified in response to these events. The proficient nurse can now recognize when the expected normal picture does not materialize. This holistic understanding improves the proficient nurse's decision making; it becomes less labored because the nurse now has a perspective on which of the many existing attributes and aspects in the present situation are the important ones. The proficient nurse uses maxims (maxims reflect nuances of the situation) as guides, which reflect what would appear to the competent or novice performer as unintelligible nuances of the situations; they can mean one thing at one time and quite another thing later. Once one has a deep understanding of the situation overall, however, the maxim provides direction as to what must be taken into account.

Stage 5: Expert

The expert performer no longer relies on an analytic principle (rule, guideline, and maxim) to connect his or her understanding of the situation to an appropriate action. The expert nurse, with an enormous background of experience, now has an intuitive grasp of each situation and zeroes in on the accurate region of the problem without wasteful consideration of a large range of unfruitful, alternative diagnoses and solutions. The expert operates from a deep understanding of the total situation. The performer is no longer aware of features and rules, his or her performance becomes fluid and flexible and highly proficient. This is not to say that the expert never uses analytic tools. Highly skilled and analytic ability is necessary for those situations with which the nurse has had no previous experience. Analytic tools are also necessary for those times when the expert gets a wrong grasp of the situation and then finds that events and behaviors are not occurring as expected.

Novice to expert theory was the guide in developing practice change. Within this framework are three aspects of skill acquisition that were used to guide the desired outcomes and help nurses adjust to their role in the ICU. The first is movement from reliance on abstract principles to use of past experiences. Secondly, change in the learner's perception of the situation in terms of equally relevant bits of information to a complete whole in which only certain parts are relevant. Lastly, passage from detached observer to involved performer (Morris et al., 2007).

Evidence-Based Practice Model for Change

Critical thinking skills and evidence-based methods for making clinical decisions are essential for maximizing the quality and cost-effectiveness of care (Rosswurm & Larrabee, 1999). The Rosswurm and Larrabee (1999) EBP model was developed and used to adapt the existing medical EBP to an approach that incorporated a focus on nursing phenomena with the goal of teaching nurses EBP while evaluating changing clinical practice (Pipe, Wellik, Buchda, Hansen, & Martyn, 2005). The six-stage model has been used in primary care settings and was adopted as a standard of care delivery in acute care settings (Melynk & Fineout-Overholt, 2005; Rosswurm & Larrabee, 1999). A description of the model is as follows:

Step 1: Assess Need for Change in Practice

Practitioners collect internal data and compare it with external data. After examining internal data, practitioners assess the need for a change in practice by comparing internal data with external data in benchmarking databases (Rosswurm & Larrabee, 1999). Benchmarking entails collecting comparable performance data and "sharing of performance information to identify operational and clinical practices that lead to the best outcomes" (Czarnecki, 1996).

Step 2: Link Problem with Interventions and Outcomes

Practitioners need to define the problem using the language of standardized classifications and then link the problem with classification of interventions and outcomes. Classification systems help to define the concepts of a science and organize the knowledge (McCloskey, 1995). They also facilitate communications among practitioners, provide standards for determining the effectiveness and cost of care, and identify needed resources (Maas & Johnson, 1998; Rosswurm & Larrabee, 1999).

Step 3: Synthesize Best Evidence

Selected interventions and outcomes are refined. The best research evidence is synthesized and combined with clinical judgment and contextual data. The problem, potential interventions, and desired outcomes become the major variables for reviewing research literature. Steps taken before conducting the literature search include clarifying the specific topic and identifying criteria for including reference in the review (Rosswurm & Larrabee, 1999; Slavin, 1995). In the critical appraisal of the literature, practitioners evaluate the strengths and weaknesses of studies and identify gaps and conflicts in the available knowledge. Practitioners need to consider the feasibility of implementing the findings in their own practice setting. The synthesis only brings together the existing evidence. It cannot create new evidence or knowledge. If the research synthesis indicates sufficient research evidence to support a change in practice with desirable benefits and minimal risks, practitioners can proceed in designing the change (Rosswurm & Larrabee, 1999).

Step 4: Design a Change in Practice

After synthesizing the best evidence, practitioners describe the process variables or detailed sequence of care activities in the change in practice, usually in the format of a protocol, procedure, or standard (Specht, Bergquist, & Frantz, 1995; Steelman, 1995). The practice environment, its resources, and feedback from stakeholders are essential considerations when designing a change. Only activities addresses in the evidence base are included in the protocol (Horsley, Crane, Crabtree, & Wood, 1983; Rosswurm & Larrabee, 1999). Likewise, the protocol is designed to guide care only for populations similar to those in evidence base. The evidence base is used to guide practitioners in identifying anticipated discipline-sensitive and interdisciplinary patient outcomes of the practice change. Those outcomes are clearly delineated as desired outcomes or reduction in undesired outcomes. The more relevant the outcomes are to the organization, the more likely the practice will be accepted (Rosswurm & Larrabee, 1999).

Step 5: Implementing and Evaluating Change in Practice

After the protocol has been in use for the designated time, patient and staff surveys and quality improvement (QI) study are conducted. Then data are analyzed and displayed in charts and bar graphs to facilitate data interpretation. Following analysis, practitioners interpret the results by deciding whether there were differences in the indicators before and after the pilot study. When considering the results, practitioners must remember that outcomes can be affected by numerous factors other than the intervention, such as characteristics of patients, staff, interpersonal aspect of care, and the setting (Rosswurm & Larrabee, 1999; Sidani & Braden, 1998). In addition to QI data, practitioners evaluate the results of staff opinion surveys at participating sites (McCollam, 1995). Endorsement by respected peers is essential for successful implementation of the change in practice (Cook, Greengold, Ellrodt, & Weingarten, 1997; Specht et al., 1995).

The decision to adapt, adopt, or reject the change is based on feedback from staff on the pilot units, managers, and pilot coordinators; QI and survey data; cost data; and recommendations from stakeholders. Feasibility, benefits, and risks are considered when evaluating data. Personnel opinions of the implemented change provide information about acceptability or the need for modifications (McCollam, 1995). QI and cost data indicate whether the care and outcomes improved at a reasonable cost to the system (McCollam, 1995; Rosswurm & Larrabee, 1999; Specht et al., 1995; Steelman, 1995).

Step 6: Integrate and Maintain Change in Practice

If the results of the study support integration of the new practice into standards of care, change strategies are initiated.

Summary

This change project builds on the learner's experiences, provides a standardized learning method, uses task-oriented problem-solving approaches to learning, and uses self-directed learning as an option when advantageous. These methods encompass Benner's model and the three aspects of skill performance, therefore encouraging nurses to advance to a higher level of clinical aptitude.

In the new health-care environment, practitioners can no longer rely solely on clinical experience, pathophysiologic rationale, and opinion-based processes. The Rosswurm and Larrabee (1999) model provides a pragmatic, theory-driven framework for empowering clinicians in the process of EBP. It guides practitioners through the entire process of EBP, beginning with the assessment of the need for change and ending with integration of an evidence-based protocol. This model was chosen for this change project because it facilitates a shift from traditional nursing practice based on intuition to one steeped in scientific evidence.

PROJECT DESIGN

Although graduate nurses have limited experience when they enter nursing practice, they are typically expected to be responsible for a standard patient assignment shortly after they complete orientation. Even if a graduate nurse is not required immediately to care for a severely ill patient, the nurse must at least have the skills to solve urgent and emergent situations that occur unexpectedly in critical care. The purpose of this EBP is to ensure graduate nurses receive a clinical orientation that meets their needs as new nurses and gives them a strong basic foundation in critical care.

Organizational readiness for change was assessed using their Center for Nursing Excellence (CEN). The Center currently has a nursing orientation based on the theoretical framework of Patricia Benner's *From Novice to Expert* (Benner, 1984). They have a nurse "internship" program that lasts 10 weeks but due to current wars lack enough staff to implement it efficiently. The stakeholders considered switching to a standardized competency-based program to reduce the load of the staff educator and scheduling conflicts and to increase reliability (ability of two different educators to teach an identical session with equal results) of the information taught.

No immediate risks are associated with this practice change. The hospital/organization has agreed to absorb the financial costs involved and facilitate space for computerized learning/group sessions. The benefits to the organization are numerous and range from decrease attrition rates to improved patient outcomes.

This evidence-based project will be using a descriptive survey design. The 20 new graduate nurses took a pre- and posttest to validate that they learned the information of the orientation program and took three 2-week post-orientation surveys to assess stress levels, burnout, and turnover intention.

Measurement for adoption of a standardized orientation program to promote competent and safe nursing care in specialized units will be a paper-and-pencil pretest before implementation of the Competency Based Orientation and Credentialing Program for the Registered Nurse in the Perianesthesia Setting (CBO) program, a prospective paper-and-pencil posttest after completion of orientation and completion of three post-orientation surveys to assess stress level, burnout, and turnover intention in this group.

The pre- and posttest originate from the CBO, are made up of CBO chapter quizzes, and are identical with established reliability and validity (American Society of

PeriAnesthesia Nurses [ASPAN], 2011). The post-orientation surveys to be used in the study are the Maslach Burnout Inventory-Human Services Survey (MBI-HSS), the Extended Nurses Stress Scale (ENSS), and the Measure of Job Satisfaction/Intent to Leave Questionnaire (MJS).

The postanesthesia care unit (PACU) also called the *recovery room* is actually a short-term critical care unit (Katz, 2008). Due to the multiple studies currently being undertaken in the critical care unit at the institution, the PACU unit was chosen for this project. Descriptions of the elements of the practice change are as follows.

Orientation Program

This practice change used the CBO program and its corresponding unit assessments. The CBO is a comprehensive, standardized guide to competency and skill development for PACU nurses. It integrates knowledge, skills, and behaviors required to maintain consistent standards of care. The latest and most validated knowledge base for perianesthesia nursing is provided in this product (ASPAN, 2011). Written by perianesthesia experts, the manual can be used to orient the new PACU nurse, or selected chapters can be used for audited skills and annual updates for the entire PACU staff (ASPAN, 2011).

It is a system/concept-based learning program that consists of eight system- and unit-based modules: cardiovascular, airway management, neurological, renal, hypothermia/malignant hyperthermia, moderate sedation/analgesia, nausea/vomiting, multisystem, and EBP (Fig. 16.1). Various media formats are used in CBO, including texts, hands-on demonstration animation, and tests (ASPAN, 2011). The goal of the

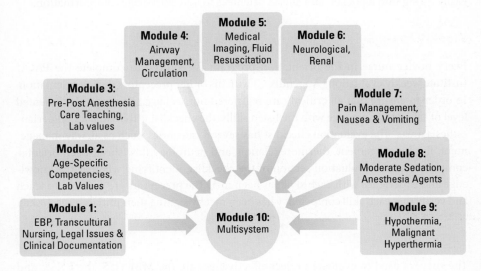

FIGURE 16.1. Structure of PACU Institute.

manual is to provide the perianesthesia nurse with a framework of essential performance criteria. The unique performance criteria establish basic competencies needed
to practice in diverse perianesthesia settings (ASPAN, 2011).

Knowledge Testing

The exam developed from the CBO is a standardized test used to measure basic
knowledge in perianesthesia nursing (Appendix A). It is accepted as one standard
for measuring basic knowledge in PACU nursing. The test is made up of all the CBO
chapter quizzes, and it has 182 items that are divided into 10 subscales based on
the modules. The CBO exam can be used prior to orientation classes in critical care
nursing to identify needed content for the classes and as a pretest and/or posttest to
measure learning in a group of nurses.

Case Studies/Reference Materials

The collection of case studies, with increasing levels of complexity, was developed by
the investigator and the educators (Appendix B). Each case situation contains relevant
patient data and a series of questions with answers so that the educator can easily guide
an orientee to the correct answers. It also contains a blank copy of the situation without
answers so that the orientee can complete it independently and review it later with the
educator. In addition, a collection of critical care reference materials such as normal
and abnormal pulmonary artery and intracranial pressure waveforms, normal ranges
of results of laboratory tests, dysrhythmias, and acid–base disturbances will be given
to each orientee. It was sized to accommodate data fitting on 3 in. $\times$ 5 in. index cards,
easily fitting into a pocket, and allows orientees to add extra pages of information.

Weekly Evaluations

Every novice nurse in the orientation program is required to complete the PACU
Institute weekly evaluation (Appendix C) with his or her preceptors during orientation.
In order to ensure that all critical care registered nurses have achieved a documented
level of safe PACU practice with the listed skills, the checklist is the same for all perianesthesia areas. The evaluation checklist has several categories, such as airway management, fluid management, thermoregulation, and neurology flow sheet. Each orientee
completes the self-evaluation section of the checklist, identifying whether the knowledge and experience with each skill has been met. The preceptors are required to teach
and verify that each skill competency has been met by signing their initials by each skill.

Surveys/Instruments

The surveys used to evaluate project effectiveness are the MBI-HSS, the ENSS, and
the MJS/Intent to Leave Questionnaire.

Maslach Burnout Inventory-Human Services Survey—Measured the Independent Variable of Job Burnout

The MBI-HSS is designed to assess the three components of the burnout syndrome: emotional exhaustion, depersonalization, and reduced personal accomplishment (Appendix D). There are 22 items, which are divided into the aforementioned three subscales. The items are written in the form of statements about personal feelings or attitudes (e.g., "I feel burned out from my work," "I don't really care what happens to some patients."). The items are answered in terms of the frequency with the participant experiences these feelings on a 7-point, fully anchored scale (ranging from 0 [*never*] to 6 [*every day*]) (Zalaquett & Wood, 1997).

Internal consistency was estimated by Cronbach coefficient alpha ($n = 1,316$). The reliability coefficients for the subscales were the following: .90 for emotional exhaustion, .79 for depersonalization, and .71 for personal accomplishment. The standard error of measurement for each subscale is as follows: 3.80 for emotional exhaustion, 3.16 for depersonalization, and 3.73 for personal accomplishment. Convergent validity was demonstrated in several ways. First, an individual's MBI scores were correlated with behavioral ratings made independently by a person who knew the individual well (i.e., spouse or coworkers). Second, MBI scores were correlated with the presence of certain job characteristics that were expected to contribute to experienced burnout. Third, MBI scores were correlated with measures of various outcomes that had been hypothesized to be related to burnout. All three sets of correlations provided substantial evidence for the validity of the MBI (Maslach et al., 1996).

Extended Nurse Stress Scale—Measured the Independent Variable of Job Stress

The ENSS is an expanded and updated revision of the classic NSS developed by Gray-Toft and Anderson (1981) (Appendix E). It contains 57 items in nine subscales: (1) death and dying, (2) conflict with physicians, (3) inadequate emotional preparation, (4) problems relating to peers, (5) problems relating to supervisors, (6) work load, (7) uncertainty concerning treatment, (8) patients and their families, and (9) discrimination. The responses are (1) "never stressful," (2) "occasionally stressful," (3) "frequently stressful," (4) "extremely stressful," and (5) "does not apply." (French, Lenton, Walters, & Eyles, 2000).

Internal consistency reliability was assessed using Cronbach coefficient alpha. The 57-item ENSS demonstrated improved reliability (.96) (French et al., 2000) over the original NSS (.89) (Gray-Toft & Anderson, 1981). Individual subscale reliability ranged from .88 (problems with supervisors) to .65 (discrimination). Discriminant validity of the ENSS was examined by computing product moment correlations with overall life stress ($r = .17$, $p < .001$) and health problems index ($r = .34$, $p < .01$) (French et al., 2000).

Measure of Job Satisfaction/Intent to Leave Questionnaire—Measured the Independent Variable of Job Satisfaction and Intent to Leave

The MJS is a multidimensional instrument designed for use in acute nursing (Appendix F). It has 44 items on eight subscales: (1) personal satisfaction, (2) satisfaction with workload, (3) satisfaction with professional support, (4) satisfaction with training, (5) satisfaction with pay, (6) satisfaction with prospects, (7) satisfaction with standards of care, and (8) intent to leave. The stem question is, "How satisfied are you this aspect of your job?" Respondents are asked to rate their degree of job satisfaction on a 5-point Likert scale, ranging from "very satisfied" to "very dissatisfied," including a neutral response choice (Traynor & Wade, 1993).

Reliability was assessed using Cronbach alpha. The 44-item test showed good reliability ranging from .85 to .95, and internal consistency is .93. For validation, Traynor and Wade (1993) correlated the instrument with a Price Waterhouse instrument, an instrument that covers work factors such as work volume, working relations, career development, etc.—convergent validity is .83 (Van Saane, Sluitter, Verbeek, & Frings-Dresen, 2003).

Summary

This practice change was designed to systematically incorporate concepts from the previous weeks so that the orientee gradually assimilates to the knowledge required in the PACU environment. A survey design was used to test the independent variables of stress, burnout, and intent to leave employment in a sample of 20 newly graduated nurses working in the PACU. The variables were measured with the MBI-HSS, ENSS, and MJS, which all have adequate reliability and validity. This project design was chosen because it would best illustrate the outcomes using tests to measure knowledge, along with the surveys measuring stress, burnout, and turnover intention.

IMPLEMENTATION PROCEDURES AND PROCESS

The quality and safety of care is associated with various factors within a nursing system and nursing work preparedness—the combination of which influences the type of quality and safety of care provided by nurses (Hughes, 2008; Institute of Medicine, 2004). Structures, processes, and outcomes are interdependent, where specific attributes of one influence another according to the strength of the relationship. When organizational structure within nursing supports the care processes and enables collaboration to change antiquated processes, nurses as a result are more satisfied with their jobs, and patients receive higher quality care. The effectiveness of individuals and teamwork is dependent on leadership, shared understanding of goals and individuals roles, effective and frequent communication, and being empowered by the organization (Hughes, 2008). The procedures and processes of this project were built on communication, teamwork, and intraprofessional collaboration and are as follows.

Plan

The planning stage lasted from January 10, 2011 until May 16, 2011. The memorandum of understanding (MOU) was facilitated through Pat Markham of Chatham University's nursing department and signed by Walter B. Fowler, vice president of finance and administration, and Admiral (Dr.) M. L. Nathan. The first meeting was on January 17, 2011 with my preceptor LCDR Angela Stanley, NP-clinical nurse specialist of pediatrics—discussed Chapters 1 and 2 of capstone and subsequent meetings with nursing administrators. The second meeting was on January 24, 2011 with Captain C. K. Gallagher, NP, department head for programs of nursing excellence—discussed nursing departments desired to revise their current nursing orientation (called the *nursing internship program*) to include the CBO program. The third meeting was on January 31, 2011 with LCDR Rhonda Hines, General Education office, to get credentialed and obtain security clearance. The fourth meeting was on February 1, 2011 with LCDR Bridgette Ferguson, NP, manager of nurse internship program. The nurse internship program was further discussed in detail. During the meeting, ideal placement for implementation of the project was determined to be postanesthesia care unit (PACU) and approval was given by Capt. Gallagher. The fifth meeting was on February 8, 2011 with CDR Deborah Jenkins, RN, Department Head of PACU—discussed the scope of PACU and her views on the problems with new graduate nurses on the unit. The sixth meeting was on February 16, 2011 with Lt. Aron Bowlin, clinical nurse specialist (CNS) of the PACU. In our meetings, we reviewed authors' capstone project to date and decided on the best design and implementation strategy. The initial design was discussed with LCDR Angela Stanley (preceptor) and presented to Capt. Gallagher and CDR Jenkins on April 4, 2011. It was preliminarily approved for implementation on April 4, 2011. The author and Lt. Bowlin developed 10 case studies to use in the weekly group sessions.

Process

After several meetings with the directors, managers, and staff educators from the PACU, project approval was given on May 16, 2011. It was decided to call this project the PACU Institute (Fig. 16.2). The project was implemented until May 30, 2011, when a request for a more detailed project review by the Scientific Review Panel (SRP) put the project on hold. The orientation program continued through a joint effort between the chief nurse executive (CNE) and the PACU unit. After completing the review process, SRP approval was granted on June 22, 2011, and the project resumed on June 28, 2011.

All nurses had already completed general hospital/nursing orientation and signed the participant consent form (Appendix G) before starting the courses. A CBO pretest was given to all nurses prior to starting the orientation program. Beginning in week 1, the graduate nurses in PACU began learning PACU concepts with the CBO program. Each week, a new module was introduced with a fluid approach, progressively

Date (s)	Weeks	Module	Group Sessions
May 23–27, 2011	Week 1	EBP, Transcultural Nursing, Legal Issues and Clinical Document	PACU Documentation
May 30–June 3, 2011	Week 2	Age-Specific Competencies, Lab Values	Recognizing Lab Values
June 6–10, 2011	Week 3	Pre/Post Care Teaching, Lab Values	Perianesthesia History and Assessment
June 13–17, 2011	Week 4	Airway Management, Circulation	Hemodynamic Monitoring/ Waveforms
June 20–24, 2011	Week 5	Medical Imaging, Fluid Resuscitation	Fluid Resuscitation
June 27–July 1, 2011	Week 6	Neurological, Renal	Neurological and Renal Changes
July 4–8, 2011	Week 7	Pain Management, Nausea/ Vomiting	Pain Assessment and Intervention
July 11–15, 2011	Week 8	Moderate Sedation/Analgesia, Anesthesia Agents	General Inhalation/ Intravenous Agents
July 18–22, 2011	Week 9	Hypothermia, Malignant Hyperthermia	Hypothermia/Hyperthermia in PACU Patients
July 25–29, 2011	Week 10	Multisystem	Multisystem Disorders

FIGURE 16.2. PACU Institute timeline.

building on the prior week. The nurses attended at least one group session focused on application of the critical care information reviewed in the corresponding module. During the clinical group sessions, PACU concepts (e.g., airway management module—managing a patient with an artificial airway) were illustrated in case study discussions with the nurse educators, simulated demonstrations, and teaching rounds in the PACU (see Fig. 16.2).

At the conclusion of the 6-week didactic orientation program, all the participants were given the CBO posttest and required to have a score of at least 80% to verify the

TABLE 16.1. Gender Analysis

		Frequency	Percentage	Valid Percentage	Cumulative Percentage
Valid	Male	7	35.0	35.0	35.0
	Female	13	65.0	65.0	100.0
	Total	**20**	**100.0**	**100.0**	

minimum amount of knowledge gained. If a score of 80% was achieved, the participant was then paired with a preceptor to begin working with patients. Two weeks after passage of the posttest, the nurses were asked to complete the three surveys to assess if the orientation program prepared them enough to decrease levels of stress, burnout, and decreased turnover intention.

Summary

The planning phase of this project used intraprofessional collaboration to effectively use EBP research to change novice nurse orientation. Changes in the "status quo" of nursing are needed to realize quality and safety improvements. Errors, particularly adverse events, are caused by the cumulative effects of smaller errors within nursing structures and processes of care. Focusing on a systemic approach of change focuses on those factors in the chain of events leading to errors and adverse events (Reason, 1997).

From a "systems" approach in tackling nursing orientation, avoidable errors are targeted through key strategies such as a standardized orientation program, longer didactic orientation time frame, and intraprofessional communication—all of which has the potential to institutionalize a culture of safety, provide nurse-sensitive but patient-centered care, and use EBP with the objective of managing uncertainty (i.e., stress, burnout, and turnover intention) and the goal of improvement (better patient outcomes).

EVALUATION AND OUTCOMES OF PRACTICE CHANGE INITIATIVE

The purpose of this EBP change was to increase didactic nursing orientation to a minimum of 10 weeks using a standardized orientation program, thereby reducing the levels of stress, burnout, and turnover intention among new graduate nurses. Based on prior research, the author chose the CBO program and used three surveys to analyze stress, burnout, and turnover intention in the participants. This section will discuss the evaluation and outcomes of a 10-week orientation program on stress, burnout, and turnover intention.

Demographics

The participants of this project were 20 new graduate nurses ($N = 20$), all graduates of 4-year program, who accepted employment in the PACU unit(s). In the sample of 20 nurses, 7 (35%) were male and 13 (65%) were female (Table 16.1).

There was a wide assortment of ages among the participants in this project. The ages ranged from 25 to 44 years of age. Eighteen participants (90%) who comprised the highest percentage of participants were 34 years of age or younger. Due to military age restrictions for this branch of service, the age limit for enlistment/officer

TABLE 16.2. Age Analysis

		Frequency	Percentage	Valid Percentage	Cumulative Percentage
Valid	Under 25	10	50.0	50.0	50.0
	25–34	8	40.0	40.0	90.0
	35–44	2	10.0	10.0	100.0
	Total	**20**	**100.0**	**100.0**	

commissioning is 34 years old; the two participants (10%) who were older than age 34, received commissioning waivers for prior enlistment (Table 16.2).

Orientation Program Analysis

In order to participate in the project, all of the nurses had to complete a pre- and post-knowledge testing. The knowledge testing was used to assess baseline PACU knowledge and post-CBO program knowledge retention. A score of 80% was required in order to achieve passing on the exam. The average overall percentage on the pretest was 55.6%, whereas the average overall percentage of the posttest was 85% after completion of the orientation program (Table 16.3). The parametric procedure for testing differences in groups, the paired t test, was used to determine the statistical significance of the practice change intervention. The standard deviation (SD) of the scores ranged from 5.76 to 12.60, and the results of the test showed a p value of .0001, significance beyond the 0.1 level, which signifies statistical significance of the practice change intervention.

Survey Analysis

To determine the impact of the CBO program on the novice nurses stress/burnout levels and turnover intention, a descriptive survey design was used. Two weeks post-orientation, all the participants completed the three surveys to assess how the CBO program prepared them for the practice of PACU nursing. Three different

TABLE 16.3. Statistical Analysis of Orientation Program

		Mean	N	Standard Deviation	Statistical Significance
Pair 1	Pretest	55.5500	20	12.59689	
	Posttest	85.1000	20	5.76651	
	p Value				**0.0001**

methods of analyzing the data were employed for this project. Frequency distribution was used to show a systematic arrangement of values for each question from the lowest to highest; together with a count of number of times, each value was obtained. Cross tabulation was used in determining the number of cases occurring when two variables are considered simultaneously. Lastly, Pearson's r was used to determine if the relationships between two variables were statistically significant.

Maslach Burnout Inventory-Human Services Survey

The MBI was scored by adding the sum of the responses on the Likert scale. High burnout is determined by a score of 27 or over, moderate burnout is determined by a score of 17 to 26, and low burnout is determined by a score of 0 to 16. Results showed that 16 of the participants (80%) had low burnout levels, 3 participants (15%) had moderate burnout levels, and 1 participant (5%) had high burnout levels (Table 16.4).

Extended Nurses Stress Scale

Three out of nine subscales where analyzed for this project: the subscales of inadequate preparation, workload, and uncertainty concerning treatment were used. To compute the total stress score, all items of the scale are added together, and the higher the score, the greater the frequency of stress on the subscale. The question of each item is the header of each table. Analyses of the scores according to the subscales are as follows:

Inadequate Preparation Subscale (Items 3, 11, and 19). Eighty-five percent to 95% of the participants found their preparation caused no or occasional stress (Tables 16.5 to 16.7).

Workload (Item 57). All the participants found that having to make quick patient decisions was particularly stressful (Table 16.8).

Uncertainty Concerning Treatment (Items 18, 29, 33, 39, and 43). Eighty percent to 100% of the participants felt little to no stress when having to make decisions on patient care (Tables 16.9 to 16.13).

TABLE 16.4. Maslach Burnout Inventory-Human Services Survey Analysis

		Frequency	Percentage	Valid Percentage	Cumulative Percentage
Valid	High burnout	1	5.0	5.0	5.0
	Moderate burnout	3	15.0	15.0	20.0
	Low burnout	16	80.0	80.0	100.0
	Total	**20**	**100.0**	**100.0**	

TABLE 16.5. Item 3: Feeling Inadequately Prepared to Help with the Emotional Needs of a Patient's Family

		Frequency	Percentage	Valid Percentage	Cumulative Percentage
Valid	Never stressful	4	20.0	20.0	20.0
	Occasionally stressful	15	75.0	75.0	95.0
	Frequently stressful	1	5.0	5.0	100.0
	Total	**20**	**100.0**	**100.0**	

TABLE 16.6. Item 11: Being Asked a Question by a Patient for Which I Do Not Have a Satisfactory Answer

		Frequency	Percentage	Valid Percentage	Cumulative Percentage
Valid	Occasionally stressful	7	35.0	35.0	35.0
	Frequently stressful	10	50.0	50.0	85.0
	Always stressful	3	15.0	15.0	100.0
	Total	**20**	**100.0**	**100.0**	

TABLE 16.7. Item 19: Feeling Inadequately Prepared to Help with the Emotional Needs of a Patient

		Frequency	Percentage	Valid Percentage	Cumulative Percentage
Valid	Never stressful	10	50.0	50.0	50.0
	Occasionally stressful	7	35.0	35.0	85.0
	Frequently stressful	3	15.0	15.0	100.0
	Total	**20**	**100.0**	**100.0**	

TABLE 16.8. Item 57: Having to Make Decisions under Pressure

		Frequency	Percentage	Valid Percentage	Cumulative Percentage
Valid	Occasionally stressful	11	55.0	55.0	55.0
	Frequently stressful	9	45.0	45.0	100.0
	Total	**20**	**100.0**	**100.0**	

TABLE 16.9. Items 18: Fear of Making a Mistake in Treating a Patient

		Frequency	Percentage	Valid Percentage	Cumulative Percentage
Valid	Occasionally stressful	1	5.0	5.0	5.0
	Frequently stressful	7	35.0	35.0	40.0
	Always stressful	12	60.0	60.0	100.0
	Total	**20**	**100.0**	**100.0**	

TABLE 16.10. Item 29: Feeling Inadequately Trained for What I Have to Do

		Frequency	Percentage	Valid Percentage	Cumulative Percentage
Valid	Never stressful	16	80.0	80.0	80.0
	Occasionally stressful	4	20.0	20.0	100.0
	Total	**20**	**100.0**	**100.0**	

TABLE 16.11. Item 33: Not Knowing What a Patient or a Patient's Family Ought to Be Told about the Patient's Condition and Its Treatment

		Frequency	Percentage	Valid Percentage	Cumulative Percentage
Valid	Never stressful	6	30.0	30.0	30.0
	Occasionally stressful	14	70.0	70.0	100.0
	Total	**20**	**100.0**	**100.0**	

TABLE 16.12. Item 39: Being in Charge with Inadequate Experience

		Frequency	Percentage	Valid Percentage	Cumulative Percentage
Valid	**Does not apply**	**20**	**100.0**	**100.0**	**100.0**

TABLE 16.13. Item 43: Uncertainty Regarding the Operation and Functioning of Specialized Equipment

		Frequency	Percentage	Valid Percentage	Cumulative Percentage
Valid	Never stressful	10	50.0	50.0	50.0
	Occasionally stressful	10	50.0	50.0	100.0
	Total	**20**	**100.0**	**100.0**	

TABLE 16.14. Job Satisfaction/Attrition

		Frequency	Percentage	Valid Percentage	Cumulative Percentage
Valid	No	19	95.0	95.0	95.0
	Yes	1	5.0	5.0	100.0
	Total	**20**	**100.0**	**100.0**	

Measure of Job Satisfaction/Intent to Leave Questionnaire

Only one question was analyzed for the practice change. The question asked intent to leave and overall job satisfaction. Ninety-five percent of the participants had no intention of leaving the unit and were satisfied with their orientation (Table 16.14).

Discussion

The basic concept is that stress relates to both an individual's perception of the demands being made on them and to their perception of their capability to meet those demands (McVicar, 2003). The nurses in the study were analyzed based on their perception of the orientation program and how it affected the level of stress, burn-out, and turnover intention. The results showed longer and standardized orientation seemed to positively affect job satisfaction and intent to leave in nurses that participated in this study. Question 29 of the ENSS, *feeling inadequately trained for what I have to do*, best accurately depicts the nurses' opinion of the orientation program, and 80% responded with no stress in feeling adequately prepared. When this question is correlated with job satisfaction and turnover intent, it shows a statistical significance of $r = 0.05$ (Table 16.15).

TABLE 16.15. Extended Nurses Stress Scale Question 29 and Job Satisfaction/Attrition Correlation

		Question 29	Job Satisfaction/Intent to Leave
Question 29	Pearson correlation	1	.459*
	Significance (2-tailed)		.042
	N	20	20
Job Satisfaction/Attrition	Pearson correlation	.459*	1
	Significance (2-tailed)	.042	
	N	20	20

*Correlation is significant at the 0.05 level (2-tailed).

TABLE 16.16. Burnout and Job Satisfaction/Attrition Correlation

		Job Satisfaction/ Intent to Leave	Burnout
Job Satisfaction/Attrition	Pearson correlation	1	−.749*
	Significance (2-tailed)		.000
	N	20	20
Burnout	Pearson correlation	−.749*	1
	Significance (2-tailed)	.000	
	N	20	20

*Correlation is significant at the 0.01 level (2-tailed).

When Question 29, *feeling inadequately trained for what I have to do*, is positively correlated with burnout, it shows a statistical significance of $r = 0.01$ (Table 16.16).

When analyzing the data through cross tabulation, it was clear that 95% of the nurses, who passed the orientation program, felt little to no stress when questioning their level of PACU knowledge and had low to moderate levels of burnout (Table 16.17).

In the current research, the relationships between job stress, job satisfaction, and intent to leave were not examined within the same analysis model, although the correlations between these outcome variables were all found to be significant. This result is consistent with several models of turnover in nursing literature and includes job satisfaction as a significant predictor of turnover (Irvine & Evans, 1995; Parasuraman, 1989; Tourangeau & Cranley, 2006). When adding the mediator of an orientation program, studies show it improves role clarity, enhances organizational commitment, increases job satisfaction, and decreases attrition (Butt et al., 2002; Crimlisk, McNulty, & Fancione, 2002; Meyer, 1997; Snow, 2002).

TABLE 16.17. Job Satisfaction/Attrition (Question 29) and Burnout Cross Tabulation

Burnout			Question 29		Total
			Never stressful	Occasionally stressful	
High burnout	Job Satisfaction/Attrition	Yes		1	1
	Total			1	1
Moderate burnout	Job Satisfaction/Attrition	No	3		3
	Total		3		3
Low burnout	Job Satisfaction/Attrition	No	13	3	16
	Total		13	3	16

Summary

This section presented the statistical analysis of the data collected from the CBO exams, MBI-HSS, ENSS, and MJS scales. The setting, age, and sex of the nurses had no bearing on the outcome of this project. After analyzing the data obtained from this EBP change, results showed that novice nurses benefit from a standardized orientation program. The end result of an adequate orientation program is evidenced by decreased stress and burnout levels and decreased attrition. Thus, this practice change contributes to the current evidence on the importance of an adequate orientation program for novice nurses.

IMPLICATIONS, LIMITATIONS, AND RECOMMENDATIONS OF PRACTICE CHANGE

This section presents the implications of this change initiative in nursing practice, administration, and education. Recommendations are discussed for each area.

Nursing Administration

For nurse administrators, using EBP research to understand the best practices in PACU nursing orientation could provide information on how best to meet the needs of all nurses regardless of specialty. Comparison of the correlations among the variables indicates that reducing stress may not be as important as increasing job satisfaction and staff retention. In this sample, job stress did not correlate with either job satisfaction or with intent to leave employment. However, nurses who demonstrated higher job satisfaction had less intent to leave their current employment. Because these units require specialized skills and orientation, replacement of staff can prove difficult and costly. Retention of staff is a primary strategy in the current and future nursing shortage and ensuring quality of care.

Nursing Practice

Nurses in clinical practice need to be aware of the impact that an adequate or inadequate nursing orientation has on levels of stress and satisfaction in their specialties. The effort given in obtaining standard level knowledge bases in orientation has the potential to reduce overall stress (on the unit), raise the level of expertise, and promote retention and group cohesiveness. It can also result in both increased quality of work environment and quality of care.

Nursing Education

For nurse educators and clinical nurse specialists, the results of the study suggest that they may need to teach skills in areas that increase nurse satisfaction.

Offering an EBP, standardized orientation program that increases and updates their clinical skills is important for nurses to feel prepared for their area of practice. However, consideration should also be given to teaching skills that promote working relationships including communication, conflict management, group interaction, and leadership and emotional preparation for difficult patient and family interactions.

Summary

In examining stress, burnout, and turnover intention among new graduate nurses in specialized units, there was a relationship between these concepts when assessing new graduate orientation. Today's hospital environment with its high-acuity patients and an increasingly novice nursing workforce necessitates tailored orientation programs that account for the unique learning needs of advanced beginner graduate nurses, giving the nurses a solid foundation in application of concepts and as much practice with clinical and time management skills as possible. Nursing education and administration should realize, if only from the evidence, that a change from traditional didactic orientations (less than 4 weeks) to one that has clear expectations, incremental learning, and consistent knowledge verification (lasting more than 10 weeks) will meet the needs of all graduate nurses.

SUMMARY

There is nothing like working on a specialized unit—the pace of change is accelerating, bombarding nurses in acute and critical care with new technology and medications, evolving care delivery models, expanded nursing roles, integrated computerized systems, and various ethical issues and challenges. Amidst all this change is a growing international nursing shortage. Coupled with a heavy physical workload, an emotionally draining environment and the need to maintain unrelenting, vigilant watch over their patients, today's acute and critical care nurses often fail to question their practices, holding tightly to traditions.

EBP is the key to this problem. Research has shown without current best evidence, practice is rapidly outdated, often to the detriment of patients. This practice change serves as evidence to indicate that health-care providers who use an evidence-based approach on delivering patient care experience higher levels of satisfaction than those who deliver care steeped in tradition. With the results of this practice change, recent reports of pervasive burnout among health-care professionals and the pressure that many influential health-care organizations exert on providers to deliver high-quality, safe care under increasingly heavy patient loads; the use and teaching of EBP may be a key not only on providing outstanding care to patients and saving health-care dollars but also on reducing the escalating turnover rate in health-care professions.

The foundation that the PACU Institute has provided will prove importance in areas of the hospital other than specialized units; it can also serve as a template for major changes to the way orientation is provided in other nursing units. Using standardized orientation programs will allow nurse administrators, nurse educators, and organizations to address some of the challenges facing new graduate critical care/PACU nurses. Using programs such as the CBO will result in a more coordinated, consistent orientation experience for all stakeholders involved. Comprehensive didactic programs could help prepare each graduate nurse to be not only a nurse who gives safe care but also a nurse who will soon be able to anticipate complications and rescue patients.

REFERENCES

Aiken, L. H., Clarke, S. P., Sloane, D. M., Sochalski, J., & Silber, J. H. (2002). Hospital nurse staffing and patient mortality, nurse burnout, and job dissatisfaction. *Journal of the American Medical Association, 288*(16), 1987–1993.

Altmann, T. K. (2007). An evaluation of the seminal work of Patricia Benner: Theory or philosophy? *Contemporary Nurse, 25,* 114–123.

American Society of PeriAnesthesia Nurses. (2011). *A competency based orientation and credentialing program for the registered nurse in the perianesthesia setting-2009 edition.* Cherry Hill, NJ: Author.

Archibald, L. K., Manning, M. L., Bell, L. M., Banerjee, S., & Jarvis, W. R. (1997). Patient density, nurse-patient ratio and nosocomial infection risk in a pediatric cardiac intensive care unit. *Pediatric Infectious Disease Journal, 16*(11), 1045–1048.

Badger, J. M. (2008). Critical care nurse intern program: Addressing psychological reactions related to critical care nursing. *Critical Care Nursing Quality, 31*(2), 184–187.

Batcheller, J., Burkman, K., Armstrong, D., Chappell, C., & Carelock, J. L. (2004). A practice model for patient safety. *Journal of Nursing Administration, 34*(4), 200–205.

Beecroft, P. C., Dorey, F., & Wenten, M. (2007). Turnover intention in new graduate nurses: A multivariate analysis. *Journal of Advanced Nursing, 62*(1), 41–52.

Benner, P. (1984). *From novice to expert: Excellence and power in clinical nursing practice.* Menlo Park, CA: Addison-Wesley.

Benner, P., Tanner, C., & Chesla, C. (1992). From beginner to expert: Gaining a differentiated clinical world in critical care nursing. *Advance Nursing Science, 14,* 13–28.

Blegen, M. A., Goode, C. J., & Reed, L. (1998). Nurse staffing and patient outcomes. *Nursing Residency, 47*(1), 43–50.

Blegen, M. A., & Vaughn, T. A. (1998). A multisite study of nurse staffing and patient occurrences. *Nursing Economics, 16*(4), 196–203.

Boswell, S., & Wilhoit, K. (2004). New nurses' perceptions of nursing practice and quality patient care. *Journal of Nursing Care Quality, 19*(1), 76–81.

Butt, M., Baumann, A., O'Brien-Pallas, L., Deber, R., Blythe, J., & DiCenso, A. (2002). The learning needs of nurses experiencing job change. *Journal of Continuing Education in Nursing, 33*(2), 67–73.

Cangelosi, J. D., Markham, F. S., & Bounds, W. T. (1998). Factors related to nurse retention and turnover: An updated study. *Health Marketing Quarterly, 15*(3), 25–43.

Cook, D. J., Greengold, N. L., Ellrodt, A. G., & Weingarten, S. R. (1997). The relation between systematic reviews and practice guidelines. *Annuals of Internal Medicine, 127*(3), 210–216.

Crimlisk, J. R., McNulty, M. J., & Fancione, D. A. (2002). New graduate RNs in a float pool: An inner-city hospital experience. *Journal of Nursing Administration, 32*(4), 211–217.

Czarnecki, M. T. (1996). Benchmarking: A data-oriented look at improving health care performance. *Journal of Nursing Care Quality, 10*(3), 1–6.

Davies, W. (2008). Mindful meditation: Healing burnout in critical care nursing. *Holistic Nurse Practice, 22*(1), 32–36.

Dunn, D. (2005). Substance abuse among nurses—Defining the issue. *Journal of American Operating Room Nurses, 82*(4), 572–596.

Elbright, P., Urden, L., Patterson, E., & Chalko, B. (2004). Themes surrounding novice nurse near miss and adverse-event situations. *Journal of Nursing Administration, 34*(11), 531–538.

Foley, B. J., Kee, C. C., Minick, P., Harvey, S. S., & Jennings, B. M. (2002). Characteristics of nurses and hospital work environments that foster satisfaction and clinical expertise. *Journal of Nursing Administration, 32*(5), 273–281.

French, S. E., Lenton, R., Walters, V., & Eyles, J. (2000). An empirical evaluation of an expanded nursing stress scale. *Journal of Nursing Measurement, 8*(2), 161–178.

Fridkin, S. K., Pear, S. M., Williamson, T. H., Galgiani, J. N, & Jarvis, W. R. (1996). The role of understaffing in central venous catheter-associated bloodstream infections. *Infection Control in Hospital Epidemiology, 17*(3), 150–158.

Gray-Toft, P., & Anderson, J. G. (1981). The nursing stress scale: Development of an instrument. *Journal of Behavioral Assessment, 3*(1), 11–23.

Greco, P., Laschinger, H. K., & Wong, C. (2006). Leader empowering behaviors, staff nurse empowerment and work engagement/burnout. *Nursing Leadership, 19*(4), 41–56.

Hamel, E. J. (1990). *An interpretive study of the professional socialization of neophyte nurses into the nursing subculture* (Unpublished doctoral dissertation). University of San Diego, CA.

Hampton, D. C., Griffith, D., & Howard, A. (2005). Evidence-based clinical improvement for mechanically ventilated patients. *Rehabilitation Nursing, 30*, 160–165.

Hart, P., & Davis, N. (2011). Effects of nursing care and staff skill mix on patient care outcomes within acute care nursing units. *Journal of Nursing Care Quality, 26*(2), 161–168.

Hassmiller, S. B., & Cozine, M. (2006). Addressing the nurse shortage to improve the quality of patient care. *Health Affairs, 25*(1), 268–274.

Horsley, J., Crane, J., Crabtree, M. K., & Wood, D. (1983). *Using research to improve nursing practice: A guide.* New York, NY: Grune & Straton.

Hughes, R. G. (Ed.). (2008). *Patient safety and quality: An evidence-based handbook for nurses.* Rockville, MD: Agency for Healthcare Research and Quality.

Ihelenfeld, J. T. (2005). Hiring and mentoring graduate nurses in the intensive care unit. *Dimensions in Critical Care Nursing, 24*(4), 175–178.

Institute of Medicine. (1999). *To err is human: Building a safer health system.* Washington, DC: Author.

Institute of Medicine. (2004). *Keeping patients safe: Transforming the work environment of nurses.* Washington, DC: National Academies Press.

Irvine, D. M., & Evans, M. G. (1995). Job satisfaction and turnover among nurses: Integrating research findings across studies. *Nursing Research, 44*(4), 246–253.

Jasper, M. (1996). The first year as a staff nurse: The experiences of a first cohort of Project 2000 nurses in a demonstration district. *Journal of Advanced Nursing, 24*, 771–778.

Jones, C. B. (2005). The costs of nurse turnover, Part 2: Application of the nursing turnover cost calculation method. *Journal of Nursing Administration, 35*, 41–49.

Katz, M. J. (2008). *Post anesthesia care of adults.* Comptche, CA: Wild Iris Medical Education.

Kelly, B. (1996). Hospital nursing: "It's a battle!" A follow-up study of English graduate nurses. *Journal of Advance Nursing, 24*(5), 1063–1069.

Kelly, M., & Mynatt, S. (2000). Addiction among nurses: Does the health care industry compound the problem? *Health Care Management Review, 15,* 3–42.

Kim, H. K., Ji, H. S., Ryu, E. K., Lee, H. J., Yun, S. E., Jeon, M. K, et al. (2005). Factors influencing on burnout of the nurses in hospitals. *Clinical Nursing Research, 10*(2), 7–18.

Kirchhoff, K. T., & Dahl, N. (2006). American Association of Critical Care Nurses' national survey of facilities and units providing critical care. *American Journal of Critical Care, 15,* 13–27.

Kovner, C., & Gergen, P. (1998). Staffing levels and adverse events following surgery in U.S. hospitals. *Image, 30*(1), 315–321.

Lang, T. A., Hodge, M., Olson, V., Romano, P. S., & Kravitz, R. L. (2004). Nurse-patient ratios. *Journal of Nursing Administration, 34*(7–8), 326–337.

Laschinger, H., & Leiter, M. (2006). The impact of nursing work environments on patient safety outcomes: The mediating the role of burnout/engagement. *The Journal of Nursing Administration, 36*(5), 259–267.

Lazarus, R. S., & Folkman, S. (1984). Stress, appraisal, and coping. New York, NY: Springer.

Maas, M., & Johnson, M. (1998). Nursing outcomes accountability. *Outcomes Management for Nursing Practice, 2*(1), 3–5.

Maslach, C., Jackson, S. E., & Leiter, M. P. (1996). *The Maslach Burnout Inventory* (3rd ed.). Palo Alto, CA: Consulting Psychologists Press.

Mathews, J. J., & Nunley, C. (1992). Rejuvenating orientation to increase more satisfaction and retention. *Journal of Nursing Staffing Development, 8,* 159–164.

McCall, J. A. (2002). Progressive critical care education-in our unit. *Critical Care Nursing, 22*(4), 87–88.

McCloskey, J. C. (1995). Help to make nursing visible. *Image: Journal of Nursing Scholarship, 27,* 170–175.

McCollam, M. E. (1995). Evaluation and implementation of a research-based falls assessment innovation. *Nursing Clinics of North America, 30*(3), 507–514.

McGillis-Hall, L., Doran, D., Baker, G. R., Pink, G. H., Sidani, S., O'Brien-Pallas L., & Donner, G. J. (2003). Nurse staffing models as predictors of patient outcomes. *Medical Care, 41*(9), 1069–1109.

McGillis-Hall, L., Doran, D., & Pink, G. H. (2004). Nurse staffing models, nurse hours, and patient safety outcomes. *Journal of Nursing Administration, 34*(1), 41–45.

McGirr, M., & Bakker, D. A. (2000). Shaping positive work environments for nurses: The contributions of nurses at various organizational levels. *Canada Journal of Nursing Leadership, 13*(1), 7–14.

McVicar, A. (2003). Workplace stress in nursing: A literature review. *Journal of Advanced Nursing, 44*(6), 633–642.

Melynk, B. M., & Fineout-Overholt, E. (2005). *Evidence-based practice in nursing and healthcare.* Philadelphia, PA: Lippincott Williams & Wilkins.

Melynk, B. M., Fineout-Overholt, E., Stillwell, S., & Williamson, K. (2010). The seven steps of evidence-based practice. *American Journal of Nursing, 110*(1), 51–53.

Meyer, K. A. (1997). An educational program to prepare acute care nurses for a transition to home health care nursing. *Journal of Continuing Education in Nursing, 28*(3), 124–129.

Mirski, M. A., Chang, C. W. J., & Cowan, C. (2001). Impact of a neuroscience intensive care unit on neurosurgical patient outcomes and cost of care. *Journal of Neurosurgery and Anesthesiology, 13*(2), 83–92.

Morris, L. L., Pfeifer, P. B., Catalano, R., Fortney, R., Hilton, E. L., McLaughlin, J., . . . Goldstein, L. (2007). Designing a comprehensive model for critical care orientation. *Critical Care Nurse, 27*(6), 37–60.

National League for Nursing. (2001). Impact of the nursing shortage on critical care. *Nursing and Health Care Perspectives, 22*(4), 71–72.

Needleman, J., Buerhaus, P. I., Mattke, S., Stewart, M., & Zelevinsky, K. (2002). Nurse-staffing levels and the quality of care in hospitals. *New England Journal of Medicine, 346*(22), 1715–1722.

Oermann, M. H., & Moffitt-Wolf, A. (1997). New graduates perceptions of clinical practice. *Journal of Continuing Education in Nursing, 28*(1), 20–25.

Olson, R., Nelson, M., Stuart, C., Young, L., Kleinsasser, A., Schroedermeier, R., & Newstrom, P. (2001). Nursing student residency program: A model for a seamless transition from nursing student to expert. *Journal of Nursing Administration, 31*(1), 40–48.

Parasuraman, S. (1989). Nursing turnover: An integrated model. *Research in Nursing and Health, 12*, 267–277.

Peterson, K., & Van Buren, K. (2006). Implementing essentials of critical care orientation. *Critical Care Nursing Quarterly, 29*(3), 218–230.

Pipe, T. B., Wellik, K. E., Buchda, V. L., Hansen, C. M., & Martyn, D. R. (2005). *Implementing evidence-based nursing practice: Conceptual model for translating evidence into practice.* Retrieved from http://www.medscape.com/viewarticle/514532_5

Pooler, C., Slater-MacLean, L., Simpson, N., & Giblin, C. (2005). Knowledge and skill acquisition for critical care nursing practice. *Dynamics, 16*, 20–23.

Reason, J. (1997). *Managing the risks of organizational accidents.* Aldershot, United Kingdom: Ashgate.

Reddish, V., & Kaplan, L. (2007). When are new graduate nurses competent in the intensive care unit? *Critical Care Nursing Quarterly, 30*(3), 199–205.

Rosswurm, M. A., & Larrabee, J. H. (1999). A model for change to evidence-based practice. *Clinical Scholarship, 31*(4), 317–322.

Sackett, D. L., Straus, S. E., Richardson, W. S., Rosenberg, W., & Haynes, R. B. (2000). *Evidence-based medicine: How to practice and teach EBM* (2nd ed.). London, United Kingdom: Churchill Livingstone.

Sidani, S., & Braden, C. J. (1998). *Evaluating nursing interventions: A theory-driven approach.* Thousand Oaks, CA: Sage.

Slavin, R. (1995). Best evidence synthesis: An intelligent alternative to meta-analysis. *Journal of Clinical Epidemiology, 48*(1), 9–18.

Snow, J. L. (2002). Enhancing work climate to improve performance and retain valued employees. *Journal of Nursing Administration, 32*(7–8), 393–397.

Sovie, M. D., & Jawad, A. F. (2001). Hospital restructuring and its impact on outcomes: Nursing staff regulations are premature. *Journal of Nursing Administration, 31*(12), 588–600.

Specht, J. P., Bergquist, S., & Frantz, R. A. (1995). Adoption of a research-based practice for treatment of pressure ulcers. *Nursing Clinics of North America, 30*(3), 553–563.

Speedling, E., Ahmade, K., & Kuhn-Weissman, G. (1981). Encountering reality: Reactions of newly hired RNs to the world of the medical center. *International Journal of Nursing Students, 18*, 217–225.

Steelman, V. M. (1995). Latex allergy precautions: A research based protocol. *Nursing Clinics of North America, 30*(3), 475–493.

Stevens, K. R., & Staley, J. M. (2006). The quality chasm reports, evidence-based practice, and nursing's response to improve healthcare. *Nursing Outlook, 54*, 94–101.

Stone, P. W., Tourangeau, A. E., Duffield, C. M., Hughes, F., Jones, C. B., O'Brien-Pallas, L., & Shamian, J. (2003). Evidence of nurse working conditions: A global perspective. *Policy, Politics and Nursing Practice, 4*(2), 120–130.

Symes, L., Krepper, K. R., Lindy, C., Byrd, M. N., Jacobus, C., & Throckmorton, T. (2005). Stressful life events among new nurses: Implications for retaining new graduates. *Nursing Administration Quarterly, 29*(3), 292–296.

Thomason, T. (2006). ICU nursing orientation and postorientation practices—A national survey. *Critical Care Nursing Quality, 29*(3), 237–245.

Tourangeau, A. E., & Cranley, L. A. (2006). Nurse intentions to remain employed: Understanding and strengthening determinants. *Journal of Advanced Nursing, 55*(4), 497–509.

Tourangeau, A. E., Giovanetti, P., Tu, J. V., & Wood, M. (2002). Nursing related determinants of 30-day mortality for hospitalized patients. *Canadian Journal Nursing Residency, 33*(4), 71–88.

Traynor, M., & Wade, B. (1993). The development of a measure of job satisfaction for the use in monitoring morale in nurses in four trusts. *Journal of Advanced Nursing, 18*, 127–136.

Van Saane, N., Sluitter, J. K., Verbeek, J. H. A. M., & Frings-Dresen, M. H. W. (2003). Reliability and validity of instruments measuring job satisfaction—A systematic review. *Occupational Medicine, 53*(3), 191–200.

Wells, N., Free, M., & Adams, R. (2007). Nursing research internship: Enhancing evidence-based practice among staff nurses. *Journal of Nursing Administration, 37*(3), 135–143.

Whitman, G. R., Kim, Y., Davidson, L. J., Wolf, G. A., & Wang, S. L. (2002). The impact of staffing on patient outcomes across specialty units. *Journal of Nursing Administration, 32*, 633–639.

Winter-Collins, A., & McDaniel, A. (2000). Sense of belonging and new graduate job satisfaction. *Journal of Nurses Staff Development, 16*(3), 103–111.

Zalaquett, C. P., & Wood, R. J. (1997). Evaluating stress: A book of resources. Lanham, MD: Scarecrow Press.

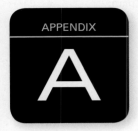

Pre/Post Comprehensive Based Orientation
Program Exam

Perianesthesia Care: Testing Competency

1. A 70-year-old female presents for perianesthesia testing, scheduled for a right total hip arthroplasty in 1 week. She has a history of hypertension, is a borderline diabetic, and takes several medications "for her heart." Tests you would expect to be ordered include:

    a. ECG, glucose, CXR
    b. ECG, Hgb & Hct, Basic Metabolic Panel, Type and Screen
    c. Hgb & Hct, Type and Screen, CXR
    d. PT and PTT, ECG, Basic Metabolic Panel

2. A 27-year-old female comes in on the day of surgery for a D & C for a miscarriage. Tests needed for this patient include:

    a. Hgb and/or Hct, possibly Type and Screen
    b. ECG, Hgb and/or Hct, Glucose
    c. Basic Metabolic Screen, Type and Screen
    d. CXR, Hgb and/or Hct

3. A 65-year-old male comes in for testing, scheduled for a radical prostatectomy in 3 days. He has a 45 pack-year history of smoking. He also takes some medicine for "heart palpitations." Tests needed for this patient include:

    a. Hgb and/or Hct, CXR, Comprehensive Metabolic Panel
    b. ECG, CXR, Hgb and/or Hct, Basic Metabolic Panel, Type and Screen
    c. Glucose, ECG, Hgb and/or Hct, Type and Crossmatch
    d. Hgb and/or Hct, Basic Metabolic Panel, CXR

4. Which of the following elective tests obtained during a perianesthetic evaluation is most likely to provide you useful information that will assist in the clinical decision making prior to an elective repair of an inguinal hernia?

    a. A chest X-ray on an asthmatic 40-year-old woman
    b. An electrocardiogram on a hypertensive 72-year-old man
    c. A pregnancy testing on an amenorrheic 18-year-old woman
    d. A prothrombin time on an anemic 55-year-old man

5. The educator, when preparing an effective teaching plan:

   a. Uses principles of learning
   b. Uses age-appropriate guidelines for children
   c. Uses a standard teaching plan
   d. a and b

6. For perianesthesia teaching to be effective, it must:

   a. Be tailored to the patient's identified needs
   b. Be presented in a manner in which the patient can understand
   c. Be modified to overcome sensory and language barriers
   d. Use simple phrases, repetition, and return demonstrations
   e. All of the above

7. The best way to encourage patient feedback/participation is to:

   a. Use open-ended questions
   b. Explain everything so that there are no questions
   c. Leave out valuable information so the patient will ask questions
   d. b and c

8. Teaching that focuses on an individual's needs increases:

   a. Comprehension
   b. Compliance
   c. A positive experience
   d. All of the above

9. Teaching is most effective when the following techniques are used:

   a. Quiet atmosphere
   b. Eye contact
   c. Nontechnical language
   d. Repetition and return demonstration
   e. All of the above

10. The following areas are usually discussed with a patient preoperatively:

    a. NPO status/medications to take/hold
    b. Transportation home
    c. Responsible adult help at home
    d. Expectations as a result of the planned procedure
    e. All of the above

11. The following statements about pain management apply:

    a. Preoperative discussion about pain expectations/management can decrease anxiety
    b. Discussion should start in the physician's office
    c. The patient has a role in his or her management of pain and comfort
    d. All of the above

12. Home support/after care is key in the safe recovery of the patient.

    a. True
    b. False

13. Documentation of all teaching serves as a:

    a. Reference for the patient to review
    b. Checklist for the nurse to review
    c. Legal and chart auditing purposes
    d. All of the above

14. The primary goal of perianesthesia assessment includes:

    a. Obtaining a comprehensive health history
    b. Performing a complete physical assessment
    c. Identifying risk factors
    d. Collaboration with other disciplines
    e. All of the above

15. The perianesthesia comprehensive health history includes all the following except:

    a. Past surgeries
    b. Age-related factors
    c. Vital signs
    d. Cardiovascular system review
    e. Psychosocial issues

16. The perianesthesia nurse completes a physical examination that includes:

    a. Bilateral blood pressures
    b. Baseline O_2 saturation
    c. Height and weight
    d. Lung sounds
    e. All of the above

17. The perianesthesia nurse recognizes the following medication as a potential risk factor for surgery and/or anesthesia:

    a. Cefazolin sodium
    b. Warfarin sodium
    c. Acetaminophen
    d. Glycopyrrolate
    e. All of the above

18. The perianesthesia nurse notifies the anesthesiologist of the following physical findings:

    a. Fever
    b. Productive cough
    c. Pale color
    d. All the above
    e. a and b

19. Identification of the responsible caregiver and assuring safe discharge for the patient begins:

    a. In PACU
    b. In pre-op holding
    c. On initial contact
    d. On admission
    e. At discharge

20. During the patient interview, which of the following would need to be reported to an anesthesia provider?

    a. Recent cardiac surgery
    b. Myocardial infarction within the last 6 months
    c. Discharge 3 weeks ago with congestive heart failure
    d. Chest pain 2 weeks ago
    e. All of the above

21. Patients checking into the facility for surgery later that day can have their anxiety level reduced by which nursing actions?

    a. Sending the family immediately to the waiting room
    b. Outlining the day's schedule for the patient and family
    c. Saying, "Here are your roommates, get undressed and I will be right back."
    d. Introducing yourself and other caregivers present
    e. b and d
    f. a and b

22. Serious surgical complications can be prevented by the proper:

    a. Selection of surgeons
    b. Scheduling the surgery for the first case of the day
    c. Marking of the surgical site according to facility policy
    d. Reassuring the patient that "everything will be okay"

23. The perianesthesia nurse's goal of preoperative preparation for the patient is:

    a. To decrease the potential for complications
    b. To reduce anxiety in the patient
    c. To impart accurate and timely communication to the health-care team
    d. All of the above

24. Preoperatively, the patient is under the perianesthesia nurse's care until:

    a. The surgery consent is signed
    b. The IV is in and the preoperative medication has been given
    c. The patient's chart is completed
    d. Handoff has occurred between the circulating/procedural nurse and the anesthesia care provider, and the patient is transferred to the OR

25. Pain management for the patient should begin:

    a. In PACU as the patient arouses
    b. In the preoperative area after the IV is started
    c. In the Phase II recovery area before the patient starts to ambulate
    d. At the first contact with the patient, either in preadmission testing or on admission prior to leaving for surgery

26. Airway sounds associated with laryngospasm may include all of the following except:

    a. Absence of breath sounds
    b. Continuous musical rhonchi
    c. Crowing respirations
    d. Diminished breath sounds

27. Early signs of hypoxemia in the adult immediately after anesthesia may include:

    a. Twelve to 16 respirations per minute
    b. Pulse oximetry measurement of 92% to 96% saturation
    c. Restlessness, confusion, and anxiety
    d. Symmetrical chest movement with normal breath sounds

28. Techniques included in basic airway management include:

    1. Chin hold, jaw lift
    2. Intubation
    3. Suctioning
    4. Insertion of oral/nasal airway

        a. 1, 2, 3
        b. 1, 3, 4
        c. 1, 2, 4
        d. None of the above

29. Which of the following are included in respiratory assessment of the patient in the immediate postoperative period?

    a. Work of breathing
    b. CBC, chemistries, ABGs
    c. Previous history of respiratory illness
    d. Location of incision site
    e. All of the above

30. Classic signs and symptoms associated with pneumothorax include:

    a. Crowing, stridor, and wheezing
    b. Hyperthermia, tachycardia, and flushing
    c. Chest pain, tracheal shift, and dyspnea
    d. None of the above

31. This type of cyanosis presents as cyanosis of the mucous membranes, earlobes, cheeks, and lips and is reflective of reduced oxygen concentration:

    a. Hypoxic cyanosis
    b. Central cyanosis
    c. Peripheral cyanosis
    d. Hypercarbic cyanosis

32. This heart sound results from the atria working harder to fill against a stiff ventricle:

    a. S1
    b. S2
    c. S3
    d. S4

33. The following rhythm is a regular rhythm that is associated with an atrial and ventricular rate of 150 to 250:

    a. ST
    b. SVT
    c. Atrial flutter
    d. Atrial fibrillation

34. The dicrotic notch of the arterial waveform is associated with closure of the:

    a. Tricuspid valve
    b. Pulmonic valve
    c. Mitral valve
    d. Aortic valve

35. Pulsus paradoxus in the PACU is most commonly associated with:

    a. Severe hypovolemia
    b. Sympathetic blockade
    c. Cardiac tamponade
    d. Tension pneumothorax

36. The most common cause of PEA in the perianesthesia setting is hypovolemia.

    a. True
    b. False

37. Risks and complications associated with central venous cannulation include:

    a. Heart block
    b. Valvular damage
    c. Ventricular tachycardia
    d. Pneumothorax

38. This naturally occurring antidiuretic hormone will act as a powerful vaso-constrictor when given at high doses:

    a. Epinephrine
    b. Ephedrine
    c. Vasopressin
    d. Voltaren

39. To avoid erroneous readings, CVP should always be measured at end-inspiration.
    a. True
    b. False

40. The most common cause of decreased CVP in the PACU is:

    a. Sepsis
    b. Sympathetic blockade
    c. Hypovolemia
    d. Lymphatic blockage

41. Checking for pupillary constriction is an assessment of the:

    a. Optic nerve
    b. Abducens nerve
    c. Oculomotor nerve
    d. Trochlear nerve

42. Narcotics can cause pupillary constriction.

    a. True
    b. False

43. A positive Babinski reflex sign is normally present in patients age:

    a. 3 years old
    b. 18 years old
    c. 15 months old
    d. 20 months old

44. Decorticate posturing is described as:

    a. Extension of arms across the chest
    b. Flexion of arms across the chest

45. Decerebrate posturing is described as:

    a. Extension of arms across the chest
    b. Flexion of arms across the chest

46. The Glasgow Coma Scale (GCS) is the most reliable indicator of change in LOC and neurological status.

    a. True
    b. False

47. A patient presented the following responses when assessing LOC using the GCS: opens eyes to pain, is confused, and withdraws extremities from pain. What is the patient's GCS score?

    a. 9
    b. 10
    c. 11
    d. 12

48. The normal value for ICP is:

    a. 0 to 10 mm Hg
    b. 10 to 25 mm Hg
    c. 0 to 20 mm Hg
    d. 20 to 35 mm Hg

49. Signs of increased ICP include the following:

    a. Restlessness, tachycardia, decreased blood pressure, and widening pulse pressure
    b. Restlessness, tachycardia, increased blood pressure, and widening pulse pressure
    c. Restlessness, bradycardia, decreased blood pressure, and widening pulse pressure
    d. Restlessness, bradycardia, increased blood pressure, and widening pulse pressure

50. The following position is appropriate for a supratentorial craniotomy patient:

    a. Flat in bed
    b. HOB 15° to 25°
    c. HOB 30° to 45°
    d. High Fowler position

51. The following position is appropriate for an infratentorial craniotomy patient:

    a. Flat in bed
    b. HOB 15° to 25°
    c. HOB 30° to 45°
    d. High Fowler position

52. The kidneys are located:

    a. Within the peritoneum
    b. Within the pelvis
    c. Retroperitoneally
    d. Above the thoracic vertebrae

53. Normal urine output is considered to be:

    a. 1 to 2 mL/kg/hr
    b. 0.5 to 1.0 mL/kg/hr
    c. 5 mL/kg/hr
    d. 0.5 mL/kg/hr

54. Changes in urine color may result from all but:

    a. Trauma to the kidney or bladder
    b. Drug therapy
    c. Inflammation or infection
    d. Intravenous normal saline

55. Volume intake includes:

    a. Intravenous crystalloids and colloids
    b. Intravenous blood products
    c. Autotransfusion
    d. All of the above

56. Volume output does not include:

    a. Interstitial fluid shifts
    b. Blood loss during surgery
    c. Output from nasogastric tubes or surgical drains
    d. Urine output

57. Changes in patient position may enhance or impede drainage from a suprapubic catheter.

    a. True
    b. False

58. When irrigating a ureteral catheter, one should:

    a. Irrigate vigorously to dislodge blood clots
    b. Irrigate gently with 5 to 10 mL of irrigant
    c. Use a syringe to pull back the irrigant
    d. Irrigate gently with less than 5 mL of irrigant

59. When calculating urine output with continuous bladder irrigation:

    a. Irrigant and urine output are added together
    b. Irrigant is withdrawn with a syringe
    c. Irrigant is subtracted from total output
    d. Irrigant is irrelevant

60. Symptoms of post-TURP syndrome (dilutional hyponatremia) may include:

    a. Slowed respiratory rate and lowered blood pressure
    b. Rapid respiratory rate and slowed heart rate
    c. Rapid respiratory rate and rapid heart rate
    d. Elevated serum sodium levels

61. The primary goal(s) of moderate sedation/analgesia is/are:

    a. Amnesia
    b. Elevate the pain threshold
    c. Maintain protective reflexes
    d. Allay fear and anxiety
    e. Deep sleep
    f. a, b, c, and d

62. For the adult patient, an early sign of hypoventilation which can lead to hypoxia and cardiac arrest is:

    a. Bradycardia
    b. Slow capillary refill
    c. Slow, shallow respirations
    d. Diaphoresis

63. Benzodiazepines and narcotics are the classes of drugs most often used in moderate sedation/analgesia.

    a. True
    b. False

64. The primary drug used to reverse sedation and analgesia in moderate sedation is:

    a. Physostigmine
    b. Naloxone
    c. Flumazenil
    d. Prostigmin
    e. b and c

65. Patients receiving medication to achieve moderate sedation/analgesia must have venous access maintained until discharge criteria are met.

    a. True
    b. False

66. In healthy patients, midazolam is recommended to be given:

    a. One milligram per minute until patient is completely sedated
    b. In 500 mL normal saline over 1 hour
    c. Rapid IV push over 5 seconds
    d. Titrated to desired effect with no more than 2.5 mg over 2 minutes

67. When discharge teaching, the nurse should always:

    a. Provide written discharge instruction to patient and caregiver
    b. Provide patient with telephone number to call in case of further questions
    c. Review written discharge instructions with patient and caregiver both present
    d. All of the above

68. The response of patients to verbal command during procedures performed with moderate sedation/analgesia is not reflective of their LOC.

    a. True
    b. False

69. The highest priority of assessment is:

    a. Cardiovascular
    b. Oxygenation
    c. Renal perfusion
    d. Skin integrity

70. Nurses administering moderate sedation/analgesia should follow the scope of practice as directed by:

    a. ASPAN Standards
    b. Their state board of nursing
    c. The facility's policies and procedures
    d. All of the above

71. The primary process of elimination for inhalation agents is:

    a. Hepatic
    b. Renal
    c. Pulmonary
    d. Fat cells

72. The stage of anesthesia during which the patient is at most risk to harm himself or herself is:

    a. Stage I
    b. Stage II
    c. Stage III
    d. Stage IV

73. Recovery and emergence are dependent on:

    a. The duration of anesthesia
    b. Use of additional medications
    c. Physical status of the patient
    d. All of the above

74. Characteristics of nitrous oxide include all of the following except:

    a. Depresses CNS
    b. Nonirritating to the respiratory system
    c. Can be mixed with room air
    d. Minimal cardiovascular effects

75. Characteristics of sevoflurane include all of the following except:

    a. Sweet smelling, excellent for induction
    b. Lowers ICP
    c. Useful in ambulatory settings
    d. Less airway irritation than other inhalation agents

76. Pharmacokinetic properties of inhalation agents include all except:

    a. Cardiac output
    b. Age
    c. Blood solubility
    d. Gender

77. Nursing considerations for inhalation agents include:

    a. Depression of laryngeal and pharyngeal reflexes
    b. Dysrhythmic effects
    c. Analgesic requirements
    d. All of the above

78. Postoperative shivering due to intraoperative vasodilatation is a consideration with:

    a. Halothane
    b. Desflurane
    c. Isoflurane
    d. Enflurane
    e. All of the above

79. Seizure activity may be enhanced by the administration of:

    a. Enflurane
    b. Nitrous oxide
    c. Sevoflurane
    d. Halothane

80. In normal neuromuscular transmission, the enzyme/neurotransmitter released at the neuromuscular junction resulting in depolarization is:

    a. Acetylcholinesterase
    b. Pseudocholinesterase
    c. Acetylcholine
    d. Plasma cholinesterase

81. Succinylcholine is:

    a. Easily reversed by neostigmine
    b. Easily reversed by edrophonium
    c. A non-depolarizing neuromuscular blocker
    d. Metabolized by plasma cholinesterase

82. Factor(s) that may contribute to a prolonged neuromuscular blockade is/are:

    a. Hypothermia
    b. Acidosis
    c. Renal or hepatic disease
    d. All of the above

83. A long-acting non-depolarizing muscle relaxant is:

    a. Vecuronium bromide
    b. Rocuronium bromide
    c. Pipecuronium bromide
    d. Atracurium besylate

84. Reversal agents for non-depolarizing muscle relaxants include:

    a. Glycopyrrolate
    b. Neostigmine
    c. Pyridostigmine
    d. b and c
    e. All of the above

85. Nursing considerations when caring for patients who have had a peripheral nerve block include all of the following except:

    a. Assess motor and sensory levels frequently
    b. Monitor patient for bladder distention
    c. Maintain joints in proper alignment
    d. Support the blocked extremity when changing patient's position

86. Treatment of hypotension caused by neuraxial anesthesia does not include:

    a. Transfuse packed cells
    b. Elevate patient's legs
    c. Give IV bolus
    d. Administer vasopressors

87. The incidence of postdural puncture headache is more common when:

    a. The patient moves during the procedure
    b. A sterile field is not maintained
    c. Dextrose is used
    d. A larger size needle is used

88. Blockade of nerve fibers by local anesthetic agents occurs in the following order: sensory blockade, sympathetic blockade, and motor blockade.

    a. True
    b. False

89. Vasoconstrictors such as epinephrine may be added to a local anesthetic to:

    a. Decrease the intensity of the blockade
    b. Prolong the duration of the block
    c. Increase the rate of absorption of the local anesthetic
    d. Increase systemic absorption

90. The most difficult type of nerves to block is:

    a. Sensory nerves
    b. Motor nerves
    c. Sympathetic nerves
    d. Parasympathetic nerves

91. When used for neuraxial blocks, morphine:

    a. Offers analgesia without motor or sympathetic blockade
    b. Prolongs a block's duration
    c. Offers analgesia by blocking parasympathetic nerves
    d. Increases the density of anesthesia

92. A patient who exhibits an allergy to Novocain cannot receive any local anesthetics.

    a. True
    b. False

93. Dose for dose, fentanyl is how many more times potent than morphine?

    a. 5 times
    b. 10 times
    c. 50 times
    d. 100 times

94. A patient has been given fentanyl 200 mcg. In the PACU, the patient's respirations are shallow and 6 breaths per minute. The reversal agent of choice is:

    a. Atropine 0.4 mg
    b. Antilirium
    c. Naloxone 0.4 mg
    d. None of the above

95. Midazolam has which of the following properties:

    a. Anxiolytic
    b. Hypnotic
    c. Amnesic
    d. Mood alteration
    e. All of the above

96. The reversal drug of choice for benzodiazepines is:

    a. Physostigmine
    b. Glycopyrrolate
    c. Naloxone
    d. Flumazenil

97. In outpatient surgery, a patient has had a reversal agent in Phase I PACU. Twenty minutes later, the patient is transferred to Phase II PACU. Suddenly, the patient is exhibiting the following signs and symptoms: drowsy and unarousable, respirations are 8 breaths per minute and shallow, blood pressure is 90/60 mm Hg, and the heart rate is 58 beats per minute. The initial nursing management of this patient is:

    a. Nasal cannula at 4 L/min
    b. Face mask at 6 L/min
    c. Bag-valve-mask at 15 L/min
    d. Call physician

98. Total body water in the normal adult is:

    a. 25%
    b. 70%
    c. 40%
    d. 90%

99. Hypertonic solutions:

    a. Shift fluid into the interstitium
    b. Shift fluid into the circulating plasma
    c. Keep the fluid compartments equalized
    d. None of the above

100. An example of a hypertonic solution is:

    a. 0.9% NS
    b. D5LR
    c. LR
    d. D_s1/4 NS

101. The significance of ECF deficit (hypovolemia) is:

    a. Increased CVP
    b. Shortness of breath
    c. Decreased perfusion to the brain, kidneys, liver
    d. All of the above

102. Third spacing is:

    a. Only seen in massive trauma patients
    b. A result of damage to capillary permeability
    c. When fluid shifts out of the plasma into areas normally having minimal to no fluid
    d. b and c

103. Treatment for third spacing in the PACU includes:

    a. Obtain baseline breath sounds and assess at regular intervals
    b. Administer fluids at rapid rate (200 to 1,000 mL/hr)
    c. Monitor VS, UO, lab if ordered, pressures if lines in
    d. All of the above

104. Perioperative alterations in fluid status that warrant fluid volume include:

    a. Preoperative NPO status
    b. Inhalation agents, spinal or epidural blocks
    c. Potential for third spacing
    d. All of the above

105. A 30-year-old male, 90 kg, is scheduled for a knee arthroscopy. NPO at midnight. Surgery start time 0800. OR length 1 hour. Total fluids required:

    a. 2,700 mL
    b. 1,440 mL
    c. 1,890 mL
    d. 2,450 mL

106. A 75-year-old female, 80 kg, scheduled for a total hip replacement. NPO at midnight. Surgery start time 0800. OR length 2 hours. EBL 500 mL. Total crystalloids required:

    a. 1,280 mL
    b. 1,920 mL
    c. 4,700 mL
    d. 3,650 mL

107. Potential adverse effects of administration of intravenous opioids include all of the following except:

    a. Respiratory depression/apnea
    b. Hypertension
    c. Loss of consciousness
    d. Loss of protective reflexes

108. The perianesthesia nurse should discontinue the use of intravenous opioids when there is/are:

    a. Respiratory rate of 10 breaths per minute
    b. Drowsiness
    c. BP of 90/56 mm Hg
    d. Signs of allergic reaction to the drug

109. All of the following are part of emergency treatment for the patient receiving analgesia except:

    a. Continue pump until a complete physical assessment can be made
    b. Arouse patient/encourage respirations
    c. Administer oxygen or support ventilation
    d. Titrate naloxone IV until desired effects are achieved

110. When caring for a patient who has just had a lumbar epidural catheter placed, all of the following are true except:

    a. The patient may experience pruritus due to the opioid
    b. Cold temperature fibers are blocked first and an initial sensory blockage assessment can be made using an alcohol wipe
    c. Continuous administration of the medication is appropriate with a dermatome level of T3
    d. A pain scale should be used to assess patient response to medication

111. A potential complication associated with epidural catheter usage in the perianesthesia patient includes which of the following?

    a. Sudden onset of distal extremity weakness
    b. Loss of bladder and bowel control
    c. Segmental block
    d. Spinal headache
    e. All of the above

112. All of the following are considered support measures for treatment during an epidural emergency except:

    a. Assessment of level of sympathetic blockade
    b. Administration of intravenous fluid bolus
    c. Administration of drugs such as naloxone or ephedrine
    d. Supporting ventilations with a bag-valve-mask

113. The four contexts in which comfort is experienced are:

    a. Physiological, cognitive, cultural, environmental
    b. Spiritual, physiological, cognitive, environmental
    c. Physiological, psychospiritual, sociocultural, environmental
    d. Sociocultural, cognitive, physiological, environmental

114. Pain management is the same as comfort management.

    a. True
    b. False

115. According to Kolcaba, *comfort* is defined as the immediate state of being strengthened through having met human needs for _____, _____, and _____.

    a. Pain, support, and empathy
    b. Ease, relief, and transcendence
    c. Social support, relief, and ease
    d. Transcendence, empathy, and social support

116. Comfort measures for patients in perianesthesia care include:

    a. Assisting with guided imagery
    b. Providing a soothing environment
    c. Giving emotional support
    d. All of the above

117. It is important to measure, informally or formally, your patient's comfort before and after a comfort intervention because:

    a. You want to prove to the patient that your intervention worked
    b. You want to document the effectiveness of your intervention
    c. You need the information to ask for a raise
    d. It is not important to measure your patient's comfort at all

118. An example of an informal measurement of comfort is:

    a. Asking your patient about his or her comfort
    b. Asking the patient to complete a comfort questionnaire
    c. Asking the patient to put a dot on a IO centimeter line with IO being the highest possible comfort
    d. Asking the patient to define holistic comfort

119. The feelings of being anxious or cold are called:

    a. Infantile feelings
    b. Inexperienced
    c. Pain intensifiers
    d. Unnecessary

120. An example of visible comfort behavior is:

    a. Sweating
    b. Muscular tension
    c. Being quiet and withdrawn
    d. Relaxed demeanor

121. The most reliable measure of pain in the newborn is:

    a. Continued crying without comfort
    b. Trained assessment of physiological and behavioral responses
    c. Parent(s) assessment of newborn responses
    d. Numerical pain scale

122. The behavioral activity offering the most specific indicator of pain is:

    a. Sleep/wake cycles
    b. Vocalizations
    c. Facial activity
    d. Limb withdrawal

123. The Neonatal Infant Pain Scale (NIPS) is a pain assessment tool used for assessing pain in neonates. The NIPS scale assesses:

    a. Cry, breathing patterns, and extremity movement
    b. Facial expression and psychological responses
    c. Vocalizations, state of arousal, and movement
    d. Facial expression, cry, breathing patterns, extremities, and state of arousal

124. The FLACC behavior assessment scale is used to assess pain in children who:

    a. Have attention deficit disorder
    b. Have insufficient cognitive skills/communication
    c. Have minimal pain intensity
    d. Have long-term or repeated procedure pain

125. Assessment of pain is inaccurate and unreliable in neonates and infants and questionable in the nonverbal toddler.

    a. True
    b. False

126. At 3 to 6 months of age, healthy infants can metabolize opioids similarly to other children.

    a. True
    b. False

127. It is safe and effective to use IV PCA administration in children older than 8 years of age provided they:

    a. Understand the relationship between pain and pushing the PCA button
    b. Have a parent(s) who are going to be with them in the room at all times
    c. Can manipulate the PCA button and understand how to push it correctly
    d. Have a designated primary pain manager who will control the PCA button

128. When assessing pain in a geriatric patient, the nurse may need to use a combination of pain assessment tools.

    a. True
    b. False

129. Misconceptions regarding pain in the elderly include all except:

    a. Pain is a normal part of aging
    b. Pain perception is decreased in the elderly
    c. Elderly patients can tolerate pain better than the young age
    d. Elderly patients may under report pain because they want to be a good patient

130. Consequences of inadequate pain management include:

    a. Increased oxygen demand
    b. Delayed wound healing
    c. Prolongation of the stress response
    d. All of the above

131. Metabolic issues to consider in the geriatric patient include:

    a. Decreased hepatic blood flow
    b. Decreased renal blood flow
    c. Decreased muscle mass
    d. Increased plasma proteins
    e. All of the above

132. Factors influencing nausea and vomiting are either peripheral or central in origin. Which of the following are peripheral factors?

    a. Major intraabdominal surgery and premature oral intake of fluids
    b. Anesthetic inhalation agents, especially nitrous oxide
    c. Prior history of nausea and vomiting, motion sickness
    d. None of the above

133. The chemoreceptor trigger zone–vomiting center of the brain is located in the medulla.

    a. True
    b. False

134. Which of the following affect the chemoreceptor trigger zone–vomiting center of the brain?

    a. Anesthetic agents, opioids, neuromuscular blockade
    b. Anesthetic agents, opioids, pain, motion
    c. Premature intake of oral fluids
    d. All the above

135. The best position for the prevention of aspiration is:

    a. Head of bed elevated 30° to 35°
    b. Turn head to either side
    c. Head down and left lateral
    d. Lateral or prone

136. Ondansetron, a serotonin antagonist, is best described as:

    a. Accelerating gastric emptying
    b. An antiemetic that may cause headache and sedation
    c. A CNS depressant, anticholinergic, antispasmodic
    d. None of the above

137. Every patient receiving anesthetic agents should also receive antiemetic prophylaxis.

    a. True
    b. False

138. Complications associated with nausea and vomiting include:

    a. Dehydration
    b. Electrolyte imbalance
    c. Increased length of stay
    d. All of the above

139. Malignant hyperthermia may be triggered by which agent?

    a. Pancuronium
    b. Succinylcholine
    c. Fentanyl
    d. Sodium pentothal

140. The only inhalation agent safe for use in MH–susceptible patients is:

    a. Desflurane
    b. Isoflurane
    c. Halothane
    d. Nitrous oxide

141. The most reliable laboratory test for preoperative detection of MH is:

    a. Creatinine phosphokinase
    b. Cardiac enzymes
    c. Serum electrolytes
    d. Caffeine/halothane contracture test

142. Increased end tidal CO_2 and tachycardia are early indications of an MH crisis.

    a. True
    b. False

143. The initial drug of choice for treatment of MH is:

    a. Pancuronium
    b. Lidocaine
    c. Dantrolene
    d. Sodium bicarbonate

144. Initial dosing with dantrolene is:

    a. 1 mg/kg
    b. 10 mg/kg
    c. 2.5 mg/kg
    d. 25 mg/kg

145. MH deaths may be prevented with:

    a. Proper preoperative screening
    b. Education and preparation
    c. Identification of individuals at risk
    d. All of the above

146. MH only occurs in the operating room.

    a. True
    b. False

147. Of the following, which patient is most at risk for developing intraoperative hypothermia?

    a. A 75-year-old male undergoing transurethral resection of the prostate gland
    b. A 25-year-old female undergoing a D&C
    c. A 3-year-old undergoing a tonsillectomy
    d. A 60-year-old woman undergoing a thyroidectomy

148. If a patient undergoing a major abdominal surgery is more likely to become hypothermic than another patient having a ventral hernia repair, and both surgeries take approximately 2 hours, what would be the minimum ambient room temperature?

    a. 64° F
    b. 68° F
    c. 70° F
    d. 72° F

149. A true core temperature can be measured by all methods except:

    a. An infrared tympanic thermometer
    b. An oral thermometer
    c. A pulmonary artery catheter
    d. An esophageal probe

150. Temperature assessment on admission is all that is necessary if the patient presents with a core temperature greater than 36° C (96.8° F).

    a. True
    b. False

151. Which of the following may be demonstrated by a child during hospitalization and surgery?

    a. Fear
    b. Regression in development
    c. Behavior changes
    d. Sleep disturbances
    e. All of the above

152. Bradycardia may be life-threatening in the infant/small child and requires immediate attention.

    a. True
    b. False

153. Concerns about loss of body parts, loss of control, and loss of friends are most commonly noted in which age group?

    a. 2 to 4 years
    b. 4 to 9 years
    c. 10 to 16 years

154. Your 87-year-old patient is recovering from an incisional hernia repair. The pain score verbalized is an "8" on a 0 to 10 scale, and you have orders on the chart for an injectable NSAID and IV morphine, up to 15 mg to be titrated to effect for pain. You would:

    a. Give only the NSAID
    b. Give smaller than average doses of IV morphine at 10-minute intervals
    c. Give medication(s) based on weight, current physical status, and any relevant medical history
    d. Call the physician and request that the incision be "blocked" for pain control

155. Your patient is arousing and begins to move about on the post-op stretcher. He is not responding appropriately to your questions or commands. Which of the following is NOT a recommended intervention?

    a. Frequent reorientation to time, place, event
    b. Check for hearing impairment or the need to place hearing assistive devices
    c. Try to let the patient know you need to touch him before providing care
    d. Place the patient in 4-point restraints until he can cooperate

156. You have just admitted a frail 92-year-old female to the PACU after her hip fracture repair. On assessment, you note several large flat bruised areas on her hands and arms. You:

    a. Immediately call social services and report it as elder abuse
    b. Continue your assessment by reviewing the chart
    c. Continue your assessment by receiving report from the anesthesiologist
    d. b and c

157. For perianesthesia teaching to be effective, it must:

    a. Be tailored to the patient's identified needs
    b. Be presented in a manner in which the patient can understand
    c. Be modified to overcome sensory and language barriers
    d. Use simple phrases, repetition, and return demonstration
    e. All of the above

158. The best way to encourage patient feedback/participation is to:

    a. Use open-ended questions
    b. Explain everything so that there are no questions
    c. Leave out valuable information so that the patient will ask questions
    d. a and c

159. Documentation of all teaching, both preoperative and postoperative, serves as a:

    a. Reference for the patient to review
    b. Checklist for the nurse to refer to
    c. Legal and chart auditing purposes
    d. All of the above

160. Postoperative instruction should include the following information:

    a. Prescription information and emergency phone number
    b. Activity, diet, wound care, and pain management
    c. Follow-up appointment, and other special instructions
    d. All of the above

161. Teaching that focuses on an individual's needs increases:

    a. Comprehension
    b. Compliance
    c. A positive experience
    d. All of the above

162. Teaching is most effective when the following techniques are used:

    a. Quiet atmosphere and eye contact
    b. Nontechnical language
    c. Repetition and return demonstration
    d. All of the above

163. Identify three ways to limit exposure to radiation.

    a. Increase the duration of exposure; decrease the distance from the radiation source; place an absorbent shield over the patient
    b. Decrease the time of exposure; increase the distance from the radiation source; place an absorbent shield between staff and the radiation source
    c. Decrease the duration of exposure; decrease the distance from the radiation source; place an absorbent shield over the physician

164. Treatment of severe anaphylactoid reactions to radiologic contrast material includes the following:

    a. Intravenous fluids
    b. Oxygen administration
    c. Antihistamines
    d. Bronchodilators
    e. a and c
    f. All of the above

165. Name three major complications of cardiac catheterization.

    a. Death, stroke, and cardiac perforation
    b. Death, hematoma, and contrast reaction
    c. Death, hematoma, and vasovagal reaction

166. Extracorporeal shockwave lithotripsy (ESWL) is the ideal procedure for pregnant women with gallstone disease.

    a. True
    b. False

167. Absolute contraindications for the use of MRI technology include:

   a. Pacemakers, plaster casts, contact lenses
   b. Pacemakers, implanted defibrillators, implantable drug infusers
   c. Implanted defibrillators, plaster casts, chewing gum

168. Angioplasty or stent placement for known arterial occlusions or stenosis is best performed by:

   a. Ultrasound
   b. MRI
   c. Nuclear medicine
   d. Interventional vascular radiology

169. Which of the following statements is true?

   a. Patients prone to contrast medium reactions ought to be premedicated with beta-blockers and H_2 receptor blockers
   b. Patients prone to contrast medium reactions ought to be premedicated with analgesics and steroids
   c. Patients prone to contrast medium reactions ought to be premedicated with steroids and antihistamines

170. Common causes for litigation include all of the following except:

   a. Failure to identify the patient
   b. Administration of the wrong medication
   c. Notification of the anesthesiologist with a condition change
   d. Failure to provide concise discharge instructions
   e. Abandonment

171. Documentation should include:

   a. Admission assessment
   b. Discharge assessment
   c. Identification of patient/family needs
   d. Patient education
   e. All of the above

172. Information provided to new staff during orientation should include:

   a. Hospital policies and procedures
   b. Perianesthesia policies and practices
   c. Safe Medical Device Act
   d. Advance directives
   e. All of the above

173. Maintaining patient confidentiality can be achieved by all of the following except:

    a. Keeping your voice low while giving report
    b. Writing the patient's name on a board in the outpatient unit for all to see
    c. Avoiding discussion of patients in the cafeteria
    d. Keeping the patient chart in a place with limited access to the public
    e. Avoiding discussion of a patient while caring for someone else

174. Culture does not influence a nurse's view and the nursing care that is given.

    a. True
    b. False

175. A client's religious system would fit under which phenomenon?

    a. Space
    b. Time
    c. Environmental control
    d. Biological variations

176. Culture is shaped by a system of beliefs and values, norms, and practices that are shared by:

    a. One person
    b. A group and passed down by generation
    c. A group and not passed down by generation
    d. Many ethnic groups

177. How is Madeleine Leininger's Theory of Cultural Care Diversity and Universality depicted?

    a. As a sunset
    b. As a block
    c. As a sunrise
    d. As a triangle

178. What is a potential source of cultural conflict that touches on basic values of a patient and a nurse?

    a. Language differences
    b. Attitude
    c. Religious differences
    d. Use of folk medicine

179. Evidence-based practice:

    a. Is using the best available information for clinical care
    b. Is a complex decision making that uses available evidence and clinical expertise
    c. Promotes quality clinical decisions
    d. Promotes cost-effective care
    e. All of the above

180. The most important aspect of implementing EBP is:

    a. Searching the right database
    b. Finding a model to use when evaluating the evidence
    c. Ranking the evidence
    d. Developing the right question

181. Barriers to implementing EBP include:

    a. Lack of skill set
    b. Lack of time
    c. The perception that research is too hard
    d. Lack of support to implement EBP recommendations
    e. All of the above

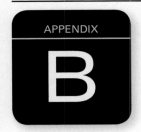

PACU Institute Case Studies

PACU Institute Case Study

What are the three phases of recovery that occur in the PACU?

What specific information do you, as a PACU nurse, expect to receive from the OR nurse?

What should the nurse remember about the patient psychological equilibrium in the PACU?

What are the PACU nurses' priority of concerns when the patient arrives from the OR?

What respiratory functions is the nurse responsible for managing?

What does the PACU nurse monitor regarding fluid status?

What does the nurse assess on the incisional site?

When can the patient leave PACU?

PACU Institute Case Study

A client recovering from surgery in the postanesthesia care unit (PACU) is difficult to arouse two hours following surgery. The nurse in the PACU has been administering morphin sulfate intravenously to the client for complaints of postsurgical pain. The client's respiratory rate is 7 per minute and demonstrates shallow breathing. The patient does not respond to any stimuli. The nurse obtains ABGs STAT.

The STAT results come back from the laboratory and show:

pH = 7.15
Pa C02 = 68 mm Hg
HC03 = 22 mEq/L

Which of the following to you suspect?

- Compensated respiratory acidosis
- Uncompensated metabolic acidosis
- Compensated metabolic alkalosis
- Uncompensated respiratory acidosis

Give the definitions for each of the above pulmonary diagnoses?

What medication should be administered immediately? And in what dose?

What is the best option for pain management in this patient?

PACU Institute Case Study

Mr. Don McMann, 42, underwent arthroscopic repair of a torn anterior cruciate ligament and arrived in the PACU about 5 minutes ago. He has no significant medical or surgical history. Reviewing his medical record, you see he received isoflurane for general anesthesia. He's receiving supplemental oxygen by nasal cannula. He is in the post anesthesia care unit when you notice muscle rigidity and see that he's becoming tachypneic and tachycardic. His blood pressure is 154/90 and his temperature, which was 98°F (37°C) preoperatively and 100°F (38°C) at PACU admission, has jumped to 104°F (40°C).

What syndrome do you suspect?

Identify the complications the patient endure if not treated properly or in a timely manner?

What should be the nurses' first response?

When the anesthesiologist arrives, she orders I.V. dantrolene. What is its correct dose?

Your colleague sees what is happened and comes to help. He immediately begins inserting a urinary catheter, orders ABGs, comprehensive metabolic panel, and CK levels . . . what is the significance of these tests?

What cardiac sequelae are you now waiting for?

Mr. Mann has now stabilized and he is being transferred to ICU. What medication are you sure to tell the nurse to give him? And for how long?

G.S. a 36-year-old secretary, was involved in a motor vehicle accident; a car drifted left of center and struck G.S. head-on, pinning her behind the steering wheel. She was intubated immediately after extrication and flown to this hospital. Her injuries were found to be extensive: bilateral flail chest, torn innominate artery, right hemo/pneumothorax, fractured spleen, multiple small liver lacerations, compound fractures of both legs, and probable cardiac contusion. She was taken to the OR where she received 36 units of PRCs, 20 units of platelets, 20 units of cryoprecipitate, 12 units of FFP, and 18L of LR. She is now in PACU.

What is your primary concern for this patient?

During your initial assessment you note SOB, crackles throughout all lung fields posteriorly and in both lower lobes anteriorly, and rhonchi over the large airways. What is the significance of crackles and rhonchi in G.S. case?

What medication(s) should you anticipate administering?

At 0500, laboratory values are as follows: Na 129 mmol/L, K 3.3 mmol/Kg, Cl 92 mmol/L, HCO3 26 mmol/L, BUN 37 mg/dL, creatinine 2.0 mg/dL, glucose 128 mg/dL, calcium 7.1 mg/dL, ABGs pm 6L 02/nc: pH 7.38, PaCO2 49 mm HG, PaO2 82 mm Hg, HCO3 36 mmol/L, BE + 2.2, SaO2 91%.

Given her fluid status and lab values, what precautions should you take before administering diuretics? What effects, if any, will it have on her breath sounds?

D.A. is a slender, active 50-year-old engineer, married with two children. He has polycystic kidney disease with renal failure and has been on dialysis for 5 years. He was admitted to the hospital for surgical repair of a ruptured sinus of Valsalva aneurysm. During the surgery a 4 mm hole for the R coronary sinus to the R atrium was discovered and repaired with a patch. There were no complications. You are caring for D.A. in the PACU after the surgery. While assessing him you note the following: VS are 90/54, 87, 12, 37.8°C. Central venous pressure averages 10 mm Hg. He has a temporary pacemaker set at 87/min, which is functioning correctly. Lungs are clear. He has been extubated and is on 02 at 2L/min by nasal cannula with a SaO2 of 99%. He has a chest tube and indwelling urinary catheter. You review his lab results, noting a BUN 120 mg/dL, creatinine 8.5 mg/dL, and K 6.2 mmol/L. His pre-op Hct was 32%; now it is 22.1%, and his Hgb is 9.0 g/dL. Other lab values are within normal ranges.

Which of the above physiologic data should cause you concern and prompt careful monitoring on your part?

When you perform your physical assessment, you should pay special attention to s/s r/t D.A.'s problems. List at least five priority assessment areas, and explain why they are important.

While in post-op, D.A. has an infectious disease consult. The consulting physician writes in the chart, "the Enterobacter infection of the sinus of valsalva is the likely cause of the aneurysm. The heart was probably seeded from a renal source. If the patch continues to harbor organisms, the patient may have future problems. I recommend starting gentamicin and cefotaxime immediately". List 3 problems D.A. might have as a result of the antibiotics (consider his renal failure and common side effects of the medications)?

What are you sure to tell the receiving floor nurse?

PACU Institute Case Study

A 47-year-old woman with no known systemic disease was admitted to the PACU after a 5-hour face-lift procedure during which she was given intravenous sedatives with monitored anesthesia care. Vital signs on admission included a blood pressure of 148/77 mm Hg, a heart rate of 90/min, spontaneous respirations of 16/min to 20/min, and oxygen saturation of 99%. The patient was sleeping and was nonresponsive to verbal or painful stimuli.

Preoperatively, no medications were given. Intraoperatively, the patient received 2 mg of midazolam intravenously, 100 µg of fentanyl intravenously, 50 to 75 µg/kg per minute of propofol via infusion, 0.625 mg droperidol intravenously, and 3 L/m of oxygen via nasal cannula. Her vital signs remained normal throughout the 5-hour operation.

After 30 minutes in the PACU, the patient remained somnolent and could not be aroused. Suddenly she began thrashing in the bed, screaming and kicking, and seemed uncontrollable. This behavior lasted approximately 2 to 3 minutes and was followed by somnolence lasting 10 to 13 minutes. Again, she began shouting profanities, then relaxed momentarily. Her demeanor was irrational and inappropriate. The certified registered nurse anesthetist and surgeon were notified of the change in status and were asked to assist. During an evaluation, the patient was unresponsive to commands. Vital signs were unchanged, and oxygen saturation remained at 98% to 100%, confirming an absence of hypoxemia.

What medications can you give to calm the patient?

Despite medication administration her behavior did not change. She continued to have intermittent episodes of the previously described inappropriate behavior that lasted approximately 1 to 3 minutes and were followed by rest periods of 1 to 15 minutes.

What do you suspect is going on?

What is one of the most important questions to ask pre-op?

Because of her unexplained behavior in the PACU, her family was called. Her husband disclosed that she was using the antidepressants fluoxetine and citalopram as well as lorazepam for sleep, all doses unknown. The bottles were sitting on her bedside table at home. Additional social history was significant for marital problems, including physical and emotional abuse and extramarital affairs.

After approximately 2 hours, the patient was awake and calm. Her vital signs remained stable, and she was deemed ready for discharge. For her safety, however, she was admitted to the hospital for observation and a psychiatric consultation

PACU Institute Case Study

You receive the following report from the OR nurse: A.J. is a 56-year-old man with a PMH of chronic bronchitis. He quit smoking 12 yrs ago. He is s/p RML and RLL lobectomy; the pathology report is pending. He is extubated, has no neuro deficits and his VS are 120s/70, 110s, 34 and 100.2. His heart RRR, +pulses, and an IV of D51/2NS at 50ml/h R forearm. He has a R midaxillary chest tube to PleurEvac drain; there's no air leak, and its draining small amts of serosanguineous fluid. He's c/o pain at the insertion site, but the site looks good, and the dressing is dry and intact. He's on 5L/O2. He is refusing pain medications. He is very nervous and anxious.

What additional information would you ask the nurse to provide at this time?

A.J. is now in his post-op bed. When you try and get him to lie down he refuses and says he has to sit up and keeps rubbing his left hand over his right chest. What issues/problems can you already identify?

List four things you would do for A.J.?

A.J states, "I have a nephew who rolled his Jeep and busted himself up real bad. He got hooked on those drugs, and I don't want any part of them". How do you response to his statement?

Why is A.J. experiencing difficulty using his R arm? Given the type of surgery he underwent, is this expected?

You administer 8 mg morphine (MSO4) IM and tell A.J. that you will return in 30 minutes; 15 minutes later, he turns on his call light. When you enter the room, A.J. says, "I think I'm going to throw up." What are the next 3 things you would do? What do you think s responsible for the sudden onset of nausea? What medications would you anticipate giving?

A.J.'s pain and nausea are under control, but 30 minutes later you note is his head bobs up and his mouth opens, like a fish taking in water, every time he inhales. He says "I just can't (breath) seen to (breath) get enough (breath) air". Identify six possible problems that would account for his behavior? What 3 actions should you take next?

B. G. is struck by a vehicle while riding his motorcycle and is transported to your hospital by ambulance. He is found to have a fractured mandible and multiple fractures for the R tibia and fibula. He is taken to the OR for intermaxillary fixation (wiring of the jaw) and pinning of the fractured tibia and fibula. He returns from surgery with his jaws wired. What patient care issues related to his wired jaw would you be concerned about postoperatively?

What precautions will you take to ensure a patent airway in B.G. if he begins vomiting while his jaws are wired?

If B.G. begins vomiting with his jaws wired, what actions should you take?

You are now calling the floor to give report, what instructions should you give the nurse (to tell B.G. at D/C) concerning oral care and safety?

C.W. is a 36-year-old woman admitted 7 days ago for IBD with SBO. She underwent surgery 3 days post admission for a colectomy and ileostomy. She underwent surgery 3 days post admission for a colectomy and ileostomy. She developed peritonitis, and 4 days later she is back in the OR for an exploratory laparotomy. The lap revealed another area of perforated bower, generalized peritonitis, and a fistula tract to the abdominal surface. Another 12 in. of ileum were resected (in addition to the 7 ft previously taken out). The peritoneal cavity was irrigated with NS, and 3 tubes were placed: a JP drain to bulb suction, a rubber catheter to irrigate the wound bed with NS, and a sump pump to remove the irrigation. An R subclavian triple lumen catheter was inserted.

C.W. returns to PACU on your shift. What do you do when her bed is rolled into the room?

You pull back the covers to inspect the abdominal dressing and find that the original surgical dressing is saturated with fresh bloody drainage. What should you do?

C.W. has a total of 4 tubes in her abdomen as well as an NGT. What information should you gather from each tube? **Note: for safety all tubes should be clearly labeled.**

The sump irrigation fluid bag is nearly empty. You close the roller clamp, thread the IV tubing through the infusion pump, check the irrigation catheter connection site to make sure it is snug, and then discover that the nearly empty liter bag infusing into C.W.'s abdomen is D5W, not NS. Does this require any action? If so, give rationale, and explain overall situation.

PACU Institute Case Study

Mr. Smith a 74-year-old male married and retired is presently in pre-op awaiting a right hemisphere colectomy. He has a 40 pack-year history of smoking. The surgeon has ordered meperidine (Demerol) 50mg IM and glycopyrrolate (Robinul) 0.35mg IM on call to surgery. His daughter asks you why her dad is getting medication before his surgery.

Describe what you would explain to the family about the drugs that were ordered for Mr. Smith.

After surgery the OR nurse calls and says Mr. Smith did well in theatre and has a midline incision with a penrose drain, and a stab wound with a Jackson pratt drain to the incision. He also has a NG tube attached to intermittent suction. He is alert and oriented ×3 and can move all four extremities. VS BP 136/76, R 16, O2 stat 6% on 2L via mask.

What are his risk factors?

What is his aldrete score?

What nursing measures can you initiate to promote oxygenation?

Fifteen minutes after he arrived to the PACU, you retake his vital signs. His temp is 95.4 and he is shivering uncontrollably. What is your first action?

His shivering has caused a distal 1cm dehiscence, what is the sequelae you are trying to prevent?

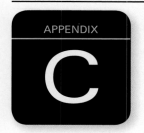

APPENDIX

C

PACU Institute Weekly Evaluations

Weekly Evaluation for PACU Institute
Year of 2011

Orientee: _____ Dates of evaluation period: _____ Week#: 1

Preceptor: #1 _____ #2 _____

Note: This form must be completed within 3 days after the report period. Completion of this form is a shared responsibility between the orientee and preceptor.

Assign the appropriate numerical value to the following statements:

Needs no supervision	Needs minimal supervision	Continuous supervision		not observed
(5)	(4)	(3)	(2) (1)	(0)

I. WORK QUALITY/QUANTITY

    a. Displays organizational skills in managing patient assignments.   _____

    b. Sets priorities according to the needs of the patient and unit.   _____

    c. Works to meet emotional/physical needs of the patient and family.   _____

    d. Documentation is organized and complete.   _____

    e. Understands theoretical information and applies to practice.   _____

    f. Identifies interventions required in actual and potential emergency situations.   _____

    g. Seeks out appropriate guidance in unfamiliar situations.   _____

    h. Reports patient changes promptly to the appropriate personnel.   _____

II. DEVELOPMENT OF TECHNICAL SKILLS AND CRITICAL THINKING

    a. States priorities in post-operative nursing care, including phase I, phase II, and Fast Track   _____

    b. Perform head to toe assessment.   _____

    c. Demonstrates ability to care for each patient despite phase of recovery and age.   _____

    d. Able to use equipment, monitors, and essentris after demonstrations and supervision.   _____

    e. Effective airway management.   _____

    f. States indications for emergency equipment and prepares for use. _____

    g. Able to differentiate normal/abnormal lab values, interpret results, and recognize appropriate interventions for abnormal ABGs, CBC, BMP, coagulation panels, cardiac enzymes, electrolyte panels, Mg, Phos, TSH. _____

    h. Implements pain and sedation management strategies for a variety of patients with pain control, sedation, including pain management via PCAs, Epidural, and Peripheral Nerve Caths _____

    i. Management of post-operative nausea, vomiting. _____

    j. Demonstrate care of the hypothermic patient. _____

    k. Able to describe indications, expected effects, adverse/side effects of PACU meds. _____

    l. Demonstrates appropriate administration of analgesics, antiarrhythmics, anxiolytics, beta blockers, calcium anatagonists, inotropes, neuromuscular blocking agents, sedatives, vasodilators, vasopressors. _____

    m. Understands and correctly assesses the Aldrete Score. _____

    n. Assess sensory level using appropriate dermatome levels. _____

    o. Takes initiative to assist with procedures and attempt new skills _____

    p. Displays knowledge of unit policies: infection control, biohazard safety, fire safety, and Crash cart. _____

III. <u>PERSONAL TRAITS</u>

    a. Displays military and professional decorum. _____

    b. Displays a positive attitude and accepts constructive guidance. _____

    c. Works cooperatively with peers and willingly offers assistance to peers and co-workers. _____

    d. Is self-motivated in enhancing his/her own personal and professional development. _____

IV. <u>ACCOMPLISHMENTS FOR WEEK 1 (To be completed by orientee).</u>
Assign the appropriate numerical value to the following statements:

    Weekly objective met   Weekly objective not met
        (1)   (0)

    a. Adult Post-operative/anesthesia care. _____

    b. Demonstrates ability to assess patient on arrival to PACU. _____

    c. Basic airway management. _____

    d. Perform a respiratory assessment on admission and upon discharge. _____

    e. Identify the signs and symptoms of respiratory distress or airway obstruction. _____

    f. Identify existing and/or select the appropriate type of airway adjunct and oxygen delivery system based on condition of patient. _____

    g. Establish Level of Consciousness (LOC). _____

    h. Initiate steps of BLS if indicated _____

    i. Demonstrate use of bag-valve-mask. _____

   j. Circulatory management. _____

   k. General anesthesia recovery. _____

   l. Regional anesthesia recovery. _____

  m. Monitored Anesthesia Care (MAC) recovery. _____

   n. Fluid management. _____

   o. Pain management. _____

   p. Nausea and vomiting management. _____

   q. Thermoregulation. _____

   r. Documentation of circulation and neurovascular checks on vital signs flow sheet. _____

   s. Documentation of dermatome levels. _____

   t. Neurology flow sheet. _____

   u. Identify location of Malignant Hyperthermia (MH) Cart. _____

   v. Assess patient for discharge criteria. _____

  w. Completes and documents recovery record. _____

   x. Demonstrate competency in the use of the i-STAT, POCT, Glucometer, PCA, and epidural pumps. _____

V. <u>GOALS FOR THE FOLLOWING WEEK (To be completed by the orientee and preceptor).</u>

_____

_____

_____

_____

_____

_____

VI. <u>PRECEPTORS COMMENTS/SUGGESTIONS (Include strengths/weaknesses)</u>

_____

_____

_____

_____

_____

_____

VIII.   ORIENTEE'S <u>COMMENTS/SUGGESTIONS</u>

_____

_____

_____

_____

_____

Preceptor's signature: _____ Date: _____

Orientee's signature: _____ Date: _____

CNS's signature: _____ Date: _____

Division Officer's signature: _____ Date: _____

Weekly Evaluation for PACU Institute
Year of 2011

Orientee: _____ Dates of evaluation period: _____ Week#: 2

Preceptor: #1 _____ #2 _____

Note: This form must be completed within 3 days after the report period. Completion of this form is a shared responsibility between the orientee and preceptor.

Assign the appropriate numerical value to the following statements:

Needs no supervision	Needs minimal supervision	Continuous supervision	not observed
(5)	(4)	(3)	(2)	(1)	(0)

I. WORK QUALITY/QUANTITY

    a. Displays organizational skills in managing patient assignments. _____

    b. Sets priorities according to the needs of the patient and unit. _____

    c. Works to meet emotional/physical needs of the patient and family. _____

    d. Documentation is organized and complete. _____

    e. Understands theoretical information and applies to practice. _____

    f. Identifies interventions required in actual and potential emergency situations. _____

    g. Seeks out appropriate guidance in unfamiliar situations. _____

    h. Reports patient changes promptly to the appropriate personnel. _____

II. DEVELOPMENT OF TECHNICAL SKILLS AND CRITICAL THINKING

    a. States priorities in post-operative nursing care, including phase I, phase II, and Fast Track _____

    b. Review surgeons versus anesthesia providers' responsibilities to the PACU patient. _____

    c. Perform head to toe assessment. _____

    d. Demonstrates ability to care for each patient despite phase of recovery and age. _____

    e. Able to use equipment, monitors, and essentris after demonstrations and supervision. _____

    f. Effective airway management. _____

    g. States indications for emergency equipment and prepares for use. _____

    h. Able to differentiate normal/abnormal lab values, interpret results, and recognize appropriate interventions for abnormal ABGs, CBC, BMP, coagulation panels, cardiac enzymes, electrolyte panels, Mg, Phos, TSH. _____

    i. Implements pain and sedation management strategies for a variety of patients with pain control, sedation, including pain management via PCAs, Epidural, and Peripheral Nerve Caths _____

    j. Management of post-operative nausea, vomiting. _____

    k. Demonstrate care of the hypothermic patient.   _____

    l. Able to describe indications, expected effects, adverse/side effects of PACU meds.   _____

    m. Demonstrates appropriate administration of analgesics, antiarrhythmics, anxiolytics, beta blockers, calcium antagonists, inotropes, neuromuscular blocking agents, sedatives, vasodilators, vasopressors.   _____

    n. Understands and correctly assesses the Aldrete Score.   _____

    o. Assess sensory level using appropriate dermatome levels.   _____

    p. Takes initiative to assist with procedures and attempt new skills   _____

    q. Displays knowledge of unit policies: infection control, biohazard safety, fire safety, and Crash cart.   _____

III. PERSONAL TRAITS

    a. Displays military and professional decorum.   _____

    b. Displays a positive attitude and accepts constructive guidance.   _____

    c. Works cooperatively with peers and willingly offers assistance to peers and co-workers.   _____

    d. Is self-motivated in enhancing his/her own personal and professional development.   _____

IV. ACCOMPLISHMENTS FOR WEEK 2 (To be completed by orientee).

Assign the appropriate numerical value to the following statements:

  Weekly objective met   Weekly objective not met
        (1)   (0)

    a. Adult Post-operative/anesthesia care.   _____

    b. Demonstrates ability to assess patient on arrival to PACU.   _____

    c. Basic airway management.   _____

    d. Perform a respiratory assessment on admission and upon discharge.   _____

    e. Identify the signs and symptoms of respiratory distress or airway obstruction.   _____

    f. Identify existing and/or select the appropriate type of airway adjunct and oxygen delivery system based on condition of patient.   _____

    g. Establish Level of Consciousness (LOC).   _____

    h. Initiate steps of BLS if indicated.   _____

    i. Demonstrate use of bag-valve-mask.   _____

    j. Circulatory management.   _____

    k. General anesthesia recovery.   _____

    l. Regional anesthesia recovery.   _____

    m. Monitored Anesthesia Care (MAC) recovery.   _____

    n. Fluid management.   _____

    o. Pain management.   _____

    p. Nausea and vomiting management.   _____

q. Thermoregulation. _____

r. Documentation of circulation and neurovascular checks on vital signs flow sheet. _____

s. Documentation of dermatome levels. _____

t. Neurology flow sheet. _____

u. Identify location of Malignant Hyperthermia (MH) Cart. _____

v. Assess patient for discharge criteria. _____

w. Completes and documents recovery record. _____

V. GOALS FOR THE FOLLOWING WEEK (To be completed by the orientee and preceptor).

_____

_____

_____

_____

_____

_____

VI. PRECEPTORS COMMENTS/SUGGESTIONS (Include strengths/weaknesses)

_____

_____

_____

_____

_____

_____

VIII. ORIENTEE'S COMMENTS/SUGGESTIONS

_____

_____

_____

_____

_____

_____

Preceptor's signature: _____ Date: _____

Orientee's signature: _____ Date: _____

CNS's signature: _____ Date: _____

Division Officer's signature: _____ Date: _____

Weekly Evaluation for PACU Institute
Year of 2011

Orientee: _____ Dates of evaluation period: _____ Week#: _3_

Preceptor: #1 _____ #2 _____

Note: This form must be completed within 3 days after the report period. Completion of this form is a shared responsibility between the orientee and preceptor.

Assign the appropriate numerical value to the following statements:

Needs no supervision	Needs minimal supervision	Continuous supervision		not observed
(5)	(4)	(3)	(2)	(1)	(0)

I. WORK QUALITY/QUANTITY

a. Displays organizational skills in managing patient assignments. _____

b. Sets priorities according to the needs of the patient and unit. _____

c. Works to meet emotional/physical needs of the patient and family. _____

d. Documentation is organized and complete. _____

e. Understands theoretical information and applies to practice. _____

f. Identifies interventions required in actual and potential emergency situations. _____

g. Seeks out appropriate guidance in unfamiliar situations. _____

h. Reports patient changes promptly to the appropriate personnel. _____

II. DEVELOPMENT OF TECHNICAL SKILLS AND CRITICAL THINKING

a. States priorities in post-operative nursing care, including phase I, phase II, and Fast Track _____

b. Perform head to toe assessment. _____

c. Demonstrates ability to care for each patient despite phase of recovery and age. _____

d. Able to use equipment, monitors, and essentris after demonstrations and supervision. _____

e. Effective airway management. _____

f. States indications for emergency equipment and prepares for use. _____

g. Able to differentiate normal/abnormal lab values, interpret results, and recognize appropriate interventions for abnormal ABGs, CBC, BMP, coagulation panels, cardiac enzymes, electrolyte panels, Mg, Phos, TSH. _____

h. Implements pain and sedation management strategies for a variety of patients with pain control, sedation, including pain management via PCAs, Epidural, and Peripheral Nerve Caths _____

i. Management of post-operative nausea, vomiting. _____

j. Demonstrate care of the hypothermic patient. _____

k. Able to describe indications, expected effects, adverse/side effects of PACU meds. _____

l. Demonstrates appropriate administration of analgesics, antiarrhythmics, anxiolytics, beta blockers, calcium anatagonists, inotropes, neuromuscular blocking agents, sedatives, vasodilators, vasopressors. _____

m. Understands and correctly assesses the Aldrete Score. _____

n. Assess sensory level using appropriate dermatome levels. _____

o. Takes initiative to assist with procedures and attempt new skills _____

p. Displays knowledge of unit policies: infection control, biohazard safety, fire safety, and Crash cart. _____

III. PERSONAL TRAITS

a. Displays military and professional decorum. _____

b. Displays a positive attitude and accepts constructive guidance. _____

c. Works cooperatively with peers and willingly offers assistance to peers and co-workers. _____

d. Is self-motivated in enhancing his/her own personal and professional development. _____

IV. ACCOMPLISHMENTS FOR WEEK 3 (To be completed by orientee).
Assign the appropriate numerical value to the following statements:

Weekly objective met   Weekly objective not met
    (1)   (0)

a. Demonstrates competency to coordinate care. _____

b. Establishes priorities and organizes nursing activities. _____

c. Promotes patient and family centered care. _____

d. Performs 12 Lead EKG. _____

e. Performs cardiovascular assessment. _____

f. Interpret cardiac rhythm. _____

g. Monitor cardiopulmonary status. _____

h. Monitor body temperature and initiate warming measures (warmed blankets, Bair Paws, Bair Hugger). _____

i. Demonstrates knowledge of and indications for the use of common PACU medications. _____

j. Provides nursing care for the patient requiring a urologic assessment. _____

k. Provides care for the patient with a urethral catheter. _____

l. Identifies indications and demonstrates use of bladder scanner. _____

m. Effectively communicates SBAR to receiving units. _____

n. TOW independently. _____

V. <u>**GOALS FOR THE FOLLOWING WEEK (To be completed by the orientee and preceptor).**</u>

_____

_____

_____

_____

_____

_____

VI. <u>**PRECEPTORS COMMENTS/SUGGESTIONS (Include strengths/weaknesses)**</u>

_____

_____

_____

_____

_____

_____

VIII. **ORIENTEE'S** <u>**COMMENTS/SUGGESTIONS**</u>

_____

_____

_____

_____

_____

Preceptor's signature: _____ Date: _____

Orientee's signature: _____ Date: _____

CNS's signature: _____ Date: _____

Division Officer's signature: _____ Date: _____

Weekly Evaluation for PACU Institute
Year of 2011

Orientee: _____ Dates of evaluation period: _____ Week#: 4

Overview for age specific competencies. Pediatric Assessment

Preceptor: #1 _____ #2 _____

Note: This form must be completed within 3 days after the report period. Completion of this form is a shared responsibility between the orientee and preceptor.

Assign the appropriate numerical value to the following statements:

Needs no supervision   Needs minimal supervision   Continuous supervision   not observed
(5)   (4)   (3)   (2)   (1)   (0)

I.   WORK QUALITY/QUANTITY

a.   Displays organizational skills in managing patient assignments.   _____

b.   Sets priorities according to the needs of the patient and unit.   _____

c.   Works to meet emotional/physical needs of the patient and family.   _____

d.   Documentation is organized and complete.   _____

e.   Understands theoretical information and applies to practice.   _____

f.   Identifies interventions required in actual and potential emergency situations. _____

g.   Seeks out appropriate guidance in unfamiliar situations.   _____

h.   Reports patient changes promptly to the appropriate personnel.   _____

II.   DEVELOPMENT OF TECHNICAL SKILLS AND CRITICAL THINKING

a.   States priorities in post-operative nursing care, including phase I, phase II, and Fast Track   _____

b.   Perform head to toe assessment.   _____

c.   Demonstrates ability to care for each patient despite phase of recovery and age.   _____

d.   Able to use equipment, monitors, and essentris after demonstrations and supervision.   _____

e.   Effective airway management.   _____

f.   States indications for emergency equipment and prepares for use.   _____

g.   Able to differentiate normal/abnormal lab values, interpret results, and recognize appropriate interventions for abnormal ABGs, CBC, BMP, coagulation panels, cardiac enzymes, electrolyte panels, Mg, Phos, TSH.   _____

h.   Implements pain and sedation management strategies for a variety of patients with pain control, sedation, including pain management via PCAs, Epidural, and Peripheral Nerve Caths   _____

i.   Management of post-operative nausea, vomiting.   _____

j.   Demonstrate care of the hypothermic patient.   _____

    k. Able to describe indications, expected effects, adverse/side effects of PACU meds. _____

    l. Demonstrates appropriate administration of analgesics, antiarrhythmics, anxiolytics, beta blockers, calcium anatagonists, inotropes, neuromuscular blocking agents, sedatives, vasodilators, vasopressors. _____

    m. Understands and correctly assesses the Aldrete Score. _____

    n. Assess sensory level using appropriate dermatome levels. _____

    o. Takes initiative to assist with procedures and attempt new skills _____

    p. Displays knowledge of unit policies: infection control, biohazard safety, fire safety, and Crash cart. _____

III. PERSONAL TRAITS

    a. Displays military and professional decorum. _____

    b. Displays a positive attitude and accepts constructive guidance. _____

    c. Works cooperatively with peers and willingly offers assistance to peers and co-workers. _____

    d. Is self-motivated in enhancing his/her own personal and professional development. _____

IV. ACCOMPLISHMENTS FOR WEEK 4 (To be completed by orientee).

Assign the appropriate numerical value to the following statements:

    Weekly objective met   Weekly objective not met

         (1)   (0)

    a. Perform a nursing assessment of the pediatric patient. _____

    b. Discuss the differences in pediatric anatomy, physiology, and development needs specific to perianesthesia interventions. _____

    c. Identify normal respirations, depressed respirations, stridor, croup, laryngospasm, obstruction, and appropriate nursing interventions for each of the assessment findings. _____

    d. Recognize indications of pain in the pediatric patient and initiate appropriate pain management techniques for age and weight. _____

    e. Identify the growth and development stage of the individual and adapt the nursing interventions to meet the unique needs of the child. _____

    f. Recognize signs and symptoms of child abuse. _____

    g. Complete earliest PALS available course ASAP. _____

V. GOALS FOR THE FOLLOWING WEEK (To be completed by the orientee and preceptor).

_____

_____

_____

_____

_____

_____

VI.   <u>PRECEPTORS COMMENTS/SUGGESTIONS (Include strengths/weaknesses)</u>

_____

_____

_____

_____

_____

VIII.   <u>ORIENTEE'S COMMENTS/SUGGESTIONS</u>

_____

_____

_____

_____

Preceptor's signature: _____ Date: _____

Orientee's signature: _____ Date: _____

CNS's signature: _____ Date: _____

Division Officer's signature: _____ Date: _____

Weekly Evaluation for PACU Institute
Year of 2011

Orientee: _____ Dates of evaluation period: _____ Week#: _5_

Advanced Airway

Preceptor: #1 _____ #2 _____

Note: This form must be completed within 3 days after the report period. Completion of this form is a shared responsibility between the orientee and preceptor.

Assign the appropriate numerical value to the following statements:

Needs no supervision	Needs minimal supervision	Continuous supervision	not observed
(5)	(4)	(3)	(2)	(1)	(0)

I. WORK QUALITY/QUANTITY

a. Displays organizational skills in managing patient assignments. _____

b. Sets priorities according to the needs of the patient and unit. _____

c. Works to meet emotional/physical needs of the patient and family. _____

d. Documentation is organized and complete. _____

e. Understands theoretical information and applies to practice. _____

f. Identifies interventions required in actual and potential emergency situations. _____

g. Seeks out appropriate guidance in unfamiliar situations. _____

h. Reports patient changes promptly to the appropriate personnel. _____

II. DEVELOPMENT OF TECHNICAL SKILLS AND CRITICAL THINKING

a. States priorities in post-operative nursing care, including phase I, phase II, and Fast Track _____

b. Perform head to toe assessment. _____

c. Demonstrates ability to care for each patient despite phase of recovery and age. _____

d. Able to use equipment, monitors, and essentris after demonstrations and supervision. _____

e. Effective airway management. _____

f. States indications for emergency equipment and prepares for use. _____

g. Able to differentiate normal/abnormal lab values, interpret results, and recognize appropriate interventions for abnormal ABGs, CBC, BMP, coagulation panels, cardiac enzymes, electrolyte panels, Mg, Phos, TSH. _____

h. Implements pain and sedation management strategies for a variety of patients with pain control, sedation, including pain management via PCAs, Epidural, and Peripheral Nerve Caths _____

i. Management of post-operative nausea, vomiting. _____

j. Demonstrate care of the hypothermic patient. _____

k. Able to describe indications, expected effects, adverse/side effects of PACU meds. _____

l. Demonstrates appropriate administration of analgesics, antiarrhythmics, anxiolytics, beta blockers, calcium anatagonists, inotropes, neuromuscular blocking agents, sedatives, vasodilators, vasopressors. _____

m. Understands and correctly assesses the Aldrete Score. _____

n. Assess sensory level using appropriate dermatome levels. _____

o. Takes initiative to assist with procedures and attempt new skills _____

p. Displays knowledge of unit policies: infection control, biohazard safety, fire safety, and Crash cart. _____

III. PERSONAL TRAITS

a. Displays military and professional decorum. _____

b. Displays a positive attitude and accepts constructive guidance. _____

c. Works cooperatively with peers and willingly offers assistance to peers and co-workers. _____

d. Is self-motivated in enhancing his/her own personal and professional development. _____

IV. ACCOMPLISHMENTS FOR WEEK 5 (To be completed by orientee).

Assign the appropriate numerical value to the following statements:

Weekly objective met   Weekly objective not met
      (1)   (0)

a. Demonstrates advanced airway management. _____

b. Demonstrate use of bag-valve mask. _____

c. Identify equipment utilized for advanced airway support. _____

d. Identify indications for advanced airway support. _____

e. Shadow anesthesia provider to observe airway management in the MOR for one day. _____

f. Shadow respiratory therapist for one day. _____

g. Tracheostomy and ventilators orientation. _____

V. GOALS FOR THE FOLLOWING WEEK (To be completed by the orientee and preceptor).

_____

_____

_____

_____

_____

_____

VI. <u>PRECEPTORS COMMENTS/SUGGESTIONS (Include strengths/weaknesses)</u>

_____

_____

_____

_____

_____

_____

VIII. <u>COMMENTS/SUGGESTIONS</u>

_____

_____

_____

_____

_____

Preceptor's signature: _____ Date: _____

Orientee's signature: _____ Date: _____

CNS's signature: _____ Date: _____

Division Officer's signature: _____ Date: _____

Weekly Evaluation for PACU Institute
Year of 2011

Orientee: _____ Dates of evaluation period: _____ Week#: _6_

<u>Wounded Warrior Care</u>

Preceptor: #1 _____ #2 _____

Note: This form must be completed within 3 days after the report period. Completion of this form is a shared responsibility between the orientee and preceptor.

<u>Assign the appropriate numerical value to the following statements:</u>
Needs no supervision   Needs minimal supervision   Continuous supervision   not observed
(5)   (4)   (3)   (2)   (1)   (0)

I.   WORK QUALITY/QUANTITY

a. Displays organizational skills in managing patient assignments.   _____

b. Sets priorities according to the needs of the patient and unit.   _____

c. Works to meet emotional/physical needs of the patient and family.   _____

d. Documentation is organized and complete.   _____

e. Understands theoretical information and applies to practice.   _____

f. Identifies interventions required in actual and potential emergency situations.   _____

g. Seeks out appropriate guidance in unfamiliar situations.   _____

h. Reports patient changes promptly to the appropriate personnel.   _____

II.   DEVELOPMENT OF TECHNICAL SKILLS AND CRITICAL THINKING

a. States priorities in post-operative nursing care, including phase I, phase II, and Fast Track   _____

b. Perform head to toe assessment.   _____

c. Demonstrates ability to care for each patient despite phase of recovery and age.   _____

d. Able to use equipment, monitors, and essentris after demonstrations and supervision.   _____

e. Effective airway management.   _____

f. States indications for emergency equipment and prepares for use.   _____

g. Able to differentiate normal/abnormal lab values, interpret results, and recognize appropriate interventions for abnormal ABGs, CBC, BMP, coagulation panels, cardiac enzymes, electrolyte panels, Mg, Phos, TSH.   _____

h. Implements pain and sedation management strategies for a variety of patients with pain control, sedation, including pain management via PCAs, Epidural, and Peripheral Nerve Caths   _____

i. Management of post-operative nausea, vomiting.   _____

    j. Demonstrate care of the hypothermic patient. _____

    k. Able to describe indications, expected effects, adverse/side effects of PACU meds. _____

    l. Demonstrates appropriate administration of analgesics, antiarrhythmics, anxiolytics, beta blockers, calcium antagonists, inotropes, neuromuscular blocking agents, sedatives, vasodilators, vasopressors. _____

    m. Understands and correctly assesses the Aldrete Score. _____

    n. Assess sensory level using appropriate dermatome levels. _____

    o. Takes initiative to assist with procedures and attempt new skills _____

    p. Displays knowledge of unit policies: infection control, biohazard safety, fire safety, and Crash cart. _____

III. PERSONAL TRAITS

    a. Displays military and professional decorum. _____

    b. Displays a positive attitude and accepts constructive guidance. _____

    c. Works cooperatively with peers and willingly offers assistance to peers and co-workers. _____

    d. Is self-motivated in enhancing his/her own personal and professional development. _____

IV. ACCOMPLISHMENTS WEEK 6 (To be completed by orientee).

Assign the appropriate numerical value to the following statements:

Weekly objective met   Weekly objective not met
       (1)   (0)

    a. PACU Wounded Warrior care assignment. _____

    b. Oriented to wound vacs. _____

    c. Increased proficiency for skills in week's I-V. _____

    d. Demonstrates ability to care for intubated patients including suctioning techniques. _____

    e. Demonstrate use of artificial airways. _____

    f. Oriented to arterial, CVP, cordis, peripheral nerve, and Swan ganz caths. _____

    g. Care for complex post-op patients. _____

V. GOALS FOR THE FOLLOWING WEEK (To be completed by the orientee and preceptor).

_____

_____

_____

_____

_____

_____

VI.   PRECEPTORS COMMENTS/SUGGESTIONS (Include strengths/weaknesses)

_____
_____
_____
_____
_____
_____

VIII.   COMMENTS/SUGGESTIONS

_____
_____
_____
_____
_____

Preceptor's signature: _____ Date: _____

Orientee's signature: _____ Date: _____

CNS's signature: _____ Date: _____

Division Officer's signature: _____ Date: _____

Weekly Evaluation for PACU Institute
Year of 2011

Orientee: _____ Dates of evaluation period: _____ Week#: 7

Preceptor: #1 _____ #2 _____

Note: This form must be completed within 3 days after the report period. Completion of this form is a shared responsibility between the orientee and preceptor.

Assign the appropriate numerical value to the following statements:

Needs no supervision   Needs minimal supervision   Continuous supervision   not observed

(5)   (4)   (3)   (2)   (1)   (0)

I. WORK QUALITY/QUANTITY

a. Displays organizational skills in managing patient assignments. _____

b. Sets priorities according to the needs of the patient and unit. _____

c. Works to meet emotional/physical needs of the patient and family. _____

d. Documentation is organized and complete. _____

e. Understands theoretical information and applies to practice. _____

f. Identifies interventions required in actual and potential emergency situations. _____

g. Seeks out appropriate guidance in unfamiliar situations. _____

h. Reports patient changes promptly to the appropriate personnel. _____

II. DEVELOPMENT OF TECHNICAL SKILLS AND CRITICAL THINKING

a. States priorities in post-operative nursing care, including phase I, phase II, and Fast Track _____

b. Perform head to toe assessment. _____

c. Demonstrates ability to care for each patient despite phase of recovery and age. _____

d. Able to use equipment, monitors, and essentris after demonstrations and supervision. _____

e. Effective airway management. _____

f. States indications for emergency equipment and prepares for use. _____

g. Able to differentiate normal/abnormal lab values, interpret results, and recognize appropriate interventions for abnormal ABGs, CBC, BMP, coagulation panels, cardiac enzymes, electrolyte panels, Mg, Phos, TSH. _____

h. Implements pain and sedation management strategies for a variety of patients with pain control, sedation, including pain management via PCAs, Epidural, and Peripheral Nerve Caths _____

i. Management of post-operative nausea, vomiting. _____

j. Demonstrate care of the hypothermic patient. _____

k. Able to describe indications, expected effects, adverse/side effects of PACU meds. _____

l. Demonstrates appropriate administration of analgesics, antiarrhythmics, anxiolytics, beta blockers, calcium antagonists, inotropes, neuromuscular blocking agents, sedatives, vasodilators, vasopressors. _____

m. Understands and correctly assesses the Aldrete Score. _____

n. Assess sensory level using appropriate dermatome levels. _____

o. Takes initiative to assist with procedures and attempt new skills _____

p. Displays knowledge of unit policies: infection control, biohazard safety, fire safety, and Crash cart. _____

III. PERSONAL TRAITS

a. Displays military and professional decorum. _____

b. Displays a positive attitude and accepts constructive guidance. _____

c. Works cooperatively with peers and willingly offers assistance to peers and co-workers. _____

d. Is self-motivated in enhancing his/her own personal and professional development. _____

IV. ACCOMPLISHMENTS WEEK 7 (To be completed by orientee).

Assign the appropriate numerical value to the following statements:

Weekly objective met   Weekly objective not met
      (1)   (0)

a. Demonstrates ability to independently provide patient care with minimal supervision from preceptor. _____

b. Complete Mosby CBT clinical skills. _____

V. GOALS FOR THE FOLLOWING WEEK (To be completed by the orientee and preceptor).

_____

_____

_____

_____

_____

_____

_____

VI.   <u>PRECEPTORS COMMENTS/SUGGESTIONS (Include strengths/weaknesses)</u>

_____

_____

_____

_____

_____

_____

VIII.   ORIENTEE'S <u>COMMENTS/SUGGESTIONS</u>

_____

_____

_____

_____

_____

Preceptor's signature: _____ Date: _____

Orientee's signature: _____ Date: _____

CNS's signature: _____ Date: _____

Division Officer's signature: _____ Date: _____

Weekly Evaluation for Institute
Year of 2011

Orientee: _____ Dates of evaluation period: _____ Week#: _8_

<u>PACU Keep Rotation/Final Orientation</u>

Preceptor: #1 _____ #2 _____

Note: This form must be completed within 3 days after the report period. Completion of this form is a shared responsibility between the orientee and preceptor.

<u>Assign the appropriate numerical value to the following statements:</u>

Needs no supervision	Needs minimal supervision	Continuous supervision	not observed
(5)	(4)	(3)	(2)	(1)	(0)

I. <u>WORK QUALITY/QUANTITY</u>

a. Displays organizational skills in managing patient assignments.   _____

b. Sets priorities according to the needs of the patient and unit.   _____

c. Works to meet emotional/physical needs of the patient and family.   _____

d. Documentation is organized and complete.   _____

e. Understands theoretical information and applies to practice.   _____

f. Identifies interventions required in actual and potential emergency situations.   _____

g. Seeks out appropriate guidance in unfamiliar situations.   _____

h. Reports patient changes promptly to the appropriate personnel.   _____

II. <u>DEVELOPMENT OF TECHNICAL SKILLS AND CRITICAL THINKING</u>

a. States priorities in post-operative nursing care, including phase I, phase II, and Fast Track   _____

b. Perform head to toe assessment.   _____

c. Demonstrates ability to care for each patient despite phase of recovery and age.   _____

d. Able to use equipment, monitors, and essentris after demonstrations and supervision.   _____

e. Effective airway management.   _____

f. States indications for emergency equipment and prepares for use.   _____

g. Able to differentiate normal/abnormal lab values, interpret results, and recognize appropriate interventions for abnormal ABGs, CBC, BMP, coagulation panels, cardiac enzymes, electrolyte panels, Mg, Phos, TSH.   _____

h. Implements pain and sedation management strategies for a variety of patients with pain control, sedation, including pain management via PCAs, Epidural, and Peripheral Nerve Caths   _____

    i. Management of post-operative nausea, vomiting. _____

    j. Demonstrate care of the hypothermic patient. _____

    k. Able to describe indications, expected effects, adverse/side effects of PACU meds. _____

    l. Demonstrates appropriate administration of analgesics, antiarrhythmics, anxiolytics, beta blockers, calcium antagonists, inotropes, neuromuscular blocking agents, sedatives, vasodilators, vasopressors. _____

    m. Understands and correctly assesses the Aldrete Score. _____

    n. Assess sensory level using appropriate dermatome levels. _____

    o. Takes initiative to assist with procedures and attempt new skills _____

    p. Displays knowledge of unit policies: infection control, biohazard safety, fire safety, and Crash cart. _____

III. PERSONAL TRAITS

    a. Displays military and professional decorum. _____

    b. Displays a positive attitude and accepts constructive guidance. _____

    c. Works cooperatively with peers and willingly offers assistance to peers and co-workers. _____

    d. Is self-motivated in enhancing his/her own personal and professional development. _____

IV. ACCOMPLISHMENTS WEEK 8 (To be completed by orientee).

Assign the appropriate numerical value to the following statements:

Weekly objective met   Weekly objective not met
      (1)   (0)

    a. Coriented to care of the PACU Keep. _____

    b. Complete Post PACU Medication Exam. _____

    c. Complete Competency Based Orientation Modules including all chapters' quizzes. _____

    d. Complete Competency Based Orientation exam achieving a score of 128/159. _____

V. GOALS FOR THE FOLLOWING WEEK (To be completed by the orientee and preceptor).

_____

_____

_____

_____

_____

_____

VI.   <u>PRECEPTORS COMMENTS/SUGGESTIONS (Include strengths/weaknesses)</u>

_____

_____

_____

_____

_____

_____

VIII.   <u>COMMENTS/SUGGESTIONS</u>

_____

_____

_____

_____

_____

Preceptor's signature: _____ Date: _____

Orientee's signature: _____ Date: _____

CNS's signature: _____ Date: _____

Division Officer's signature: _____ Date: _____

Department Head's signature: _____ Date: _____

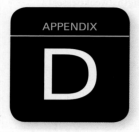

Maslach Burnout Inventory-Human Services Survey

For use by Seun Ross only. Received from Mind Garden, Inc. on June 15, 2011

MBI-Human Services Survey

Christina Maslach & Susan E. Jackson

The purpose of this survey is to discover how various persons in the human services, or helping professionals view their job and the people with whom they work closely.

Because persons in a wide variety of occupations will answer this survey, it uses the term *recipients* to refer to the people for whom you provide your service, care, treatment, or instruction. When answering this survey please think of these people as recipients of the service you provide, even though you may use another term in your work.

Instructions: On the following pages are 22 statements of job-related feelings. Please read each statement carefully and decide if you ever feel this way about *your* job. If you have *never* had this feeling, write the number "0" (zero) in the space before the statement. If you have had this feeling, indicate *how often* you feel it by writing the number (from 1 to 6) that best describes how frequently you feel that way. An example is shown below.

Example:

How often:	0	1	2	3	4	5	6
	Never	A few times a year or less	Once a month or less	A few times a month	Once a week	A few times a week	Every day

How Often 0-6	Statement:
1. _____	I feel depressed at work.

If you never feel depressed at work, you would write the number "o" (zero) under the heading "How Often." If you rarely feel depressed at work (a few times a year or less), you would write the number "1." If your feelings of depression are fairly frequent (a few times a week but not daily), you would write the number "5."

MBI-Human Services Survey

How often:	0	1	2	3	4	5	6
	Never	A few times a year or less	Once a month or less	A few times a month	Once a week	A few times a week	Every day

How Often 0-6	Statement:
1. _____	I feel emotionally drained from my work.
2. _____	I feel used up at the end of the workday.
3. _____	I feel fatigued when I get up in the morning and have to face another day on the job.
4. _____	I can easily understand how my recipients feel about things.
5. _____	I feel I treat some recipients as if they were impersonal objects.
6. _____	Working with people all day is really a strain for me.
7. _____	I deal very effectively with the problems of my recipients.
8. _____	I feel burned out from my work.
9. _____	I feel I'm positively influencing other people's lives through my work.
10. _____	I've become more callouts toward people since I took this job.
11. _____	I worry that this job is hardening me emotionally.
12. _____	I feel very energetic.
13. _____	I feel frustrated by my job.
14. _____	I feel I'm working too hard on my job.
15. _____	I don't' really care what happens to some recipients.
16. _____	Working with people directly puts too much stress on me.
17. _____	I can easily create a relaxed atmosphere with my recipients.
18. _____	I feel exhilarated after working closely with my recipients.
19. _____	I have accomplished many worthwhile things in this job.
20. _____	I feel like I'm at the end of my rope.
21. _____	In my work, I deal with emotional problems very calmly.
22. _____	I feel recipients blame me for some of their problems.

(Administrative use only)

EE: _____ cat: _____   DP: _____ cat: _____   PA: _____ cat: _____

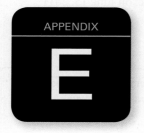

APPENDIX

E

Expanded Nurse Stress Scale

Below is a list of situations that commonly occur in a work setting. For each situation you have encountered in your **PRESENT WORK SETTING**, would you indicate **HOW STRESSFUL** it has been for you:

(Enter the number in the right-hand column that best applies to you. If you have not encountered the situation, write "0".)

Never Stressful	Occasionally Stressful	Frequently Stressful	Always Stressful	Does Not Apply
1	2	3	4	5

1. Performing procedures that patients experience as painful . . . . ___
2. Criticism by a physician . . . . ___
3. Feeling inadequately prepared to help with the emotional needs of a patient's family . . . . ___
4. Lack of opportunity to talk openly with other personnel about problems in the work setting. . . . . ___
5. Conflict with a supervisor . . . . ___
6. Inadequate information from a physician regarding the medical condition of a patient . . . . ___
7. Patients making unreasonable demands . . . . ___
8. Being sexually harassed . . . . ___
9. Feeling helpless in the case of a patient who fails to improve . . . . ___
10. Conflict with a physician. . . . . ___
11. Being asked a question by a patient for which I do not have a satisfactory answer . . . . ___
12. Lack of opportunity to share experiences and feelings with other personnel in the work setting . . . . ___
13. Unpredictable staffing and scheduling. . . . . ___
14. A physician ordering what appears to be inappropriate treatment for a patient . . . . ___
15. Patients' families making unreasonable demands . . . . ___
16. Experiencing discrimination because of race or ethnicity . . . . ___
17. Listening or talking to a patient about his/her approaching death . . . . ___
18. Fear of making a mistake in treating a patient . . . . ___

Never Stressful	Occasionally Stressful	Frequently Stressful	Extremely Stressful	Does Not Apply
1	2	3	4	5

19. Feeling inadequately prepared to help with the emotional needs of a patient . . . . ____

20. Lack of an opportunity to express to other personnel on the unit my negative feelings toward patients . . . . ____

21. Difficulty in working with a particular nurse (or nurses) in my <u>immediate</u> work setting . . . . ____

22. Difficulty in working with a particular nurse (or nurses) <u>outside</u> my immediate work setting . . . . ____

23. Not enough time to provide emotional support to the patient . . . . ____

24. A physician not being present in a medical emergency . . . . ____

25. Being blamed for anything that goes wrong . . . . ____

26. Experiencing discrimination on the basis of sex . . . . ____

27. The death of a patient . . . . ____

28. Disagreement concerning the treatment of a patient . . . . ____

29. Feeling inadequately trained for what I have to do . . . . ____

30. Lack of support of my immediate supervisor . . . . ____

31. Criticism by a supervisor . . . . ____

32. Not enough time to complete all of my nursing tasks . . . . ____

33. Not knowing what a patient or a patient's family ought to be told about the patient's condition and its treatment . . . . ____

34. Being the one that has to deal with the patients' families . . . . ____

35. Having to deal with violent patients . . . . ____

36. Being exposed to health and safety hazards . . . . ____

37. The death of a patient with whom you developed a close relationship . . . . ____

38. Making a decision concerning a patient when the physician is unavailable . . . . ____

39. Being in charge with inadequate experience . . . . ____

40. Lack of support by nursing administration . . . . ____

41. Too many non-nursing tasks required, such as clerical work . . . . ____

42. Not enough staff to adequately cover the unit . . . . ____

43. Uncertainty regarding the operation and functioning of specialized equipment . . . . ____

44. Having to deal with abusive patients . . . . ____

Never	Occasionally	Frequently	Extremely	Does Not
Stressful	Stressful	Stressful	Stressful	Apply
1	2	3	4	5

45. Not enough time to respond to the needs of patients' families. . . . . ___
46. Being held accountable for things over which I have no control . . . . . . ___
47. Physician(s) not being present when a patient dies . . . . ___
48. Having to organize doctors' work. . . . . ___
49. Lack of support from other health-care administrators . . . . ___
50. Difficulty in working with nurses of the opposite sex . . . . ___
51. Demands of patient classification system . . . . ___
52. Having to deal with abuse from patients' families . . . . ___
53. Watching a patient suffer. . . . . ___
54. Criticism from nursing administration . . . . ___
55. Having to work through breaks . . . . ___
56. Not knowing whether patients' families will report
    you for inadequate care . . . . ___
57. Having to make decisions under pressure. . . . . ___

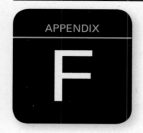

Measure of Job Satisfaction/Intent to Leave Questionnaire

The measure of job satisfaction

> This measure has been designed to assess how groups of nurses feel about different aspects of their job. Please answer LACH question by ticking ONLY ONE box and be sure to answer all questions even though some may seem similar. You do not need to give your name. All answers are absolutely confidential. You will NOT BE identified.

Adapt the first two pages to your requirements: the measure starts on page 3

Age	❏
Under 25	❏
26–34	❏
35–44	❏
45–54	❏
54+	❏
Female	❏
Male	❏

JOB TITLE – adapt as necessary

District Nurse	❏	Midwife	❏
	❏	Student Midwife	❏
School Nurse	❏	Staff Nurse	❏
Practice Nurse	❏	Student Nurse	❏
Health Visitor	❏	Healthcare Assistant	❏
Student HV	❏		❏
Nurse Manager	❏	Tutor	❏
	❏	Ward Sister/ Charge Nurse	❏
Clinical Nurse Specialist	❏	Other (please verify)	❏
		_____	

How satisfied are you with these aspects of your work:	Very satisfied	Satisfied	Neither satisfied nor dissatisfied	Dissatisfied	Very dissatisfied
1. Payment for the hours I work	❏	❏	❏	❏	❏
2. The degree to which I feel part of a team	❏	❏	❏	❏	❏
3. The opportunities I have to discuss my concepts	❏	❏	❏	❏	❏
4. My salary/pay scale	❏	❏	❏	❏	❏
5. Being funded for courses	❏	❏	❏	❏	❏
6. The time available to get through my work	❏	❏	❏	❏	❏
7. The quality of work with patients/clients	❏	❏	❏	❏	❏
8. The standards of care given to patients/clients	❏	❏	❏	❏	❏
9. The degree to which I am fairly paid for what I contribute to this organisation	❏	❏	❏	❏	❏
10. The amount of support and guidance I receive	❏	❏	❏	❏	❏
11. The way that patients/ clients are cared for	❏	❏	❏	❏	❏

	Very satisfied	Satisfied	Neither satisfied nor dissatisfied	Dissatisfied	Very dissatisfied
12. My prospects for promotion	❏	❏	❏	❏	❏
13. The people I talk to and work with	❏	❏	❏	❏	❏
14. The amount of time spent on administration	❏	❏	❏	❏	❏
15. My workload	❏	❏	❏	❏	❏
16. My prospects for continued employment	❏	❏	❏	❏	❏
17. The standard of care that I am currently able to give	❏	❏	❏	❏	❏
18. The opportunities I have to advance my career	❏	❏	❏	❏	❏
19. The extent to which I have adequate training for what I do.	❏	❏	❏	❏	❏
20. Overall staffing levels.	❏	❏	❏	❏	❏
21. The feeling of worthwhile accomplishment I get from my work	❏	❏	❏	❏	❏
22. The degree of respect and fair treatment I receive from my boss.	❏	❏	❏	❏	❏
23. The degree of time available to finish everything that I have to do.	❏	❏	❏	❏	❏
24. What I have accomplished when I go home at the end of the day.	❏	❏	❏	❏	❏
25. The amount of job security I have.	❏	❏	❏	❏	❏
26. Time off for in-service training.	❏	❏	❏	❏	❏
27. The amount of personal growth and development I get from my work.	❏	❏	❏	❏	❏
28. The extent to which my job is varied and interesting.	❏	❏	❏	❏	❏

	Very satisfied	Satisfied	Neither satisfied nor dissatisfied	Dissatisfied	Very dissatisfied
29. The support available to me in my job.	❑	❑	❑	❑	❑
30. The amount of independent thought and action I can exercise in my work.	❑	❑	❑	❑	❑
31. The opportunity to attend courses.	❑	❑	❑	❑	❑
32. The possibilities for a career in my field.	❑	❑	❑	❑	❑
33. The general standard of care given in this unit.	❑	❑	❑	❑	❑
34. The outlook for any professional group/ branch of nursing.	❑	❑	❑	❑	❑
35. The overall quality of the supervision I receive in my work.	❑	❑	❑	❑	❑
36. The amount of pay I receive.	❑	❑	❑	❑	❑
37. The hours I work.	❑	❑	❑	❑	❑
38. The extent to which I can use my skills.	❑	❑	❑	❑	❑
39. The amount of challenge in my job.	❑	❑	❑	❑	❑
40. The time available for patient/client care.	❑	❑	❑	❑	❑
41. How secure things look for me in the future of this organisation.	❑	❑	❑	❑	❑
42. The contact I have with colleagues.	❑	❑	❑	❑	❑
43. Patients are receiving the care that they need.	❑	❑	❑	❑	❑
44. Overall, how satisfied are you with your job?	❑	❑	❑	❑	❑

HAVE YOU ANSWERED EVERY QUESTION? YOU ARE INVITED TO COMMENT ON A SEPARATE PIECE OF PAPER.

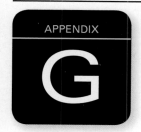

APPENDIX

G

chatham UNIVERSITY

Evidence-Based Approach to Novice Nurse Orientation in PeriAnesthesia Units

You are being asked to participate in a study about novice nurse orientation. This project is being conducted by Seun Ross a doctoral student at Chatham University. The objective of this research project is to determine if there is any relationship between the type of orientation program and stress, burnout or intent to leave. This survey is being given only to currently employed new graduate nurses working in the PeriAnesthesia units.

There are no known risks if you decide to participate in this study, nor are there any costs for participating in the study. The information you provide will add to current evidence on novice nurse orientation practices. The information collected may not benefit you directly, but what is learned from this study should provide general benefits to future new graduate nurses, hospital and institutions.

This survey is anonymous. If you choose to participate, DO NOT write your name on the questionnaire. No one will be able to identify you, nor will anyone be able to determine which survey you completed. No one will know whether you participated in this study. Nothing you say on the questionnaire will in any way influence your present or future employment with this institution.

Your participation in this study is voluntary. If you choose to participate, please place your completed questionnaire in the black box at the entrance of the unit. Questionnaires are collected each afternoon by the researcher. No one at this institution has a key to this box. If you have any questions or concerns about completing the questionnaire or about being in this study, you may contact me at (410) 293 1776 or at SRoss1@chatham.edu.

The Responsible Conduct of Research Service (RCRS) has reviewed my request to conduct this project. If you have any concerns about your rights in this study, please contact Luis Calvo of the RCRS dept at 301 295 2275 or email luis.calvo@med.navy.mil.

Thank you for your participation,

Seun Ross, RN, MSN, CRNP-F, NP-C, DNPc

CHATHAM COLLEGE FOR WOMEN · COLLEGE FOR GRADUATES STUDIES ·
COLLEGE FOR CONTINUING AND PROFESSIONAL STUDIES
Woodland Road. Pittsburgh, PA 15232. p. 412-365-1100. www.chatham.edu
Founded 1869

Index